ASAM PPC-2R

ASAM Patient Placement Criteria
for the Treatment of
Substance-Related Disorders

Second Edition-Revised

David Mee-Lee, M.D.
Editor

Gerald D. Shulman, M.A., FACATA
Marc Fishman, M.D.
David R. Gastfriend, M.D.
Julia Harris Griffith, M.A., CPHQ
Deputy Editors

American Society of Addiction Medicine, Inc.
Chevy Chase, Maryland
2001

Copyright 2001
American Society of Addiction Medicine, Inc.
4601 North Park Ave., Upper Arcade, Suite 101
Chevy Chase, Maryland 20815

ALL RIGHTS RESERVED. Unless authorized in writing by the American Society of Addiction Medicine, no part of this book may be used or reproduced in any manner, including electronic applications.

Correspondence regarding permission to reprint material from this volume should be directed to the Publications Department, American Society of Addiction Medicine, Inc., 4601 North Park Ave., Upper Arcade Suite 101, Chevy Chase, Maryland 20815.
Fax (301) 656-3815. E-mail *JGart@asam.org*.

The correct bibliographic citation for this book is Mee-Lee D, Shulman GD, Fishman M, Gastfriend DR, and Griffith JH, eds. (2001). *ASAM Patient Placement Criteria for the Treatment of Substance-Related Disorders, Second Edition-Revised (ASAM PPC-2R)*. Chevy Chase, MD: American Society of Addiction Medicine, Inc.

Library of Congress Cataloging in Publication Data
ASAM Patient Placement Criteria for the Treatment of Substance-Related Disorders, Second Edition-Revised.
    p. cm.
    Prepared by the Working Group on the PPC-2R
    of the American Society of Addiction Medicine.
    ISBN 1-880425-06-8

First printing 4,000. April 2001.
Second printing 5,000. October 2001.

Contents

Preface to the Second Edition, Revised 1

    What's New in the Second Edition-Revised? 1
    Historical Foundations of the *ASAM Patient Placement Criteria* 12
    Theoretical Foundations of the *ASAM Patient Placement Criteria* 14
    Real World Considerations in Using the *ASAM Patient Placement Criteria* 17
    Outcomes Research with the *ASAM Patient Placement Criteria* 19

Adult Patient Placement Criteria 25

    Crosswalk of the Adult Placement Criteria 27
    Continued Service and Discharge Criteria 35
    Level 0.5: Early Intervention 41
    Level I: Outpatient Treatment 45
    Level II: Intensive Outpatient Treatment/Partial Hospitalization 55
    Level III: Residential/Inpatient Treatment 71
    Level IV: Medically Managed Intensive Inpatient Treatment 127
    Opioid Maintenance Therapy 137

Dimensional Criteria

    Dimension 1 Criteria: Adult Detoxification 145

Adolescent Patient Placement Criteria 177

    Preface to the Adolescent Patient Placement Criteria 179
    Crosswalk of the Adolescent Placement Criteria 191
    Continued Service and Discharge Criteria 199
    Level 0.5: Early Intervention 205
    Level I: Outpatient Treatment 209
    Level II: Intensive Outpatient Treatment/Partial Hospitalization 217
    Level III: Residential/Intensive Inpatient Treatment 235
    Level IV: Medically Managed Intensive Inpatient Treatment 271

Appendix A: Experimental Matrix for Matching Multidimensional Risk with Type and Intensity of Service Needs—Adult 281

Appendix B: Experimental Matrix for Matching Multidimensional Risk with Type and Intensity of Service Needs—Adolescent 313

Appendix C: Dimension 5: Criteria for Relapse, Continued Use or Continued Problem Potential 341

Appendix D: Clinical Institute Withdrawal Assessment-Alcohol, Revised (CIWA-Ar) Scale 355

Appendix E: Glossary 359

Appendix F: Contributors to the Development of the *ASAM PPC-2R* 371

Dedicated to the Memory of Michael Ford

This volume is dedicated to the memory of Michael Ford, founder and first Executive Director of the National Association of Addiction Treatment Providers (NAATP) and Director of Public Policy with the National Council on Alcoholism.

It was Mr. Ford who initiated the meetings between ASAM and NAATP that ultimately led to the development of these *Patient Placement Criteria*. In this initiative as in so many aspects of his work, Mr. Ford's legacy is the notion that "with hard work, public policy change is possible."

Mr. Ford always saw the larger picture and was an outspoken champion for ASAM to lead the way in developing patient placement criteria that would be recognized and utilized by a broad spectrum of addiction treatment providers. The continued evolution and acceptance of the ASAM Criteria are the legacy of Mr. Ford's vision and leadership.

David Mee-Lee, M.D.
Editor

Gerald D. Shulman, M.A., FACATA
Marc Fishman, M.D.
David R. Gastfriend, M.D.
Julia Harris Griffith, M.A., CPHQ
Deputy Editors

Bonnie B. Wilford, M.S.
Managing Editor

Steering Committee

Candace Baker, M.S.W.
Clinical Affairs Manager
National Association of Alcoholism
  and Drug Abuse Counselors (NAADAC)
Arlington, VA

James F. Callahan, D.P.A.
Executive Vice President/CEO
American Society of Addiction Medicine (ASAM)
Chevy Chase, MD

Marc Fishman, M.D.
Department of Psychiatry and
  Behavioral Sciences
The Johns Hopkins University School of Medicine
Baltimore, MD

David R. Gastfriend, M.D.
Associate Professor of Psychiatry,
  Harvard Medical School
Director, Addiction Research Program
Massachusetts General Hospital
Boston, MA

Julia Harris Griffith, M.A., CPHQ
Managed Care Quality Assessment
  and Improvement Division
Michigan Department of Community Health
Lansing, MI

Roger W. Hartman
Office of the Assistant Secretary of Defense
  (Health Affairs)
TRICARE Management Activity
Falls Church, VA

Ronald J. Hunsicker, D.Min., FACATA
President/CEO
National Association of Addiction
  Treatment Providers (NAATP)
Lititz, PA

Ric Ohrstrom
National Council on Alcoholism and Other
  Drug Dependence (NCADD)
Greenwich, CT

Lawrence W. Osborn, M.D.
Aetna-U.S. Healthcare
Blue Bell, PA

Sam R. Segal, LPC, LADC, CBHE
Senior Clinical Officer and
Director, Addiction Services Policy
Connecticut Department of Mental Health
  and Addiction Services
Hartford, CT

Cautionary Statement

The *ASAM Patient Placement Criteria for the Treatment of Substance-Related Disorders, Second Edition-Revised (ASAM PPC-2R)* is a clinical guide to be used in matching patients to appropriate levels of care. These criteria reflect a clinical consensus of adult and adolescent treatment specialists that incorporated field review comments.

The purpose of the ASAM *Patient Placement Criteria* is to enhance the use of multidimensional assessments in making objective patient placement decisions for various levels of care. The criteria are considered evolutionary in nature and are intended to encourage further patient placement research.

It is recognized that the criteria may not encompass all of the level of service options that may be available in a changing health care field. Therefore, the criteria may not be wholly relevant to all levels and modalities of care (such as forensic treatment facilities, custodial care providers, addiction treatment programs that address concomitant developmental disability disorders) and to legal judgments concerning appropriateness of patient placement.

The *ASAM PPC-2R* is intended as a stimulus for further research and discussion of the treatment and care of substance-related disorders. The criteria are necessarily general in approach and are not intended as, and should not be used as, a standard for the treatment of any individual. The treatment of individual patients suffering from substance-related disorders requires professional evaluation and the exercise of independent judgment on a case-by-case basis.

The copyright owner, publisher and authors of the *ASAM Patient Placement Criteria for the Treatment of Substance-Related Disorders, Second Edition-Revised* expressly disclaim that application of the criteria to any particular patient will result in the appropriate level of care and expressly disclaim any and all responsibility for application of the criteria. They shall not be responsible for any action or omission by any person rendering or recommending treatment or otherwise making a patient placement decision or recommendation with respect to any particular patient. There is no warranty that the information in the *ASAM PPC-2R* is free from all errors and omissions.

Acknowledgments

Portions of the ASAM *PPC-2R* that are excerpted or reproduced from "The Cleveland Admission, Discharge and Transfer Criteria—Model for Chemical Dependency Treatment Programs, Copyright 1987, Greater Cleveland Hospital Association" are used with the permission of the Greater Cleveland Hospital Association and the Northern Ohio Chemical Dependency Treatment Directors Association. Portions that are excerpted or reproduced from the "Adult and Adolescent Alcohol and Drug Dependence Admission, Continued Stay, and Discharge Criteria, Copyright 1987, 1989, National Association of Addiction Treatment Providers" are used with the permission of the National Association of Addiction Treatment Providers.

ASAM wishes to thank . . .

- The members of the ASAM Committees on Patient Placement Criteria, Methadone Treatment, and Practice Guidelines, many of whom reviewed and improved relevant sections.

- The Massachusetts Bureau of Substance Abuse Services, which worked with the state's methadone treatment providers to develop criteria that formed the initial draft of the ASAM criteria on Opioid Maintenance Therapy.

- The federal Center for Substance Abuse Treatment (CSAT) and its Director, H. Westley Clark, M.D., J.D., M.P.H., FASAM, for providing technical expertise and material resources in support of the development of the *ASAM PPC-2R*. Special thanks go to Mady Chalk, Ph.D., Director, CSAT Office of Managed Care, and to Herman Diesenhaus, Ph.D., CSAT Public Health Analyst, for their continuing interest and support.

In addition, ASAM wishes to acknowledge the valuable comments and recommendations of the members of the Coalition for National Clinical Criteria, the members of its subcommittees and those participants who drafted material for and served as reviewers of the *ASAM PPC-2R*.

ASAM wishes to express special gratitude to those individuals who chaired the drafting committees: Marc Fishman, M.D., Chair, Work Group on Adolescent Criteria; David R. Gastfriend, M.D., Chair, Work Group on Criteria Research; Julia Harris Griffith, M.A., CPHQ, Chair, Work Group on Level 0.5/Level I; David Mee-Lee, M.D., Chair, Work Group on Co-Occurring Disorders; and Gerald D. Shulman, M.A., FACATA, Chair, Work Group on Level III. ASAM also wishes to acknowledge the important contributions of those who were engaged in drafting and reviewing the revised Adult and Adolescent Criteria (see Appendix F).

> This publication incorporates and supersedes the *Patient Placement Criteria for the Treatment of Psychoactive Substance Use Disorders*, March 1991, and the *Patient Placement Criteria for the Treatment of Substance-Related Disorders, Second Edition*, April 1996.

Preface to the Second Edition-Revised

The *ASAM Patient Placement Criteria for the Treatment of Substance-Related Disorders, Second Edition-Revised (ASAM PPC-2R)*, like the first (1991) and second (1996) editions, is published by the American Society of Addiction Medicine (ASAM).

What's New in the Second Edition-Revised?

Experience with the first and second editions of the *ASAM Patient Placement Criteria* identified areas in which the criteria required expansion or revision in order to: (a) meet the needs of patients, regardless of the availability of third-party reimbursement; (b) take a less conservative approach to detoxification, based on recent clinical research; (c) respond to the concerns of public sector treatment programs and managed care organizations; (d) develop a method of expanding the levels of care; and (e) define commonly used terms in ways that enhance communication among users of patient placement criteria. The Second Edition-Revised (PPC-2R) maintains and builds on the effort to respond to those needs.

Moreover, the continuing development and refinement of the criteria continue a shift that began with the First Edition, from:

- Unidimensional to multidimensional assessment.
- Program-driven to clinically driven treatment.
- Fixed length of service to variable length of service.
- A limited number of discrete levels of care to a continuum of care.

The *PPC-2R* has been totally reformatted to be more user-friendly and to facilitate comparisons across levels of service. More substantively, the criteria have been revised to respond to the request of users—providers, care managers, and public and private sector payers—to make the criteria more reflective of the "real world" in which providers deliver care.

On reviewing the resulting changes in this edition, the reader will note an emphasis on the following issues:

- The role of functional deficits in determining individual treatment needs.

- A shift away from identifying or describing levels of care in terms of traditional program facilities.

- A renewed emphasis on the original concept that levels of care represent intensities of service along a continuum, each of which may be provided in a variety of program types, including those that offer more than one level of care and serve multiple populations.

Providers and funders of addiction treatment, as well as certifying, licensing and regulatory authorities, are free to use the *ASAM Patient Placement Criteria* as guidelines to inform the transition away from fixed, program-driven treatment to flexible, assessment-based, clinically driven treatment.

Levels of Service Expanded

Like earlier editions, the *PPC-2R* describes treatment as a continuum marked by five basic levels of care. Roman numerals are retained to maintain a common language for describing the treatment levels of care (Levels I through IV). Thus, the *PPC-2R* provides the field with a nomenclature for describing the continuum of addiction services.

- Level 0.5: Early Intervention
- Level 1: Outpatient Treatment
- Level II: Intensive Outpatient/Partial Hospitalization Treatment
- Level III: Residential/Inpatient Treatment
- Level IV: Medically Managed Intensive Inpatient Treatment

A decimal number (ranging from .1 to .9) expresses gradations of intensity within the existing levels of care. This structure allows improved precision of description and better "inter-rater" reliability by focusing on five broad levels of service. Thus the *PPC-2R* describes gradient levels of care within each level of service. For example, a **II.1** level of care provides a benchmark for intensity at the minimum description of Level II care.

Level 0.5: Early Intervention. Professional services for early intervention were included as a level of care (Level 0.5) in the second edition and are continued in *PPC-2R*. The authors believe that early intervention constitutes a service for specific individuals who, for a known reason, are at risk of developing substance-related problems or for those for whom there is not yet sufficient information to document a substance use disorder. Consideration was given to providing criteria for Prevention/Early Intervention. Based on comments elicited by the field review, the Working Group determined that the focus on Early Intervention was the most appropriate for inclusion in this edition. The comments that led to this decision fell into two groups: first, that prevention and early intervention are different and cannot be addressed in the same criteria and, second, that primary prevention is not sufficiently clinical to support development of a separate level of care.

Where Level 0.5 is a DUI or DWI program, the length of service may be determined by program rules, and completion of the program may be a prerequisite to reinstitution of driving privileges. If the assessment of such an individual indicates a need for treatment, there are three possible options:

1. If the individual is in imminent danger, he or she should be transferred to a clinically appropriate level of care, even if that precludes completion of the mandated DUI or DWI program.

2. If the individual is not in imminent danger but does require outpatient treatment, an attempt should be made to facilitate such treatment with the services of the Level 0.5 program.

3. If the individual can wait to enter formal treatment until after the Level 0.5 program is completed, transfer to a higher level of care should be arranged as soon as possible after the Level 0.5 program is completed.

Level I: Outpatient Treatment. Level I encompasses organized services that may be delivered in a wide variety of settings. Addiction or mental health treatment personnel provide professionally directed evaluation, treatment and recovery service. Such services are provided in regularly scheduled sessions and follow a defined set of policies and procedures or medical protocols.

Level I outpatient services are designed to treat the individual's level of clinical severity and to help the individual achieve permanent changes in his or her alcohol- and drug-using behavior and mental functioning. To accomplish this, services must address major lifestyle, attitudinal and behavioral issues that have the potential to undermine the goals of treatment or inhibit the individual's ability to cope with major life tasks without the non-medical use of alcohol or other drugs.

In the *PPC-2R*, the Level I criteria have been expanded to promote greater access to care for dual diagnosis patients, unmotivated patients who are mandated into treatment, and others who previously only had access to care if they agreed to intensive periods of primary treatment. Knowledge and application of cognitive behavioral therapies such as motivational interviewing, motivational enhancement, solution-focused therapy and stages of change work have greatly increased, creating more options for those who before would have been turned away as not ready for treatment or in denial and thus in need of coerced intensive treatment. Level I now is seen as appropriate for individuals who are assessed as having high severity in Dimension 4 (readiness to change) but not in the other dimensions, because it avoids placing them at a more intensive level of care, which may only serve to harden their resistance. The expansion of Level I thus can enhance access to care and facilitate earlier engagement of patients in treatment, thereby allowing better utilization of resources and improving the effectiveness of recovery efforts.

Level II: Intensive Outpatient Treatment/Partial Hospitalization. Level II is an organized outpatient service that delivers treatment services during the day, before or after work or school, in the evening or on weekends. For appropriately selected patients, such programs provide essential education and treatment components while allowing patients to apply their newly acquired skills within "real world" environments. Programs have the capacity to arrange for medical and psychiatric consultation, psychopharmacological consultation, medication management, and 24-hour crisis services.

Level II programs can provide comprehensive biopsychosocial assessments and individualized treatment plans, including formulation of problem statements, treatment goals and measurable objectives—all developed in consultation with the patient. Such programs typically have active affiliations with other levels of care, and their staff can help patients access support services such as child care, vocational training and transportation.

Level III: Residential/Inpatient Treatment. Level III encompasses organized services staffed by designated addiction treatment and mental health personnel who provide a planned regimen of care in a 24-hour live-in setting. Such services adhere to defined sets of policies and procedures. They are housed in, or affiliated with, permanent facilities where patients can reside safely. They are staffed 24 hours a day. Mutual and self-help group meetings generally are available on-site.

Level III encompasses four types of programs:

    Level III.1: Clinically Managed Low-Intensity Residential Treatment
    Level III.3: Clinically Managed Medium-Intensity Residential Treatment
    Level III.5: Clinically Managed High-Intensity Residential Treatment
    Level III.7: Medically Monitored Inpatient Treatment.

The defining characteristic of all Level III programs is that they serve individuals who need safe and stable living environments in order to develop their recovery skills. Such living environments may be housed in the same facility where treatment services are provided or they may be in a separate facility affiliated with the treatment provider.

In the *PPC-2R*, the Level III criteria have been expanded to broaden Level III.5 so that they no longer reflect only a Therapeutic Community treatment model. The admission criteria for Level III.7 also have been realigned to match the original description of a medically monitored setting.

Level IV: Medically Managed Intensive Inpatient Treatment. Level IV programs provide a planned regimen of 24-hour medically directed evaluation, care and treatment of mental and substance-related disorders in an acute care inpatient setting. They are staffed by designated addiction-credentialed physicians, including psychiatrists, as well as other mental health- and addiction-credentialed clinicians. Such services are delivered under a defined set of policies and procedures and has permanent facilities that include inpatient beds.

Level IV programs provide care to patients whose mental and substance-related problems are so severe that they require primary biomedical, psychiatric and nursing care. Treatment is provided 24 hours a day, and the full resources of a general acute care hospital or psychiatric hospital are available. The treatment is specific to mental and substance-related disorders; however, the skills of the interdisciplinary team and the availability of support services allow the conjoint treatment of any co-occurring biomedical conditions that need to be addressed.

Opioid Maintenance Therapy. The first edition of the *Patient Placement Criteria* was criticized because it did not directly address opioid maintenance therapy (OMT). The second edition rectified this situation by explicitly addressing opioid maintenance therapy. The *PPC-2R* maintains this change.

OMT (so named to broaden the service beyond methadone maintenance) is best conceptualized as a separate service that can be provided at any level of care. OMT therefore has not been included under any of the broad levels of service (I through IV). However, the OMT criteria are included in the format of a Level I outpatient service, since most opioid maintenance therapy is delivered in an ambulatory setting.

NOTE: At the time this edition was completed, the U.S. Food and Drug Administration (FDA) was considering, but had not yet approved, buprenorphine—alone or in combination with naloxone—for the treatment of opiate addiction. Because it is not yet an approved therapy, the use of buprenorphine is not addressed in the *PPC-2R*. If it is approved by the FDA, it will be included in a future edition.

Dimensional Criteria Refined

The six assessment dimensions to be evaluated in making placement decisions are essentially the same as in earlier editions of the criteria:

- Dimension 1: Acute Intoxication and/or Withdrawal Potential
- Dimension 2: Biomedical Conditions and Complications
- Dimension 3: Emotional, Behavioral or Cognitive Conditions and Complications
- Dimension 4: Readiness to Change (formerly "Treatment Acceptance/Resistance")
- Dimension 5: Relapse, Continued Use or Continued Problem Potential
- Dimension 6: Recovery/Living Environment

The *ASAM PPC-2R* expands these assessment dimensions in subtle but significant ways. For example:

Dimension 1: Acute Intoxication and/or Withdrawal Potential. The goals of care in Dimension 1 remain the same as in the first and second editions of the *Patient Placement Criteria*, with some important additions:

1. Avoidance of the potentially hazardous consequences of discontinuation of alcohol and other drugs of dependence;

2. Facilitation of the patient's completion of detoxification and linkages and timely entry into continued medical, addiction or mental health treatment or self-help recovery as indicated; and

3. Promotion of patient dignity and easing of patient discomfort during the withdrawal process.

Assessment considerations include: What risk is associated with the patient's current level of acute intoxication? Is there significant risk of severe withdrawal symptoms or seizures, based on the patient's previous withdrawal history, as well as the amount, frequency, chronicity and recency of discontinuation of (or significant reduction in) alcohol or other drug use? Are there current signs of withdrawal? Does the patient have supports to assist in ambulatory detoxification, if medically safe?

While the First Edition of the *Patient Placement Criteria* addressed only inpatient detoxification services, which are considered Level IV, or sometimes Level III, the *PPC-2R* incorporates criteria developed for the Second Edition, which match a patient's severity of illness along Dimension 1 (Acute Intoxication and/or Withdrawal Potential) with five intensities of detoxification service, described herein as Level I-D, Level II-D, Level III.2-D, Level III.7-D, and Level IV-D. The qualifier "D" is used to designate a detoxification service within the broad division (such as III.2-D, Clinically Managed Residential Detoxification services or Social Setting Detoxification).

A particular detoxification service can be provided separately ("unbundled") from other treatment services. When such services are provided separately, a sufficiently comprehensive biopsychosocial screening assessment and linkage to non-detoxification services are essential to avoid the syndrome in which alcoholics and drug addicts revolve through acute care facilities in repeated cycles of recovery and relapse (the "revolving door syndrome").

For detoxification provided in conjunction with treatment for additional problems identified in the comprehensive biopsychosocial screening assessment, the *PPC-2R* calls for the patient to be placed in the level of care appropriate to the most acute problem.

While the *PPC-2R* describes five levels of detoxification, staffing at any given level may be structured to provide a range of intensities of service. For example, detoxification of some patients can be carried out in the office (Level I-D) or in more structured outpatient settings (Level II-D) without the use of beds or intensive nursing monitoring. Other patients may need to be monitored for a period of time before an appropriate determination can be made. (Such monitoring can, at times, be carried out in an outpatient setting, but may require an even more structured setting, such as a "23-hour observation bed".) Some programs that are described as Level III may have the capacity for more or less intensive medical monitoring of detoxification. For example, Level III.2-D includes Social Setting Detoxification, which may provide minimal medical monitoring.

The number of hours allocated to other treatment services at Level I and Level II is separate from, and does not include, those to be allocated for detoxification in an ambulatory setting. Hence the intensity of detoxification services need not match the intensity of other treatment services in Level I or Level II.

For patients who require a higher level of care because of assessments in other dimensions, it may be more expedient to carry out detoxification in that higher level of care. On the other hand, some patients who enter treatment do not require detoxification. Nevertheless, they should be assessed in Dimension 1, Acute Intoxication and/or Withdrawal Potential.

Dimension 2: Biomedical Conditions and Complications. There are no changes in Dimension 2 from the Second Edition.

Assessment considerations include: Are there current physical illnesses, other than withdrawal, that need to be addressed because they create risk or may complicate treatment? Are there chronic conditions that affect treatment?

Dimension 3: Emotional, Behavioral or Cognitive Conditions and Complications *(such as psychiatric conditions, psychological or emotional/behavioral complications of known or unknown origin, poor impulse control, changes in mental status, or transient neuropsychiatric complications).* In the *PPC-2R*, Dimension 3 has been expanded to encompass cognitive conditions and complications, reflecting the fact that there are clinical presentations that are not captured by emotional or behavioral descriptors alone. New subdomains of assessment have been added to address co-occurring mental and substance-related disorders or dual diagnosis issues in more detail.

Assessment considerations include: Are there current psychiatric illnesses or psychological, behavioral, emotional or cognitive problems that need to be addressed because they create risk or complicate treatment? Are there chronic conditions that affect treatment? Do any emotional, behavioral or cognitive problems appear to be an expected part of the addictive disorder, or do they appear to be autonomous? Even if connected to the addiction, are they severe enough to warrant specific mental health treatment? Is the patient able to manage the activities of daily living? Can he or she cope with any emotional, behavioral or cognitive problems?

It is important to note that, in assessing co-occurring disorders, a mental health or substance-related disorder should be considered secondary only if it shows improvement as a result of stabilization in the other disorder.

Dimension 4: Readiness to Change. Dimension 4 has been retitled "Readiness to Change" to reflect Prochaska and DiClemente's Stages of Change model (Prochaska, DiClemente & Norcross, 1992; Prochaska, Norcross & DiClemente, 1994), thus moving the criteria beyond the concepts of denial and resistance. This is based on the concept that an individual's emotional and cognitive awareness of the need to change and his or her level of commitment to and readiness for change indicate his or her degree of cooperation with treatment, as well as his or her awareness of the relationship of alcohol or other drug use to negative consequences.

In fact, resistance to treatment is not unexpected and does not automatically exclude a patient from receiving treatment. Rather, it is the *degree* of readiness to change that helps to determine the setting for and intensity of motivating strategies needed, rather than the patient's eligibility for treatment itself. Moreover, acceptance or resistance to treatment are more subjective and less easily measured than readiness to change. They also are subject to greater variation in interpretation, based on clinician and program ideology, clinician knowledge and skill in engagement strategies, availability of a variety of motivational enhancement therapies and levels of service, and the degree of commitment to patient-centered, participatory treatment planning.

Dimension 5: Relapse, Continued Use or Continued Problem Potential. Dimension 5 has been retitled "Relapse, Continued Use or Continued Problem Potential" to encompass mental health problems. For example, a psychotic, paranoid individual who is fearful of being poisoned and thus fails to take his or her medications would be described as having a high "Relapse or Continued

Problem Potential." This indicates that the patient is at high risk for becoming acutely psychotic and/or increasingly paranoid. Such a patient also is at high risk of relapse to substance use. The assignment of a level of care after a patient has relapsed should be made on the basis of both history and an assessment of current problems, and not merely history alone. The patient is not automatically assumed to require a higher level of care than the one at which relapse occurred.

Dimension 5 also is better understood through expanded constructs offered to assist in assessment. There are four domains that are not inconsistent with earlier versions of Dimension 5, but which offer a conceptually clearer sequence of factors that contribute to relapse potential. The sequence involves the historical phenomenon of relapse, the acute pharmacologic response to substance(s), second-order behavioral responsivity that may mediate the preceding factors, and third-order personality or learned responses that may modify the preceding factors.

Assessment considerations include: Is the patient in immediate danger of continued severe mental health distress and/or alcohol or drug use? Does the patient have any recognition or understanding of, or skills in coping with, his or her addictive or mental disorder in order to prevent relapse, continued use or continued problems such as suicidal behavior? How severe are the problems and further distress that may continue or reappear if the patient is not successfully engaged in treatment at this time? How aware is the patient of relapse triggers, ways to cope with cravings to use, and skills to control impulses to use or impulses to harm self or others?

Dimension 6: Recovery/Living Environment. There are no significant changes in Dimension 6. At Level 0.5, Dimension 6 has been retitled "Living Environment" to reflect the fact that, at this level, an individual has not been assessed as in need of treatment and may need only education and advice on managing risk.

Assessment considerations include: Do any family members, significant others, living situations, or school or work situations pose a threat to the patient's safety or engagement in treatment? Does the patient have supportive friendships, financial resources, or educational or vocational resources that can increase the likelihood of successful treatment? Are there legal, vocational, social service agency or criminal justice mandates that may enhance the patient's motivation for engagement in treatment? Are there transportation, child care, housing or employment issues that need to be clarified and addressed?

Continued Service and Discharge Criteria

In a departure from earlier editions, the *PPC-2R* contains only admission criteria for each level of care. With this edition, the specific criteria for continued service and transfer or discharge have been replaced by general guidelines to inform the judgment of the treatment professional. This change was made in recognition of the fact that, in the process of patient assessment, certain problems and priorities are identified as justifying admission to a particular level of care. The resolution of those problems and priorities determines when a patient can be treated at a different level of care or discharged. The appearance of new problems may require services that can be provided effectively at the same level of care, or transfer of the patient to a more or less intensive level of care.

Integration of Criteria for Co-Occurring Disorders

When the first edition of the *ASAM Patient Placement Criteria* (*ASAM PPC-1*) was published in 1991, the criteria generally were designed for programs that offered only addiction treatment services. However, the *PPC-1* also acknowledged that some patients come to treatment with medical (Dimension 2) and psychiatric (Dimension 3) disorders that coexist with their substance-related problems. Clinical reality suggests that programs and practitioners who are committed to meeting the total needs of the patients they serve must be able to meet the needs of these "dual diagnosis" patients. This concept is particularly relevant today, as the range of patient needs and clinical variability continues to broaden.

Factors contributing to this clinical reality include the expansion of substance use and substance-related disorders in younger populations; greater sensitivity to substance use problems in the mental health, welfare and criminal justice systems; and increased commitment to earlier intervention in substance use disorders in preference to fragmented services and incarceration. A major factor has been the growing body of scientific evidence pointing to addictive disorders as diseases of the brain; another is the development of pharmacotherapies for addiction. Greater understanding of the uses and effects of psychosocial and cognitive-behavioral strategies also has heightened awareness of a broadened range of modalities to meet individual needs.

The *ASAM PPC-2R* takes a further step toward enhancing the ability of the ASAM criteria to meet these diverse patient needs by incorporating criteria that address the large subset of individuals who present for treatment with co-occurring Axis I substance-related disorders and Axis I/Axis II mental disorders. Individuals with such co-occurring disorders (often referred to as "dual diagnoses") can be conceptualized as belonging to one of two general categories:

- *Moderate Severity Disorders:* Such persons present with stable mood or anxiety disorders of moderate severity (including resolving bipolar disorder), or with personality disorders of moderate severity (although some persons with severe levels of antisocial personality disorder may be appropriately placed in this group), or with signs and symptoms of a mental health disorder that are not so severe as to meet the diagnostic threshold.

- *High Severity Disorders:* Such persons present with schizophrenia-spectrum disorders, severe mood disorders with psychotic features, severe anxiety disorders, or severe personality disorders (such as fragile borderline conditions).

Individuals whose co-occurring mental disorders best fit within the category of moderate severity disorders are appropriately treated in programs designed to treat primary substance use disorders. Those with concurrent high severity mental disorders, on the other hand, generally are best managed in dual diagnosis specialty programs that can offer integrated mental health and addiction treatment approaches. Some patients may require immediate stabilization of their psychiatric symptoms before they can be engaged in ongoing addiction treatment and recovery. Depending on the severity of their symptoms, such patients may require referral to medical and/or psychiatric services outside the *PPC-2R* levels of care.

Once stabilization has been achieved, the initial placement for recovery services should reflect an assessment of the patient's status in all six *PPC-2R* dimensions. The principle here is that the highest severity problem (particularly those in Dimensions 1, 2 or 3) should determine the patient's initial placement. Subsequent resolution of this problem creates an opportunity to transfer the patient to a less intensive level of care. Addressing the individual's recovery needs thus may involve a sequence of services across several levels of care (involving a "step-down" or "step-up process"). For example, a patient who is assessed in Dimension 2 as dangerously hypertensive should be placed in a Level III.7 or Level IV program to stabilize his or her medical condition, before being transferred to a Level I program for treatment of the addictive disorder.

What should be avoided is the notion of "averaging" severity across dimensions to arrive at a placement determination.

Patients whose biomedical or psychiatric disorders are so severe that stabilizing them is the highest priority are most appropriately treated in a medical or psychiatric facility or unit before addiction treatment is initiated.

A Note on Terminology

The addiction and mental health fields have not yet reached consensus on terminology to describe individuals who are experiencing simultaneous addictive and mental health disorders. Terms currently in use include "dual diagnosis," "dual disorders," "mentally ill chemically addicted" (MICA), "chemically addicted mentally ill" (CAMI), "mentally ill substance abusers" (MISA), "mentally ill chemically dependent" (MICD), "co-occurring disorders," "coexisting disorders," "comorbid disorders," and "individuals with co-occurring psychiatric and substance symptomatology" (ICOPSS).

Clearly, this issue requires further discussion and consensus-building. In the interim, the *PPC-2R* has adopted the term "co-occurring mental and substance-related disorders" in formal titles so as to remain consistent with the *Diagnostic and Statistical Manual of Mental Disorders* of the American Psychiatric Association (1994). Throughout the text, however, the term "dual diagnosis" is used for the sake of simplicity and because it appears to have the widest acceptance nationally. (The authors recognize that "dual diagnosis" is an inexact term and that it fails to accommodate populations other than those with mental and substance-related disorders—such as persons with coexisting addictive and biomedical or developmental disorders—but the advantages of simplicity and wide acceptance were judged to outweigh these deficits. This decision will be revisited in future editions of the *Patient Placement Criteria*.)

Throughout the adult criteria in the *PPC-2R*, treatment programs are described as generally of two types—Dual Diagnosis Capable or Dual Diagnosis Enhanced—to reflect their ability to address co-occurring substance-related and mental disorders.

- *Dual Diagnosis Capable* programs have a primary focus on the treatment of substance-related disorders, but also are capable of treating patients who have relatively stable diagnostic or subdiagnostic co-occurring mental health problems related to an emotional, behavioral or cognitive disorder.

- *Dual Diagnosis Enhanced* programs, by contrast, are designed to treat patients who have more unstable or disabling co-occurring mental disorders in addition to their substance-related disorders.

Dual Diagnosis Capable Programs. These programs typically meet the needs of patients whose psychiatric disorders are stable and who are capable of independent functioning, so that their mental disorders do not interfere significantly with their participation in addiction treatment. Such patients may have severe and persistent mental illnesses that are in a relatively stable phase at the time that they need addiction treatment. Other patients may have difficulties in mood, behavior or cognition as the result of a psychiatric or substance-induced disorder, or their emotional, behavioral or cognitive symptoms may not rise to the level of a diagnosable mental disorder. Such patients need counseling and coordinated mental health interventions so that primary therapy can be focused on their substance-related disorders.

Dual Diagnosis Capable programs typically address dual diagnosis in their policies and procedures, assessment, treatment planning, program content, and discharge planning. They have arrangements in place for coordination and collaboration with mental health services. They also can provide psychopharmacologic monitoring and psychological assessment and consultation, either on site or through coordinated consultation off site. Program staff are able to address the interaction of the substance-related and mental disorders in assessing the patient's readiness to change, relapse risk and recovery environment. Nevertheless, the primary focus of such programs is on addiction treatment rather than dual diagnosis concerns.

Dual Diagnosis Enhanced Programs. These programs are appropriate for patients who need primary addiction treatment but who are more symptomatic and/or functionally impaired as a result of their co-occurring mental disorder than are patients treated in Dual Diagnosis Capable programs. Patients in need of Dual Diagnosis Enhanced programs typically are unstable or disabled to such a degree that specific psychiatric and mental health support, monitoring and accommodation are necessary in order for the individual to participate in treatment.

Patients in Dual Diagnosis Enhanced programs generally are not so acute or impaired as to present a significant danger to self or others, nor do they require 24-hour psychiatric supervision. For example, a typical patient may have a severe and persistent mental illness that is mildly or moderately unstable in addition to a substance-related disorder. Or the patient may have significant difficulties in mood, behavior or cognition as a result of a psychiatric or substance-related disorder. Or he or she may evidence emotional, behavioral or cognitive symptoms that do not rise to the level of a diagnosed mental disorder, but which are sufficiently severe that the patient needs concurrent addiction treatment and mental health interventions to stabilize both disorders.

Dual Diagnosis Enhanced program services are delivered by psychiatric and mental health clinicians and addiction treatment professionals in a setting where all staff are cross-trained. Such programs tend to have relatively high ratios of staff to patients and provide close monitoring of patients who demonstrate psychiatric instability or disability.

Dual Diagnosis Enhanced programs typically have policies, procedures, assessment, treatment and discharge planning that accommodate patients with dual diagnoses. Dual diagnosis-specific and mental health symptom management groups are incorporated into the addiction treatment. Motivational enhancement therapies specifically designed for those with co-occurring mental and substance-related disorders are more likely to be available (particularly in outpatient settings) and, ideally, there is close collaboration or integration with a mental health program that provides crisis back-up services and access to mental health case management and continuing care. In contrast to Dual Diagnosis Capable programs, Dual Diagnosis Enhanced programs have a primary focus on dual diagnosis patients and integrate dual diagnosis staff, services and program content.

Addiction-Only Programs. A third category describes programs that, either by choice or for lack of resources, cannot accommodate patients who have psychiatric illnesses that require ongoing treatment, however stable the illness and however well-functioning the patient.

The policies, procedures and services of addiction-only programs do not accommodate co-occurring mental disorders. Individuals who need psychotropic medications generally are not accepted by such programs, which typically have no formal coordination or collaboration with mental health services, and mental health issues are not addressed in treatment planning or content. Individuals who are appropriately placed in addiction-only programs have needs that can be met through a focus solely on the treatment of substance-related disorders.

Because the number and proportion of persons entering addiction treatment with co-occurring mental disorders is increasing, the *PPC-2R* anticipates that most addiction treatment programs are at least Dual Diagnosis Capable. Indeed, many treatment programs may be able to provide addiction treatment and a variety of mental health services in the same facility, so as to meet the needs of a diverse patient population. Other programs may be unable to or choose not to provide such a broad array of services.

The *ASAM Patient Placement Criteria* anticipate that:

- All individuals, programs and health systems that provide treatment for addictive disorders should be prepared to serve the needs of dual diagnosis patients, at least to the extent described here as Dual Diagnosis Capable.

- All health care delivery systems should be able to deliver the services needed by patients with co-occurring mental and substance-related disorders. Provider networks should include facilities that can deliver Dual Diagnosis Enhanced services at Levels I through IV, as described in the *ASAM PPC-2R*.

Essential Elements. Certain elements must be in place in any treatment program that accepts patients with co-occurring mental and substance-related disorders:

- M.D. and Ph.D. level staff are skilled in the diagnosis of psychopathology.

- A majority of staff are cross-trained to deal with both mental and substance-related disorders.

- Psychoeducational components of treatment address both mental and substance-related disorders.

- A psychiatrist is available on site in acute settings and through coordination in all other settings.

- Medication management is integrated into the treatment plan.

- Counselors are trained to monitor and promote compliance with pharmacotherapies.

- In programs that work with persons who are severely mentally ill, intensive case management and assertive community treatment services are available.

Linking Services. Specific policies and procedures enhance the linkage of services required by patients with co-occurring mental and substance-related disorders:

1. Formal memoranda of understanding specify what is expected of each provider, as well as expectations for ongoing monitoring and patient transfer and other aspects of care.

2. Staff are trained in admission procedures and common obstacles encountered by patients, as well as in identification of key persons to be contacted if problems should arise.

3. The program has a case manager who is trained to handle linkages. If the program does not have a formally designated case manager, there is at least clear delineation of responsibility for coordination with other service providers.

4. Procedures are in place for notification in emergencies (involving a patient who is suicidal or hospitalized, for example) when the primary counselor is absent from the program.

5. Staff adhere to clearly spelled out confidentiality regulations. Training on this subject is provided to all staff who work with dual diagnosis patients.

The Concept of "Imminent Danger"

The concept of "imminent danger" often is used to describe problems that can lead to grave consequences to the individual patient (and possibly others), some of which may be the basis for the legal commitment of an individual to treatment. However, the authors of the criteria believe that its application should be broader. In fact, it is the three components in combination that constitute imminent danger: (a) a strong probability that certain behaviors (such as continued alcohol or drug use or relapse) will occur, (b) the likelihood that such behaviors will present a significant risk of serious adverse consequences to the individual and/or others (as in a consistent pattern of driving while intoxicated), and (c) the likelihood that such adverse events will occur in the very near future.

On the one hand, the concept of imminent danger *does not* encompass the universe of possible adverse events, and its evaluation should be restricted to the three factors listed above. On the other hand, the interpretation of imminent danger should not be restricted to acute suicidality, homicidality, or medical or psychiatric problems that create an immediate, catastrophic risk.

Future Directions Matrix

As a first step toward a future configuration of the criteria, a "matrix" format is presented in Appendix A. This Future Directions Matrix takes a significantly different approach to assessment, treatment planning and placement. It emphasizes risk ratings, specifies types of services and modalities needed, and indicates the intensity of services and levels of service and settings where the patient's needs can best be met. The goal is to promote improved assessment and treatment of dual diagnosis patients by taking a more holistic, multidimensional approach that matches specific needs to services, rather than matching in a broader way to a level of care.

The matrix that matches multidimensional risk with the type and intensity of service is designed to be of assistance in the assessment and placement of an individual whether presenting to an addiction or mental health treatment service. It is hoped that patients will receive a similar quality of assessment and care when criteria and guidelines are used that promote a common language of assessment and placement within mental health and addiction treatment systems.

Adolescent Criteria

The Adolescent Criteria have been completely revised in this edition. See the Preface to the Adolescent Criteria for a discussion of specific changes.

Historical Foundations of the ASAM Patient Placement Criteria

The present ASAM criteria have their roots in three efforts to develop patient placement criteria:

Cleveland Criteria

Developed at the request of the Northern Ohio Chemical Dependency Treatment Directors Association, the "Cleveland Criteria" were designed by a team of consultants coordinated by the Chemical Abuse Treatment Outcome Registry (CATOR). Members of the steering committee that guided the project represented treatment programs and other interested organizations in northern Ohio. The authors of the Cleveland Criteria were Norman G. Hoffmann, Ph.D., James A. Halikas, M.D., and David Mee-Lee, M.D. As documented in the seminal 1990 report of the Institute of Medicine of the National Academy of Sciences, *Broadening the Base of Treatment for Alcohol Problems*, the Cleveland Criteria were a significant contribution to the addiction field and provided a springboard for treatment evaluation and assessment studies to follow.

NAATP Criteria

In the second effort, a work group composed of providers and consultants, coordinated by Richard D. Weedman, M.S.W., FACATA, of Healthcare Network, Inc., used all criteria sets available at the time to produce the National Association of Addiction Treatment Providers (NAATP) *Patient Placement Criteria*. These criteria were used by approximately 210 publicly and privately funded addiction treatment programs to enhance their internal utilization review and case management systems and to guide their clinical decision-making processes.

By the end of the 1980s, 40 to 50 sets of criteria were in use by various insurers and utilization management firms in the private sector. Many of these criteria varied sharply in their guidance as to assessment and placement, and some even directly contradicted others. This patchwork caused confusion where consensus was desperately needed.

NAATP-ASAM Collaboration

This work led to a third project in which NAATP and the American Society of Addiction Medicine recruited a representative group of addiction experts to develop adult and adolescent criteria based on the Cleveland Criteria and the NAATP Criteria. The project resulted in the identification and description of four levels of treatment, which were differentiated from each other by the following characteristics:

- Degree of direct medical management provided;
- Structure, safety and security provided; and
- Intensity of treatment services provided.

The drafters also identified and described six patient dimensions that could be used to differentiate patient needs for services across the four levels of care. The result of these efforts were compiled in the *Patient Placement Criteria for the Treatment of Psychoactive Substance Use Disorders*, which was published by the American Society of Addiction Medicine in 1991.

Coalition for National Clinical Criteria

The next step in criteria development occurred when, recognizing the need to broaden stakeholder participation in developing patient placement criteria, ASAM in 1991 convened a meeting of providers, payers, managed care professionals and policymakers. Out of this session emerged a consensus that the field ought to work toward one national set of criteria that could be accepted by employers, purchasers and providers of care in both the public and private sectors. The group also identified desirable characteristics of clinical criteria guidelines.

Participants concluded that consensus criteria should be developed with input from all stakeholders, which they defined as (a) those who use the criteria to make decisions about patient care, utilization review and payment, and (b) those who suffer the consequences if such criteria are not used or are used inappropriately.

In November 1992, ASAM again convened representatives of all the stakeholder groups to build on the work of the first conference. At this meeting, an *ad hoc* entity called the Coalition for National Clinical Criteria was formed to continue the consensus-building process. Four Task Forces were created to carry forward the commitment to national criteria: the ASAM Criteria Implementation Task Force, the Clinical Criteria Revision Task Force, the Treatment Access and Reimbursement Task Force, and the Criteria Research Task Force.

The Coalition initially met annually and has continued its influence through a Steering Committee comprised of major stakeholders who have either endorsed use of the ASAM criteria and/or actively promote their use in care provision and care management. Work groups composed of its members and associated organizations served as drafters and field reviewers of the *ASAM PPC-2R*.

Theoretical Foundations of the ASAM Patient Placement Criteria

Goals of Treatment

Treatment should be tailored to the needs of the individual and guided by an individualized treatment plan that is developed in consultation with the patient. Such a plan should be based on a comprehensive biopsychosocial assessment of the patient and, when possible, a comprehensive evaluation of the family as well. The plan should list problems (such as obstacles to recovery, knowledge or skill deficits, dysfunction or loss), strengths (such as readiness to change, a positive social support system, and a strong connection to a source of spiritual support) and priorities (such as obstacles to treatment or risks, identified within the list of problems and arranged according to severity), goals (a statement to guide realistic, achievable, short-term resolution or reduction of the problems), and methods or strategies (the treatment services to be provided, the site of those services, staff responsible for delivering treatment, and a timetable for follow-through with the treatment plan that promotes accountability). The plan should be written so as to facilitate measurement of progress. As with other disease processes, length of service should be linked directly to the patient's response to treatment (for example, attainment of the treatment goals and degree of resolution regarding the identified clinical problems).

The goals of intervention and treatment (including safe and comfortable detoxification; motivational enhancement to accept the need for recovery; the attainment of skills to maintain abstinence, and the like) determine the methods, intensity, frequency and types of services provided. The health care professional's decision to prescribe a type of service, and subsequent discharge of a patient from a level of care, needs to be based on how that treatment and its duration will not only influence the resolution of the dysfunction, but also positively alter the prognosis for long-term outcome for that individual patient. Thus, in addiction treatment, the treatment may extend beyond simple resolution of observable biomedical distress to the achievement of overall healthier functioning. The patient demonstrates a response to treatment through new insights, attitudes and behaviors. Addiction treatment programs have as their goal not simply stabilizing the patient's condition but altering the course of the patient's disease.

Informed Consent

Health care requires informed consent, indicating that the patient has been made aware of the proposed modalities of treatment, the risks and benefits of such treatment, appropriate alternative treatment modalities and the risks of treatment versus no treatment.

Medical Necessity

Central to judgments concerning appropriateness of care is the concept of "medical necessity." Because substance-related disorders are biopsychosocial in etiology and expression, treatment and care management are most effective if they, too, are biopsychosocial. The six assessment dimensions identified in the ASAM *Patient Placement Criteria* encompass all pertinent biopsychosocial aspects of addiction that determine the severity of the patient's illness and level of function. Medical necessity pertains to necessary care for biopsychosocial severity and is defined by the extent and severity of problems in all six multidimensional assessment areas of the patient. It should not be restricted to narrow medical concerns (such as severity of withdrawal risk) or psychiatric issues (such as imminent suicidality).

Progress Through the Levels of Service

As the patient moves through treatment in any level of service, his or her progress in all six dimensions should be continually assessed. Such multidimensional assessment ensures comprehensive treatment. In the process of patient assessment, certain problems and priorities are identified as justifying admission to a particular level of care. The resolution of those problems and priorities determines when a patient can be treated at a different level of care or discharged from treatment. The appearance of new problems may require services that can be effectively provided at the same level of care, or that require a more or less intensive level of care.

As the patient's response to treatment is assessed, new priorities for recovery are identified. The intensity of the strategies of the treatment plan helps determine the most efficient and effective level of service that can safely provide the care articulated in the individualized treatment plan. Patients may, however, worsen or fail to improve in a given level of care or with a given type of program within a level of care or service. At such time, changing the level of care or changing the program should be based upon a reassessment of the treatment plan with modifications to achieve a better therapeutic response.

In cases where some extenuating circumstances must be considered, further justification and presentation of rationale should substantiate the level of care or type of service chosen.

Exceptions to the Patient Placement Criteria

In making treatment placement decisions, three important factors override the patient-treatment match with regard to levels of service:

1. Lack of availability of appropriate, criteria-selected care;

2. Failure of a patient to progress at a given level of care, so as to warrant a reassessment of the treatment plan with a view to modification of the treatment approach. Such situations may require transfer to a specialized program at the same level of care or to a more intensive or less intensive level of care to achieve a better therapeutic response; and

3. State laws regulating the practice of medicine or licensure of a facility requiring criteria different from these.

While these criteria are intended to be as specific as possible, unique clinical presentation or extenuating circumstances may dictate some flexibility in application of the criteria to ensure the safety and welfare of the patient.

Principles Guiding Development of the ASAM Patient Placement Criteria

Several important principles have guided development of the ASAM *Patient Placement Criteria*:

Objectivity. The criteria are as objective, measurable and quantifiable as possible. Certain aspects of the criteria require subjective interpretation. In this regard, the assessment and treatment of substance-related disorders is no different from biomedical or psychiatric conditions in which diagnosis or assessment and treatment is a mix of objectively measured criteria and experientially based professional judgments.

Choice of Treatment Levels. Referral to a specific level of care must be based on a careful assessment of the patient with an alcohol or other drug dependence problem. The goal that underlies the criteria is the placement of the patient in the most appropriate level of care. For both clinical and financial reasons, the preferred level of care is the least intensive level that meets treatment objectives, while providing safety and security for the patient. Moreover, while the levels of service are presented as discrete levels, in reality they represent benchmarks or points along a continuum of treatment services that could be used in a variety of ways depending on a patient's needs and response. A patient can begin at a more intensive level and move to a more or less intensive level of care, depending on his or her individual needs.

Continuum of Care. Treatment is delivered across a continuum of services that reflect the varying severity of illnesses treated and the intensity of services required. It is understood that reimbursement needs to match this continuum of care and intensity of service. Many providers of addiction treatment offer only one of the many levels of service described. In such situations, movement between levels might mean referring the patient out of the provider's own network of care. ASAM believes that description of patient needs and treatment levels will assist the treatment field in developing the continuum of care necessary for effective and efficient treatment. While lack of reimbursement for some levels of care, or lack of availability of other levels of care, may render this impossible at present, the goal of these criteria is to stimulate the development of efficient and effective treatment services that can be made available to all patients.

Treatment Failure. Another concern is the concept of "treatment failure," which has been used by some reimbursement or managed care organizations as a prerequisite for approving admission to a higher level of care (for example, "failure" in outpatient treatment as a prerequisite for admission to inpatient treatment). In fact, the requirement that a person "fail" in outpatient treatment before inpatient treatment is approved is no more rational than treating every patient in an inpatient program or using a fixed length of stay for all. It also does not recognize the obvious parallels between addictive disorders and other chronic diseases such as diabetes or hypertension.

Such a strategy potentially puts the patient at risk because it delays a more appropriate level of treatment, and potentially increases health care costs if restricting the appropriate level of treatment allows the addictive disorder to progress.

Length of Stay. Outcomes research in addiction treatment is still relatively new, and has not yet provided a scientific basis for determining precise lengths of stay for optimum results. Addiction treatment professionals are moving in that direction, but have not yet arrived. However, the research does show a positive correlation between longer treatment and better outcomes.

Twelve Step, Mutual Help and Self-Help Recovery Groups. Recovery groups such as Alcoholics Anonymous, Narcotics Anonymous, Cocaine Anonymous or Smart Recovery® do not constitute formal treatment programs. Clinicians see the value of such groups in their presence as a lifelong support system, and believe that an individual's chances of a successful outcome are significantly enhanced by involvement in recovery groups. Because of the importance of these fellowships, most providers integrate the philosophy of Twelve Step recovery groups into the treatment services themselves. Thus, participation in mutual or self-help groups is a crucial element of *all* levels of care.

As valuable as they are, however, these groups do *not* constitute a treatment level. Rather, it is best to consider them "self problem identification, help-seeking options." To refer an individual to self-help groups based solely on cost considerations is analogous to referring a person with diabetes to a diabetes support group rather than to formal treatment. On the other hand, there are situations in which a person may be evaluated for a substance-related disorder and, based on a conclusion that no condition exists that warrants formal treatment, he or she may be referred to a Twelve Step recovery or other mutual help or self-help group.

Significant consideration was given to inclusion of spiritual parameters as they relate to placement criteria. Although spiritual concepts, ideas, and relationships are integral to all levels of care and, to a certain degree, even transcend each level of care, they are difficult to define acceptably in objective, behavioral and measurable terms. Nevertheless, spirituality is implied in all dimensions and in all levels of care.

Treatment Outcomes. As the knowledge base expands, each identified problem and level of severity, with corresponding treatment recommendations, is expected to be supported by adequate documentation in the medical-scientific literature to provide guidance to the clinician in making a prognosis and in planning appropriate care.

Real World Considerations in Using the ASAM Patient Placement Criteria

Clinical versus Reimbursement Considerations

The criteria presented in the *PPC-2R* have been developed to describe a wide range of levels and types of care for substance use problems. Not all of these services are available in all locations, nor are they covered by all payers. Clinicians who make placement decisions are expected to amplify the criteria with their clinical judgment, their knowledge of the patient, and their knowledge of the available resources. The *PPC-2R* is not intended as a reimbursement guideline, but rather as a clinical guideline for making the most appropriate placement recommendation for an individual patient with a specific set of symptoms and behaviors. If the criteria only covered the levels of care commonly reimbursable by private insurance carriers, they would not address many of the resources of the public sector and, thus, would tacitly endorse limitations on a complete continuum of care.

The Concept of "Unbundling"

While the first edition of the *Patient Placement Criteria* "bundled" clinical services with environmental supports in fixed levels of care, there is increasing recognition that clinical services can be and often are provided separately from environmental supports. Indeed, many managed care companies and public treatment systems are suggesting that treatment modality and intensity be "unbundled" from the treatment setting. Unbundling is a practice that allows any type of clinical service (such as psychiatric consultation) to be delivered in any setting (such as a therapeutic community). With unbundling, the type and intensity of treatment are based on the patient's needs and not on limitations imposed by the treatment setting. The unbundling concept thus is designed to maximize individualized care and to encourage the delivery of necessary treatment in any clinically feasible setting. As a first step toward "unbundled" criteria, the second edition incorporated criteria for five levels of detoxification care as a clinical service separate from the environmental supports. The PPC-2R continues such "unbundled" criteria.

The ASAM Criteria and State Licensure or Certification

The ASAM criteria contain descriptions of treatment programs at each level of care, including the setting, staffing, support systems, therapies, assessments, documentation and treatment plan reviews typically found at that level. This information should be useful to providers who are preparing to serve a particular group of patients, as well as to clinicians who are making placement decisions. Nevertheless, the descriptions are not requirements and are not intended to replace or supercede the relevant statutes, licensure or certification requirements of any state.

Placement Impediments and Dilemmas

In the real world, issues surrounding access, reimbursement, funding, resource allocation and availability may affect the patient placement decision.

Logistical Impediments. Logistical problems can arise anywhere, but are found most frequently in rural and underserved inner-city areas. When logistical considerations prove an impediment to the indicated services (for example, lack of available transportation is a barrier to access to an indicated outpatient program), an outpatient service combined with unsupervised/minimally supervised housing may be an appropriate treatment intervention. In cities or towns, such a domiciliary option might be found in a group living situation (such as a Salvation Army program, motel accommodations, YMCA/YWCA or mission). In rural and other underserved areas, options would include: (a) the creation of a supervised housing situation by using unused treatment beds; (b) assertive community treatment models in which the treatment is brought to rural areas (such as Native American settlements) and provided in weekend intensive models such as day treatment to both the identified patient and family members, utilizing as sites community resources such as churches; (c) vans that are sent out to pick up individuals and bring them to a treatment site or (d) conducting counseling sessions on-site, using a van or motor home as an office or group therapy room. In situations in which the primary problems are logistical (as with a patient who has no access to public transportation, automobile or valid driver's license), a combination of Level II.5 services with a domiciliary or supportive living component is the most appropriate placement.

Need for a Safe Environment. When a patient lives in a recovery environment that is so toxic as to preclude recovery efforts (as through victimization or exposure to an active addict) and a Level I or II outpatient service is indicated, the patient may need referral to a safe place to live while in treatment (that is, a domiciliary facility) as well as to treatment itself.

Assessment of Imminent Danger. If an individual has problems in Dimensions 4 and 5 that require 24-hour supervision and treatment interventions (such as boundary setting), without which treatment services cannot be effectively delivered, and/or the individual is in imminent danger, then the mere addition of room and board in a domiciliary facility would be inadequate to meet the individual's needs. Such a patient needs placement in a residential program that offers clinical staff and services 24 hours a day in order to respond to the patient's issues involving imminent danger. The assessment of risk can guide the decision.

If, in place of a Level III service, Level II.1 or II.5 services are combined with a domiciliary/ supportive living component, there are a variety of ways in which domiciliary services can be provided. The living environment may be in the same facility as the treatment services or they may be in a separate facility. Patients may be housed at the treatment program or live at a mission, Salvation Army program, halfway house, or in another supportive living environment. In the latter case, the relationship between the living environment and treatment services must be sufficiently direct to allow specific aspects of the individual treatment plan to be addressed in both facilities.

Inpatient and residential services are two qualitatively different intensities of service. Both provide 24-hour support and structure for individuals who are not stable enough to effectively utilize outpatient services no matter how intensive, and both groups of patients/residents appropriate for this level of service present issues of imminent danger, defined as "high probability of significant risk in the near future" that exist in any of the six dimensions.

Inpatient services differ from residential services in the need for access to and availability of 24-hour treatment for problems that exist in Dimensions 1, 2 or 3 and require medical and/or nursing interventions. Individuals in residential services need access to and availability of 24-hour treatment for problems that exist in Dimensions 4, 5 or 6 and thereby require clinical rather than medical and/or nursing interventions.

Mandated Level of Care or Length of Stay. In some cases, an individual is referred for treatment at a specific level of care and/or for a specific length of stay (for example, an offender in the criminal justice system may be given a choice of a prison term or fixed length of stay in a treatment center). Such mandated or court-ordered referrals may not be based on clinical considerations and thus may be inconsistent with a placement decision arrived at through the ASAM criteria. In such a case, the provider should make reasonable attempts to have the order amended to reflect the assessed clinical level or length of service.

If the court order or other mandate cannot be amended, the individual may be continuing treatment at a level of care or for a length of stay greater than is clinically indicated. The resident's readiness for discharge or transfer and the staff's attempts to implement a clinically appropriate placement should be noted in the clinical record, and the treatment plan should be updated in a manner that provides the resident with the opportunity to continue the recovery process at the same level of care even though it could be continued at a less intensive level of care.

Interactions Across Dimensions in Assessing for Level of Care. The ASAM criteria function best when individuals are assessed in each dimension independently and also in terms of the interaction across dimensions. For example, when assessing an individual for severity, a history of moderate or severe withdrawal *without* any current intoxication or withdrawal, or current intoxication without a history of significant withdrawal problems should generate a lesser level of concern than a combination of a history of moderate or severe withdrawal *with* current symptoms of intoxication or withdrawal.

In reality, there is considerable interaction across dimensions. For example, significant problems with readiness to change (Dimension 4), coupled with a poor recovery environment (Dimension 6) or moderate problems with relapse or continued use (Dimension 5), may increase the risk of relapse. Another commonly seen combination involves problems in Dimension 2 (such as chronic pain that distracts the patient from the recovery process) coupled with problems in Dimensions 4, 5 or 6.

The converse also is true. For example, problems with relapse potential (Dimension 5) may be offset by a high degree of readiness to change (Dimension 4) or a very supportive recovery environment (Dimension 6). The interaction of these factors may result in a lower level of severity than is seen in any dimension alone.

The lesson here is that assessments are most accurate when they take into account all of the factors (dimensions) that affect each individual's receptivity and ability to engage in treatment at a particular point in time.

Outcomes Research with the ASAM Patient Placement Criteria

ASAM expects the *Patient Placement Criteria* to continue to evolve as a result of research findings and further experience with their use. Thus it would be a mistake to wait for a "final" set of criteria before adopting and using the ASAM *PPC-2R*. The development of the present and future editions of the criteria should be approached in the same way clinicians approach the American Psychiatric Association's *Diagnostic and Statistical Manual of Mental Disorders*, which is now in its fifth version—that is, as a work in progress.

Over the past five years, the *Patient Placement Criteria* have been subjected to the crucial process of research testing. The ultimate goal of this work is for future editions of the criteria to be developed not simply through the current expert consensus process, but also through a nationwide system of data gathering, quantitative analysis and feedback. The literature offers numerous studies showing that constructs such as the dimensions of the *Patient Placement Criteria* predict treatment success (Gastfriend & McLellan, 1997). The *Patient Placement Criteria* now are a tested treatment planning methodology. There are at least seven known studies of the ASAM criteria, supported by funding from two of the National Institutes of Health (the National Institute on Drug Abuse and the National Institute on Alcohol Abuse and Alcoholism), as well as the Center for Substance Abuse Treatment of the Substance Abuse and Mental Health Services Administration. Grant funds specifically designated by the U.S. government for PPC research now exceed seven million dollars.

In the earliest evaluation, counselors used a simple, one-page summary of *PPC-1* in the Boston Target Cities Central Intakes (Plough et al., 1996). Compared to conventional intake without criteria at treatment sites, patients who were referred to inpatient detoxification using PPC-guided assessment were 38% more likely to transition to continuing treatment within 30 days (as in outpatient care following detoxification) (odds ratio = 1.55, $p<.005$) and were significantly less likely to return for detoxification within 90 days (odds ratio = .57, $p<.005$). This result suggested that even a coarse version of the ASAM criteria is associated with improved treatment retention.

A pilot study by Morey et al. (1996) retrospectively applied an abbreviated *PPC-1* algorithm to telephone survey data. The results showed a good degree of face validity and level of care utilization patterns that suggested a degree of concurrent validity (Morey, personal communication). A retrospective study by McKay et al. (1997) implemented only the psychosocial dimensions of the *PPC-1* with a degree of brevity that may not have been adequate. Support was found for predictive validity for some aspects of dependence, but not others. Ease of use and feasibility, however, were concerns of several research groups (Gastfriend, 1999). In a 1998 West Virginia Office of Behavioral Health Services adaptation of the first edition, "even staff who received extensive training report that their ability to determine a patient's readiness for a particular level of care is made more difficult due to (a) long and often ambiguous text/format and (b) the lack of clear directions on the use of the cross-walks provided in these instruments" (May, 1998).

A solution has been developed to address the problem of interviewer ease of use of PPC. This solution has now been tested in three prospective studies. It consists of a comprehensive implementation designed by Gastfriend et al. to offer the counselor a sequence of questions and scoring options on the screen of a microcomputer (Turner et al., 1999). This instrument has been shown to have good inter-rater reliability (intraclass correlation coefficient = 0.77) (Gastfriend et al., ASAM Annual Medical-Scientific Meeting, Chicago IL, April 2000). In a naturalistic study of 95 VA patients, *PPC-1* was found to be associated with improved hospital service utilization. Male veterans treated in Level III (residential care) but who met *PPC-1* criteria for the more intensive Level IV (hospital level of care) required nearly twice as many hospital bed days over the subsequent year as those who qualified for only Levels II (such as day treatment) or III (residential care) ($p<.05$). This finding did not appear to be merely explained by premorbid differential chronicity ($p=n.s.$) (Gastfriend et al., in press 2000).

In another naturalistic study using this computerized algorithm, Magura et al. studied 258 subjects admitted to a New York City treatment center. Patients who received a lower level of care than recommended by the *PPC-1* had poorer alcohol use outcomes than those who were correctly matched to treatment according to the *PPC-1* (Magura S, ASAM Annual Medical-Scientific Meeting, Chicago IL, April 2000).

Finally, in the only random controlled trial of placement criteria to date, Gastfriend et al., have reported good concurrent validity (Gastfriend, 1999; Turner et al., 1999) and predictive validity in a multi-site of the ASAM criteria in eastern Massachusetts. An interim analysis was performed of the first 155 subjects who were randomized to Level II or III treatment, that is, either matched or mismatched. Patients who were mismatched to lower level of care than recommended by the *PPC-1* algorithm showed less or slower improvement on several dimensions of addiction severity (Gastfriend et al., ASAM Annual Medical-Scientific Meeting, Chicago IL, April 2000).

Given these early studies showing adequate reliability, good concurrent validity and even some degree of predictive validity, the ASAM criteria appear to be clinically meaningful and suitable for research evaluation at a high level of scientific rigor. Undoubtedly, much work remains to be done. For example, the *PPC-2R* increase the levels of care through the use of sublevels for dual diagnosis enhancement.

These offer opportunities for greater individualization of care. For example, Dimension 5 has been given a new chapter in this volume, in which we propose how assessment of relapse risk may be expanded to take into account the various research constructs that have shown good predictive validity. Examples of assessment tools are included so that programs may evaluate reliable, quantitative questionnaires for assessing this dimension.

New technologies also will advance the ASAM criteria. Based on the successful replication of validity studies using the computerized algorithm of Gastfriend et al. at Massachusetts General Hospital (Gastfriend et al., in press 2000), a user-friendly software product has been exclusively authorized by ASAM for wide-scale distribution. This *PPC-2R* assessment software presents the opportunity, for the first time, to permit both providers and researchers throughout the field to speak the same language, and arrive at the same level of care determinations. The software includes the additional feature of confidential data uploads to an ASAM-authorized central data repository, which will provide aggregate analyses of the placements, utilizations and outcomes of patients who are rated according to *PPC-2R*. This new repository will have two simultaneous benefits for the field. It will permit treatment programs to understand their utilization patterns and needs. At the same time, the data repository will offer research groups a close, quantitative look at the validity of the ASAM criteria. This will establish an ongoing field trial process that will be reported back to the National Coalition on Patient Placement Criteria, so that future revisions can be driven by empirical data.

References

Allen JP & Columbus M, eds. (1995). *Assessing Alcohol Problems--A Guide for Clinicians and Researchers*. Bethesda, MD: National Institute on Alcohol Abuse and Alcoholism.

American Psychiatric Association (1994). *Diagnostic and Statistical Manual of Mental Disorders, Fourth Edition (DSM-IV)*. Washington, DC: American Psychiatric Press.

California Department of Alcohol and Drug Programs (1994). *Evaluating Recovery Services: The California Drug and Alcohol Assessment (CALDATA)*. Sacramento, CA: The Department.

Campbell EJM, Scadding JG & Roberts RS (1979). The concept of disease. *British Medical Journal* 2:757-762.

De Leon G (1995). Therapeutic communities for addictions: A theoretical framework. *International Journal of the Addictions* 30(12):1603-1645.

Donovan DM (1988). Assessment of addictive behaviors: Implications of an emerging biopsychosocial model. In DM Donovan and GA Marlatt (eds.) *Assessment of Addictive Behavior*. New York, NY: Guilford Press.

Gartner L & Mee-Lee D, eds. (1995). *The Role and Current Status of Patient Placement Criteria in the Treatment of Substance Use Disorders* (Treatment Improvement Protocol No. 13). Rockville, MD: Center for Substance Abuse Treatment.

Gastfriend DR (1994). Anticipated problems facing ASAM patient placement criteria. Presented at the CSAT TIP Meeting, April 21, 1994.

Gastfriend DR (1999). Placement Matching: Challenges and Technical Progress. Proceedings of the AAAP Tenth Annual Meeting & Symposium, pp. 19-20.

Gastfriend DR & McLellan AT (1997). Treatment matching: Theoretic basis and practical implications. *Medical Clinics of North America* 81(4):945-966.

Gastfriend DR, Najavits LM & Reif S (1994). Assessment instruments. In N Miller (ed.) *Principles of Addiction Medicine, First Edition.* Chevy Chase, MD: American Society of Addiction Medicine.

Gastfriend DR, Sharon E, Turner W, Desai N & Penk W (in press 2000). Validity of multidimensional substance abuse treatment matching using the ASAM Patient Placement Criteria.

Harbin H, Marques C, Book J, Silverman C & Lizanich-Aro S (1994). On the use of ASAM's and Green Spring's alcohol and drug detoxification and rehabilitation criteria for utilization review. Unpublished analysis.

Harrison PA, Hoffmann NG, Hollister CD & Luxenberg MG (1988). Determinants of chemical dependency treatment placement: Clinical, economic, and logistic factors. *Psychotherapy* 25:356-364.

Hoffmann NG, DeHart SS & Gogineni A (1998). Alcohol dependence as a chronic health problem among older adults. *The Southwestern Journal on Aging* 14:57-64.

Hoffmann NG, Floyd AS, Zywiak WH & DeHart SS (1999). Strategies for Case-Mix Adjustments in Addictions Treatment Evaluations: Prognostic Indicators in Public Sector Populations. Report prepared for the State of Wisconsin under CSAT Contract 270-95-0023.

Hoffmann NG & Longabaugh R (1999). Final Report: Developing a Foundation for Outcomes Based Addictions Treatment. Submitted to the Robert Wood Johnson Foundation.

Hoffmann NG, Mee-Lee D & Arrowood AA (1993). Treatment issues in adolescent substance use and addictions: Options, outcome, effectiveness, reimbursement and admissions criteria. *Adolescent Medicine: State of the Art Reviews* 4(2):371-390.

Hsieh S, Hoffmann NG & Hollister CD (1998). The relationship between pre-, during-, and post-treatment factors and adolescent substance abuse behaviors. *The Journal of Addictive Behaviors* 23:1-12.

Institute for Health Policy (1993). *Substance Abuse: The Nation's No. 1 Health Problem: Key Indicators for Policy.* Princeton, NJ: Robert Wood Johnson Foundation.

Institute of Medicine (1990). *Broadening the Base of Treatment for Alcohol Problems.* Washington, DC: National Academy Press.

Institute of Medicine (1989). *Controlling Cost and Changing Patient Care: The Role of Utilization Management*. Washington, DC: National Academy Press.

Lettieri D, Sayers M & Nelson J, eds. (1985). *Alcoholism Treatment Assessment Instruments*. Bethesda, MD: National Institute on Alcohol Abuse and Alcoholism.

Lettieri D, Sayers M & Nelson J, eds. (1985). *Summaries of Alcoholism Treatment Assessment Research*. Bethesda, MD: National Institute on Alcohol Abuse and Alcoholism.

May WW (1998). A field application of the ASAM Placement Criteria in a 12-step model of treatment for chemical dependency. *Journal of Addictive Diseases* 17(2):77-91.

McKay JR, Cacciola JS, McLellan AT, Alterman AI & Wirtz PW (1997). An initial evaluation of the psychosocial dimensions of the American Society of Addiction Medicine criteria for inpatient vs. intensive outpatient substance abuse rehabilitation. *Journal of Studies on Alcohol* 58(5):239-252.

McLellan AT & Alterman AI (1991). Patient-treatment matching: A conceptual and methodological review, with suggestions for future research. In RW Pickens, CG Leukefeld & CR Schuster (eds.) *Improving Drug Abuse Treatment* (Research Monograph 106). Rockville, MD: National Institute on Drug Abuse.

McLellan AT, Kushner H & Metzger D (1992). The fifth edition of the Addiction Severity Index. *Journal of Substance Abuse Treatment* 93(3):199-213.

Mee-Lee D (1988). An instrument for treatment progress and matching: The Recovery Attitude and Treatment Evaluator (RAATE). *Journal of Substance Abuse Treatment* 5:183-186.

Mee-Lee D (1995). Matching in addictions treatment: How do we get there from here? In *Alcoholism Treatment Quarterly*, Special issue on Treatment of the Addictions: Applications of Outcome Research for Clinical Management 12(2).

Mee-Lee D (1994). Placement criteria and patient-treatment matching. In N Miller (ed.) *Principles of Addiction Medicine, First Edition*. Chevy Chase, MD: American Society of Addiction Medicine.

Mee-Lee D & Hoffmann NG (1992). *Loci-Level of Care Index: A Concise Summary of ASAM Criteria's Factors to Document the Need for Placement, Continued Stay, and Discharge*. St. Paul, MN: New Standards, Inc.

Miller WR & Rollnick S (1991). *Motivational Interviewing: Preparing People to Change Addictive Behavior*. New York, NY: The Guilford Press, 1991.

Morey L (1996). Patient placement criteria: Linking typologies to managed care. *Alcohol Health & Research World* 20(1):36-44.

Morse RM, Flavin DK et al. (1992). The definition of alcoholism. *Journal of the American Medical Association* 268:1012-1014.

National Institute on Drug Abuse (1999). *Principles of Drug Addiction Treatment—A Research Based Guide*. Rockville, MD: NIDA (NIH Publication # 99-4180).

National Institute on Drug Abuse (1994). *Mental Health Assessment and Diagnosis of Substance Abusers* (Clinical Report Series). Rockville, MD: NIDA (NCADI #BKD148).

National Institute on Drug Abuse (1997). *Treatment of Drug-Dependent Individuals With Comorbid Mental Disorders* (Research Monograph 172). Rockville, MD: NIDA (GPO #017-024-01605).

Payte JT & Zweben JE (1998). Opioid replacement therapies. In AW Graham & TK Schultz (eds.) *Principles of Addiction Medicine, Second Edition*. Chevy Chase, MD: American Society of Addiction Medicine.

Plough A, Shirley L, Zaremba N, Baker G, Schwartz M & Mulvey K (1996). *CSAT Target Cities Demonstration Final Evaluation Report*. Boston, MA: Office for Treatment Improvement.

Prochaska JO, DiClemente CC & Norcross JC (1992). In search of how people change: Applications to addictive behaviors. *American Psychologist* 47:1102-1114.

Prochaska JO, Norcross JC & DiClemente CC (1994). *Changing for Good*. New York, NY: Avon Books.

Rawson RA & Ling W (n.d.). *American Society of Addiction Medicine Patient Placement Criteria for the Treatment of Psychoactive Substance Use Disorders: An Analysis*. Unpublished paper prepared for the California Office of Alcohol and Drug Programs.

Rinaldi RC, Steindler EM, Wilford BB & Goodwin D (1988). Clarification and standardization of substance abuse terminology. *Journal of the American Medical Association* 259:555-557.

Shulman GD (1993). The ASAM Criteria: A benefit to EAPs. *EAP Digest* 13(4):26-28.

Turner WM, Turner KH, Reif S, Gutowski WE & Gastfriend DR (1999). Feasibility of multidimensional substance abuse treatment matching: Automating the ASAM Patient Placement Criteria. *Drug and Alcohol Dependence* 55:35-43.

Weedman RD (1987). *Admission, Continued Stay and Discharge Criteria for Adult Alcoholism and Drug Dependence Treatment Services*. Irvine, CA: National Association of Addiction Treatment Providers.

Zywiak WH, Hoffmann NG & Floyd AS (1999). Enhancing alcohol treatment outcomes through aftercare and self-help groups. *Medicine & Health/Rhode Island* 82(3):87-90.

Adult Patient Placement Criteria

Crosswalk of the Adult Placement Criteria
Levels 0.5 through IV

Criteria Dimensions	Levels of Care				
	Level 0.5 Early Intervention	OMT Opioid Maintenance Therapy	Level I Outpatient Treatment	Level II.1 Intensive Outpatient	Level II.5 Partial Hospitalization
DIMENSION 1: Alcohol Intoxication and/or Withdrawal Potential	The patient is not at risk of withdrawal.	The patient is physiologically dependent on opiates and requires OMT to prevent withdrawal.	The patient is not experiencing significant withdrawal or is at minimal risk of severe withdrawal.	The patient is at minimal risk of severe withdrawal.	The patient is at moderate risk of severe withdrawal.
DIMENSION 2: Biomedical Conditions and Complications	None or very stable.	None or manageable with outpatient medical monitoring.	None or very stable, or the patient is receiving concurrent medical monitoring.	None or not a distraction from treatment. Such problems are manageable at Level II.1.	None or not sufficient to distract from treatment. Such problems are manageable at Level II.5.
DIMENSION 3: Emotional, Behavioral or Cognitive Conditions and Complications	None or very stable.	None or manageable in an outpatient structured environment.	None or very stable, or the patient is receiving concurrent mental health monitoring.	Mild severity, with the potential to distract from recovery; the patient needs monitoring.	Mild to moderate severity, with the potential to distract from recovery; the patient needs stabilization.

ASAM Patient Placement Criteria, Second Edition–Revised

Crosswalk of the Adult Placement Criteria
Levels 0.5 through IV

Criteria Dimensions	Level 0.5 Early Intervention	OMT Opioid Maintenance Therapy	Level I Outpatient Treatment	Level II.1 Intensive Outpatient	Level II.5 Partial Hospitalization
DIMENSION 4: Readiness to Change	The patient is willing to explore how current alcohol or drug use may affect personal goals.	The patient is ready to change the negative effects of opiate use, but is not ready for total abstinence.	The patient is ready for recovery, but needs motivating and monitoring strategies to strengthen readiness. Or there is high severity in this dimension but not in other dimensions. The patient therefore needs a Level I motivational enhancement program.	The patient has variable engagement in treatment, ambivalence, or lack of awareness of the substance use or mental health problem, and requires a structured program several times a week to promote progress through the stages of change.	The patient has poor engagement in treatment, significant ambivalence, or lack of awareness of the substance use or mental health problem, requiring a near-daily structured program or intensive engagement services to promote progress through the stages of change.
DIMENSION 5: Relapse, Continued Use or Continued Problem Potential	The patient needs an understanding of, or skills to change, his or her current alcohol and drug use patterns.	The patient is at high risk of relapse or continued use without OMT and structured therapy to promote treatment progress.	The patient is able to maintain abstinence or control use and pursue recovery or motivational goals with minimal support.	Intensification of the patient's addiction or mental health symptoms indicate a high likelihood of relapse or continued use or continued problems without close monitoring and support several times a week.	Intensification of the patient's addiction or mental health symptoms, despite active participation in a Level I or II.1 program, indicates a high likelihood of relapse or continued use or continued problems without near-daily monitoring and support.

ASAM Patient Placement Criteria, Second Edition–Revised

Crosswalk of the Adult Placement Criteria
Levels 0.5 through IV

Criteria Dimensions	Levels of Care				
	Level 0.5 Early Intervention	OMT Opioid Maintenance Therapy	Level I Outpatient Treatment	Level II.1 Intensive Outpatient	Level II.5 Partial Hospitalization
DIMENSION 6: Recovery Environment	The patient's social support system or significant others increase the risk of personal conflict about alcohol or drug use.	The patient's recovery environment is supportive and/or the patient has skills to cope.	The patient's recovery environment is supportive and/or the patient has skills to cope.	The patient's recovery environment is not supportive but, with structure and support, the patient can cope.	The patient's recovery environment is not supportive but, with structure and support and relief from the home environment, the patient can cope.

ASAM Patient Placement Criteria, Second Edition–Revised

Adult Admission Criteria
Crosswalk of Levels 0.5 through IV (continued)

Levels of Care

Criteria Dimensions	Level III.1 Clinically Managed Low-Intensity Residential Services	Level III.3 Clinically Managed Medium-Intensity Residential Treatment	Level III.5 Clinically Managed High-Intensity Residential Treatment	Level III.7 Medically Monitored Intensive Inpatient Treatment	Level IV Medically Managed Intensive Inpatient Treatment
DIMENSION 1: Alcohol Intoxication and/or Withdrawal Potential	The patient is not at risk of withdrawal, or is experiencing minimal or stable withdrawal. The patient is concurrently receiving Level I-D (minimal) or Level II-D (moderate) services.	The patient is not at risk of severe withdrawal, or moderate withdrawal is manageable at Level III.2-D.	The patient is at minimal risk of severe withdrawal at Levels III.3 or III.5. If withdrawal is present, it meets Level III.2-D criteria.	The patient is at high risk of withdrawal, but it is manageable at Level III.7-D and does not require the full resources of a licensed hospital.	The patient is at high risk of withdrawal and requires the full resources of a licensed hospital.
DIMENSION 2: Biomedical Conditions and Complications	None or stable, or the patient is receiving concurrent medical monitoring.	None or stable, or the patient is receiving concurrent medical monitoring.	None or stable, or the patient is receiving concurrent medical monitoring.	The patient requires 24-hour medical monitoring but not intensive treatment.	The patient requires 24-hour medical and nursing care and the full resources of a licensed hospital.

ASAM Patient Placement Criteria, Second Edition–Revised

Adult Admission Criteria
Crosswalk of Levels 0.5 through IV (continued)

Criteria Dimensions	Level III.1 Clinically Managed Low-Intensity Residential Services	Level III.3 Clinically Managed Medium-Intensity Residential Treatment	Level III.5 Clinically Managed High-Intensity Residential Treatment	Level III.7 Medically Monitored Intensive Inpatient Treatment	Level IV Medically Managed Intensive Inpatient Treatment
DIMENSION 3: Emotional, Behavioral or Cognitive Conditions and Complications	None or minimal; not distracting to recovery. If stable, a Dual Diagnosis Capable program is appropriate. If not, a Dual Diagnosis Enhanced program is required.	Mild to moderate severity; the patient needs structure to focus on recovery. If stable, a Dual Diagnosis Capable program is appropriate. If not, a Dual Diagnosis Enhanced program is required. Treatment should be designed to respond to the resident's cognitive deficits.	The patient demonstrates repeated inability to control impulses, or a personality disorder requires structure to shape behavior. Other functional deficits require a 24-hour setting to teach coping skills. A Dual Diagnosis Enhanced setting is required for the patient who is severely and persistently mentally ill.	Moderate severity; the patient needs a 24-hour structured setting. If the patient has a co-occurring mental disorder, he or she requires concurrent mental health services in a medically monitored setting.	Because of severe and unstable problems, the patient requires 24-hour psychiatric care with concomitant addiction treatment (Dual Diagnosis Enhanced).

ASAM Patient Placement Criteria, Second Edition–Revised

Adult Admission Criteria
Crosswalk of Levels 0.5 through IV (continued)

Criteria Dimensions	Level III.1 Clinically Managed Low-Intensity Residential Services	Level III.3 Clinically Managed Medium-Intensity Residential Treatment	Level III.5 Clinically Managed High-Intensity Residential Treatment	Level III.7 Medically Monitored Intensive Inpatient Treatment	Level IV Medically Managed Intensive Inpatient Treatment
DIMENSION 4: Readiness to Change	The patient is open to recovery, but needs a structured environment to maintain therapeutic gains.	The patient has little awareness and needs interventions available only at Level III.3 to engage and stay in treatment. Or there is high severity in this dimension but not in other dimensions. The patient therefore needs a Level I motivational enhancement program.	The patient has marked difficulty with or opposition to treatment, with dangerous consequences. Or there is high severity in this dimension but not in other dimensions. The patient therefore needs a Level I motivational enhancement program.	The patient's resistance is high and impulse control poor, despite negative consequences; he or she needs motivating strategies available only in a 24-hour structured setting. Or, if a 24-hour setting is not required, the patient needs a Level I motivational enhancement program.	Problems in this dimension do not qualify the patient for Level IV services.

Adult Admission Criteria
Crosswalk of Levels 0.5 through IV (continued)

Criteria Dimensions	Level III.1 Clinically Managed Low-Intensity Residential Services	Level III.3 Clinically Managed Medium-Intensity Residential Treatment	Level III.5 Clinically Managed High-Intensity Residential Treatment	Level III.7 Medically Monitored Intensive Inpatient Treatment	Level IV Medically Managed Intensive Inpatient Treatment
DIMENSION 5: Relapse, Continued Use or Continued Problem Potential	The patient understands relapse but needs structure to maintain therapeutic gains.	The patient has little awareness and needs interventions available only at Level III.3 to prevent continued use, with imminent dangerous consequences, because of cognitive deficits or comparable dysfunction.	The patient has no recognition of the skills needed to prevent continued use, with imminently dangerous consequences.	The patient is unable to control use, with imminently dangerous consequences, despite active participation at less intensive levels of care.	Problems in this dimension do not qualify the patient for Level IV services.
DIMENSION 6: Recovery Environment	The patient's environment is dangerous, but recovery is achievable if Level III.1 24-hour structure is available.	The patient's environment is dangerous and he or she needs 24-hour structure to learn to cope.	The patient's environment is dangerous and he or she lacks skills to cope outside of a highly structured 24-hour setting.	The patient's environment is dangerous and he or she lacks skills to cope outside of a highly structured 24-hour setting.	Problems in this dimension do not qualify the patient for Level IV services.

Note: This overview of the Adult Admission Criteria is an approximate summary to illustrate the principal concepts and structure of the criteria.

ASAM Patient Placement Criteria, Second Edition–Revised

Continued Service and Discharge Criteria
Adult Patient Placement Criteria

In the process of patient assessment, certain problems and priorities are identified as justifying admission to a particular level of care. The resolution of those problems and priorities determines when a patient can be treated at a different level or discharged from treatment. The appearance of new problems may require services that can be provided effectively at the same level of care, or they may require a more or less intensive level of care.

After the admission criteria for a given level of care have been met, the criteria for continued service, discharge or transfer from that level of care are as follows:

Continued Service Criteria

It is appropriate to retain the patient at the present level of care if:

1. The patient is making progress, but has not yet achieved the goals articulated in the individualized treatment plan. Continued treatment at the present level of care is assessed as necessary to permit the patient to continue to work toward his or her treatment goals;

   or

2. The patient is not yet making progress, but has the capacity to resolve his or her problems. He or she is actively working toward the goals articulated in the individualized treatment plan. Continued treatment at the present level of care is assessed as necessary to permit the patient to continue to work toward his or her treatment goals;

   and/or

3. New problems have been identified that are appropriately treated at the present level of care. This level is the least intensive at which the patient's new problems can be addressed effectively.

To document and communicate the patient's readiness for discharge or need for transfer to another level of care, each of the six dimensions of the ASAM criteria should be reviewed. If the criteria apply to the patient's existing or new problem(s), the patient should continue in treatment at the present level of care. If not, refer to the Discharge/Transfer Criteria, below.

> **Examples:** Typical findings in each of the six dimensions follow:

Dimension 1, Acute Intoxication/Withdrawal Potential: Signs and symptoms indicate the continued presence of the intoxication or withdrawal problem that required admission to the present level of care. The problem requires monitoring or detoxification services that can be provided effectively only at the present level of care.

> **Example (Continued Service Criterion #1):** A patient in a Level III.7-D program has withdrawal anxiety, tremors, pulse rate and blood pressure, which are improving. However, the patient continues to require detoxification medications and nurse monitoring every 8 hours. Therefore, continued treatment can be provided effectively only in a Level III.7-D service.

Dimension 2, Biomedical Condition and Complications: The physical health problem that required admission to the present level of care, or a new problem, requires biomedical services that can be provided effectively only at the present level of care.

> **Example (Continued Service Criterion #2):** A patient in a Level III.7 program is following through with the treatment plan strategies. However, the patient has unstable blood pressure, headaches and temporary ischemic attacks associated with co-occurring cerebrovascular disease, and his or her hypertension has not stabilized. Thus, the patient requires further medical monitoring and 24-hour nurse management, monitoring of blood pressure and mental status that can be provided effectively only in a Level III.7 program. He or she is not ready for transfer to a less intensive level of care.

Dimension 3, Emotional, Behavioral or Cognitive Conditions and Complications: The emotional, behavioral and/or cognitive problem that required admission to the present level of care continues, or a new problem has appeared. This problem requires interventions than can be provided effectively only at the present level of care.

> **Example (Continued Service Criterion #2):** A patient in a Level II.5 program has depressive symptoms and suicidal ideation that have persisted beyond what might be expected with cocaine withdrawal. The patient thus requires consistent monitoring of depression and suicidal ideation at a frequency that can be provided effectively only in a Level II.5 program.

> **Example (Continued Service Criterion #3):** Following a methamphetamine binge, a patient in a Level II.5 setting has cognitive and impulse control problems beyond what might be seen as self-limiting or substance-induced. The patient thus requires consistent behavioral interventions at a frequency that can be provided effectively only in a Level II.5 program.

Dimension 4, Readiness to Change: The patient continues to demonstrate a need for engagement and motivational enhancement that can be provided effectively only at the present level of care.

> **Example (Continued Service Criterion #1):** A patient in a Level II.1 program is attending group sessions and has articulated increasing awareness that his marijuana and alcohol use has negatively affected his work performance and family relationships. However, the patient is not yet implementing recommended changes. Further family work, employer involvement, peer confrontation, education about addiction, and attempts at abstinence thus are required to increase the patient's readiness to change. These motivational enhancement strategies are of such intensity that they can be provided effectively only in a Level II.1 program.

Dimension 5, Relapse, Continued Use or Continued Problem Potential: The patient continues to demonstrate a problem, or has developed a new problem, that requires coping skills and strategies to prevent relapse, continued use or continued problems. These strategies can be provided effectively only at the present level of care.

> **Example (Continued Service Criterion #2):** A patient in a Level I program continues to experience cravings to drink on a daily basis, but is willing to continue addressing her alcohol problem. She is attending group therapy twice a week and Alcoholics Anonymous meetings four days a week. Even though there was a brief "slip" during which the patient drank two glasses of wine, she talked about it in

group and identified the relevant relapse triggers and situations. Moreover, she articulated plans to avoid the friends and the parties associated with the slip. Continued service is required and can be provided effectively at Level I.

Dimension 6, Recovery Environment: The patient continues to demonstrate a problem in his or her recovery environment, or has a new problem, that requires coping skills and support system interventions. These interventions can be provided effectively only at the present level of care.

> **Example (Continued Service Criterion #3):** Through individual, group and family work, a patient in a Level III.5 program has demonstrated a significant problem with abusive behavior and anger impulse control. As the marijuana, heroin and alcohol used by the patient have cleared, he has become increasingly agitated. Following several loud arguments with his wife on the phone and near-fights with her after a family group session, the patient responded to a staff show of force, progressive relaxation and other behavioral techniques.
>
> The individual and group strategies required to help this patient cope with his daily emotional instability and also with family, financial and work problems without reverting to substance use can be provided effectively only in a Level III.5 program. In addition, the family work is pressing and intense enough that continued care at Level III.5 is necessary until it is clear whether the patient will need placement outside the home until he is more stable in recovery and with anger management.

Discharge/Transfer Criteria

It is appropriate to transfer or discharge the patient from the present level of care if he or she meets the following criteria:

1. The patient has achieved the goals articulated in his or her individualized treatment plan, thus resolving the problem(s) that justified admission to the present level of care;

    or

2. The patient has been unable to resolve the problem(s) that justified admission to the present level of care, despite amendments to the treatment plan. Treatment at another level of care or type of service therefore is indicated;

    or

3. The patient has demonstrated a lack of capacity to resolve his or her problem(s). Treatment at another level of care or type of service therefore is indicated;

    or

4. The patient has experienced an intensification of his or her problem(s), or has developed a new problem(s), and can be treated effectively only at a more intensive level of care.

To document and communicate the patient's readiness for discharge or need for transfer to another level of care, each of the six dimensions of the ASAM criteria should be reviewed. If the criteria apply to the existing or new problem(s), the patient should be discharged or transferred, as appropriate. If not, refer to the Continued Service criteria.

Examples: Examples of findings in each of the six dimensions follow:

Dimension 1, Acute Intoxication/Withdrawal Potential: The patient's intoxication or withdrawal problem has improved sufficiently to allow monitoring or detoxification services to be provided at a less intensive level of care. Or the patient's condition has worsened to a point at which more intensive monitoring or detoxification services are required.

> **Example (Discharge/Transfer Criterion #1):** A patient in a Level II-D program exhibits sufficient improvement in her withdrawal anxiety, tremors, pulse rate and blood pressure that nurse monitoring no longer is necessary. The patient's treatment can continue in a Level I-D program.

Dimension 2, Biomedical Conditions and Complications: The patient's physical health has improved sufficiently to allow biomedical services to be provided effectively at a less intensive level of care. Or the patient's condition has worsened to a point at which more intensive biomedical services are necessary.

> **Example (Discharge/Transfer Criterion #2):** A patient in a Level III.7 program exhibits worsening blood pressure, headaches and continuing ischemic attacks, despite medication changes, behavioral medicine interventions and biofeedback. Therefore, daily medical management, 24-hour nurse monitoring and mental status observations in a Level IV program are required.

Dimension 3, Emotional, Behavioral or Cognitive Conditions and Complications: The patient's functioning has improved sufficiently to allow interventions or services to be provided effectively at a less intensive level of care. Or the patient's condition has worsened to a point at which more intensive services are necessary.

> **Example (Discharge/Transfer Criterion #3):** A patient in a Level II.5 program has not been able to resolve her depression and suicidal ideation despite behavioral, individual and group therapy. The patient now requires more specific and structured mental health interventions in addition to the addiction treatment. The medical monitoring, 24-hour nurse monitoring, medication management, other mental health services and environmental structure the patient needs can be provided effectively only in a psychiatrically oriented Level III.7 Dual Diagnosis Enhanced service.

Dimension 4, Readiness to Change: The patient's stage of readiness to change has improved sufficiently to allow interventions or strategies to be provided effectively at a less intensive level of care. Or the patient has demonstrated regression or lack of progress to such a degree that further interventions at the present level of care will be ineffective and/or decrease the patient's willingness to engage in treatment. Transfer to another level of care will permit the use of different strategies to engage the patient in treatment and enhance his or her readiness to change.

> **Example (Discharge/Transfer Criterion #2):** A patient in a Level II.5 program demonstrates an increasingly fixed belief that he does not have a drinking problem, especially while in a structured environment that is sheltered from his drinking co-workers. The patient asserts that he has no thoughts of alcohol, no urges to use, a good understanding of what alcohol can do to his life, and an awareness of his overuse in the past. However, the patient insists that these behaviors were associated with the pressures of starting a new job. Despite his wife's and the treatment team's concern that the patient has a more severe problem than he is willing to acknowledge, and despite family and workplace strategies, group

confrontation and education, the patient is convinced his problematic use was temporary and is now under control. The patient is not ready to engage in treatment, but is willing to attend a weekly group session and to abstain from alcohol for three months to demonstrate that he does not have a drinking problem. His family is willing to continue in family therapy. These services can be provided effectively in a Level I program. The patient thus can be discharged from Level II.5.

Example (Discharge/Transfer Criterion #2): A patient in a Level 0.5 program has been only minimally compliant with attendance at drinking and driving education classes. The patient's focus on his legal problems and his intense anger at being compared to his alcoholic father make it difficult for him to grasp that he has a problem and to listen attentively enough to commit to change. Transfer to a Level I outpatient program for further evaluation and motivational enhancement therapy therefore is indicated.

Example (Discharge/Transfer Criterion #3): A patient with a schizophrenic disorder who has smoked marijuana daily for almost 25 years is sporadically attending a Level II.5 Dual Diagnosis Enhanced program while residing in a Level III.1 therapeutic group home. Despite a variety of interventions, including intensive case management, assertive community treatment and motivational enhancement therapy, the patient is making no progress toward his recovery goals. He is convinced that marijuana relieves his chronic hallucinations (which have not responded to other treatment), despite clear evidence that the marijuana actually makes the hallucinations worse. The patient's chronic symptoms prevent any meaningful engagement in recovery activities.

The patient's lack of capacity to resolve his delusions requires strategies that are designed for maintenance of basic functioning and self-care. The patient thus is appropriately transferred to a Level I Dual Diagnosis Enhanced service, where the focus will be on maximizing control of the symptoms of schizophrenia and limiting his access to drugs. Ongoing Level III.1 services will focus on interventions such as simple behavioral contingencies and limiting the patient's access to marijuana through custodial supervision and confinement.

Dimension 5, Relapse, Continued Use or Continued Problem Potential: The patient's coping skills have improved sufficiently that strategies to prevent relapse or continued use can be provided effectively at a less intensive level of care. Or the patient has demonstrated regression or lack of progress so significant that further interventions at the present level of care will not enhance his or her ability to prevent relapse or continued use and/or will decrease the patient's willingness to engage in treatment. Transfer to another level of service will allow different strategies to be employed to engage the patient in treatment and enhance his or her ability to prevent relapse or continued use.

Example (Discharge/Transfer Criteria #4): A patient in a Level II.5 program has experienced intense thoughts of alcohol and other drug use, cravings and impulses to use for more than two weeks. Her ability to cope is deteriorating, despite more focused role-playing to enhance peer refusal skills, other behavioral techniques, attendance at AA meetings and increased individual sessions. Because the patient becomes depressed and suicidal when drinking and, over the past two days, has been drinking daily, she is appropriately transferred to a Level III.5 program.

Dimension 6, Recovery Environment: The patient's environment and/or ability to cope with it have improved sufficiently to allow interventions or services to be provided effectively at a less intensive level of care. Or the patient's recovery environment and/or ability to cope with it have worsened to such a degree that the patient requires transfer to another level of care, where different interventions or strategies can be provided.

> **Example (Discharge/Transfer Criterion #3):** A patient in a Level II.5 program is in a physically and emotionally abusive relationship with a drug-dealing boyfriend, who continues to use and refuses to attend family meetings. The patient is not able to cope with her anxiety and stress reactions, particularly during the month she has been drug free. Such a patient is appropriately transferred to a Level III.1 safe living environment, with concurrent Level II.5 services to strengthen her ability to cope with both her substance use problems and the stressors in her living environment.

Level 0.5
Early Intervention

Early intervention is an organized service that may be delivered in a wide variety of settings. Early intervention services are designed to explore and address problems or risk factors that appear to be related to substance use and to help the individual recognize the harmful consequences of inappropriate substance use.

Length of Service

Length of service at Level 0.5 varies according to (a) an individual's ability to comprehend the information provided and use that information to make behavior changes and avoid problems related to substance use or (b) the appearance of new problems that require treatment at another level of care.

Adult Criteria
Level 0.5: Early Intervention

CHARACTERISTIC	ESSENTIAL FEATURES
EXAMPLES	Level 0.5 program services encompass one-to-one counseling with at-risk individuals and educational programs for first-time DUI (Driving Under the Influence) offenders.
SETTING	Level 0.5 programming may be offered in any appropriate setting, including clinical offices or permanent facilities, schools, work sites, community centers or an individual's home.
SUPPORT SYSTEMS	At Level 0.5, necessary support systems include: (a) Referral for ongoing treatment of substance abuse or dependence. (b) Referral for medical, psychological or psychiatric services, including assessment. (c) Referral for community social services.
STAFF	Level 0.5 programs are staffed by trained personnel who are knowledgeable about the biopsychosocial dimensions of substance use and dependence, the recognition of substance-related disorders, alcohol and other drug education, motivational counseling, and the legal and personal consequences of inappropriate substance use.
INTERVENTIONS	Interventions offered at Level 0.5 may involve individual, group or family counseling, as well as planned educational experiences focused on helping the individual recognize and avoid harmful or inappropriate substance use.
ASSESSMENT	At Level 0.5, sufficient assessment is performed to screen for, and rule in or out, substance-related disorders.
DOCUMENTATION	Documentation standards for Level 0.5 programs include progress notes in the individual's record that clearly indicate assessment findings, attendance and significant clinical events, particularly those that require further assessment and referral.

Level 0.5 Admission Criteria
Diagnostic and Dimensional Criteria

CRITERIA	LEVEL 0.5 Early Intervention
DIAGNOSTIC ADMISSION CRITERIA	The individual who is an appropriate candidate for Level 0.5 services evidences problems and risk factors that appear to be related to substance use but do not meet the diagnostic criteria for Substance-Related Disorder as defined in the current *Diagnostic and Statistical Manual of Mental Disorders (DSM)* of the American Psychiatric Association or other standardized and widely accepted criteria.
DIMENSIONAL ADMISSION CRITERIA	The individual who is appropriately cared for at Level 0.5 meets *one* of the specifications in Dimensions 4, 5 or 6. Any identifiable problems in Dimensions 1, 2 or 3 are stable or are being addressed through appropriate outpatient medical or mental health services.
DIMENSION 1: Acute Intoxication and/or Withdrawal	See the separate Dimension 1 criteria.
DIMENSION 2: Biomedical Conditions and Complications	In Dimension 2, the individual's biomedical conditions and problems, if any, are stable or are being actively addressed and thus will not interfere with therapeutic interventions.
DIMENSION 3: Emotional, Behavioral or Cognitive Conditions and Complications	In Dimension 3, the individual's emotional, behavioral or cognitive conditions and complications, if any, are being addressed through appropriate mental health services and thus will not interfere with therapeutic interventions.
DIMENSION 4: Readiness to Change	In Dimension 4, the individual expresses willingness to gain an understanding of how his or her current use of alcohol or other drugs may be harmful or impair his or her ability to meet responsibilities and achieve personal goals.

Level 0.5 Admission Criteria
Diagnostic and Dimensional Criteria

CRITERIA	LEVEL 0.5 Early Intervention
DIMENSION 5: **Continued Problem Potential**	The individual's status in Dimension 5 is characterized by (a) *or* (b): (a) The individual does not understand the need to alter his or her current pattern of use of alcohol or other drugs to prevent harm that may be related to such use; *or* (b) The individual needs to acquire the specific skills needed to change his or her current pattern of use.
DIMENSION 6: **Living Environment**	The individual's status in Dimension 6 is characterized by (a) *or* (b) *or* (c) *or* (d): (a) The individual's social support system is composed primarily of persons whose substance use patterns prevent them from meeting social, work, school or family obligations; *or* (b) The individual's family member(s) currently is/are abusing alcohol or other drugs (or has/have done so in the past), thereby heightening the individual's risk for a substance-related disorder; *or* (c) The individual's significant other(s) expresses values concerning alcohol or other drug use that create serious conflict for the individual; *or* (d) The individual's significant other(s) condones or encourages inappropriate use of alcohol or other drugs.

Level I
Outpatient Treatment

Level I encompasses organized outpatient treatment services, which may be delivered in a wide variety of settings. In Level I programs, addiction treatment staff, including addiction-credentialed physicians, provide professionally directed evaluation, treatment and recovery services. Such services are provided in regularly scheduled sessions of (usually) fewer than nine contact hours a week. The services follow a defined set of policies and procedures or clinical protocols.

Level I services are tailored to each patient's level of clinical severity and are designed to help the patient achieve changes in his or her alcohol- or other drug-using behaviors. Treatment thus must address major lifestyle, attitudinal and behavioral issues that have the potential to undermine the goals of treatment or to impair the individual's ability to cope with major life tasks without the non-medical use of alcohol or other drugs.

Level I services are appropriate in several different situations:

- Level I may be the initial level of care for a patient whose severity of illness warrants this intensity of treatment. Such a patient should be able to complete professionally directed addiction treatment at this level, thus using only one level of care, unless (a) an unanticipated event causes a change in his or her level of functioning, leading to a reassessment of the appropriateness of this level of care, or (b) there is recurring evidence of the patient's inability to use this level of care (such as repeated episodes of drinking or non-medical drug use even after the treatment plan has been reviewed and revised).

- Level I may represent a "step down" from a more intensive level of care for a patient whose progress warrants such a transfer, assuming that he or she meets the criteria for placement in Level I.

- Level I may be used for a patient who is in the early stages of change and who is not yet ready to commit to full recovery (Dimension 4 issues). For such a patient, placement in a more intensive level of care is apt to lead to increased conflict, passive compliance or even leaving treatment.

The relationship between the severity of illness and the intensity of treatment is most clearly seen in Dimensions 1, 2 and 3. On the other hand, increasing the intensity of services solely because of Dimension 4 issues may be counterproductive. An alternative approach is to use Level I services to engage the resistant individual in treatment. If this approach proves successful, the patient may no longer require a higher intensity of service, or may be able to better use such services.

Length of Service

The duration of treatment varies with the severity of the individual's illness and his or her response to treatment.

Co-Occurring Mental and Substance-Related Disorders

Level I services are appropriate for patients with co-occurring mental and substance-related disorders *if*:

1. The patient's disorders are of *moderate severity* (as defined in the introduction to this section) and have responded to more intensive treatment services. The mental disorders have resolved to an extent that addiction treatment services are assessed as potentially beneficial. However, ongoing monitoring of the patient's mental status is required.

2. The patient's disorders are of *high severity* (as defined in the Preface) and are persistent, but have stabilized to such an extent that integrated mental health and addiction treatment services are assessed as potentially beneficial. Patients who have severe and persistent mental disorders may not have been able to achieve sobriety or to maintain abstinence for a significant period of time (months) in the past; nevertheless, they are appropriately placed at Level I because they need engagement strategies and intensive case management.

Adult Criteria
Level I: Outpatient Treatment

CHARACTERISTIC	ESSENTIAL FEATURES
EXAMPLES	**All Programs** Level I services may be delivered in office practice, health clinics, primary care clinics, addiction and mental health clinics.
SETTING	**All Programs** Level I program services may be offered in any appropriate setting that meets state licensure or certification criteria.
SUPPORT SYSTEMS	**All Programs** In Level I programs, necessary support systems include: (a) Medical, psychiatric, psychological, laboratory and toxicology services, which are available on-site or through consultation or referral. Medical and psychiatric consultation are available within 24 hours by telephone or, if in person, within a time frame appropriate to the severity and urgency of the consultation requested. (b) Direct affiliation with (or close coordination through referral to) more intensive levels of care and medication management. (c) Emergency services available by telephone 24 hours a day, 7 days a week. **Dual Diagnosis Enhanced Programs** In addition to the support systems listed above, which encompass those offered by Level I Dual Diagnosis Capable programs, Level I Dual Diagnosis Enhanced programs offer ongoing intensive case management for highly crisis-prone (and often homeless) dually diagnosed individuals. Such services are delivered by cross-trained interdisciplinary staff through mobile outreach and engagement-oriented psychiatric and substance disorders programming.
STAFF	**All Programs** Level I programs are staffed by appropriately credentialed treatment professionals (including addiction-credentialed physicians, counselors, psychologists, social workers, and others), who assess and treat substance-related disorders. Staff are able to obtain and interpret information regarding the patient's biopsychosocial needs, and are knowledgeable about the biopsychosocial dimensions of alcohol and other drug disorders, including assessment of the patient's stage of readiness to change. Program staff are capable of monitoring stabilized mental health problems and recognizing any instability of patients with co-occurring mental health problems.

Adult Criteria
Level I: Outpatient Treatment

CHARACTERISTIC	ESSENTIAL FEATURES
STAFF (continued)	**Dual Diagnosis Enhanced Programs** Staff of Level I Dual Diagnosis Enhanced programs include credentialed mental health trained personnel who are able to assess, monitor and manage the types of severe and persistent mental disorders seen in a Level I setting, as well as other psychiatric disorders that are mildly unstable. Such staff are knowledgeable about the management of co-occurring mental and substance-related disorders, including assessment of the patient's stage of readiness to change and engagement of patients who have co-occurring mental disorders.
THERAPIES	**All Programs** Therapies offered by Level I programs involve skilled treatment services, which may include individual and group counseling, motivational enhancement, opioid substitution therapy, family therapy, educational groups, occupational and recreational therapy, psychotherapy, or other therapies. Such services are provided in an amount, frequency and intensity appropriate to the patient's treatment plan. Motivational enhancement and engagement strategies are used in preference to confrontational approaches. For patients with mental health problems, the issues of psychotropic medication, mental health treatment and their relationship to substance use disorders are addressed as the need arises. **Dual Diagnosis Enhanced Programs** In addition to the therapies described above, Level I Dual Diagnosis Enhanced programs offer therapies to actively address, monitor and manage psychotropic medication, mental health treatment and the interaction with substance-related disorders. There may be close coordination with intensive case management and assertive community treatment for patients who have severe and persistent mental illnesses.
ASSESSMENT/ TREATMENT PLAN REVIEW	**All Programs** In Level I programs, the assessment and treatment plan review include: (a) An individual biopsychosocial assessment of each patient. (b) An individualized treatment plan, which involves problem formulation and articulation of short-term, measurable treatment goals and activities designed to achieve those goals. The plan is developed in collaboration with the patient and reflects the patient's personal goals. Treatment plan reviews are conducted at specified times, as noted in the plan. **Dual Diagnosis Enhanced Programs** In addition to the assessment and treatment plan review activities described above, which encompass Dual Diagnosis Capable programs, Level I Dual Diagnosis Enhanced programs provide a a review of the patient's recent psychiatric history and a mental status examination. If necessary, the review is conducted by a psychiatrist. A comprehensive psychiatric history and examination and a psychodiagnostic assessment are performed within a reasonable time, as determined by the patient's psychiatric condition.

Adult Criteria
Level I: Outpatient Treatment

CHARACTERISTIC	ESSENTIAL FEATURES
ASSESSMENT/ TREATMENT PLAN REVIEW (continued)	Level I Dual Diagnosis Enhanced programs also provide active reassessment at each visit of the patient's mental status and follow-through with mental health treatment and psychotropic medication. Patients in need of Dual Diagnosis Capable services also may require the kinds of assessment and treatment plan review offered by Dual Diagnosis Enhanced programs, but at a reduced level of frequency and comprehensiveness, because their mental health problems are more stable.
DOCUMENTATION	**All Programs** Documentation standards for Level I programs include individualized progress notes in the patient's record that clearly reflect implementation of the treatment plan and the patient's response to therapeutic interventions for all disorders treated, as well as subsequent amendments to the plan. **Dual Diagnosis Programs** In addition to the information described above, Level I Dual Diagnosis Capable and Dual Diagnosis Enhanced programs document the patient's mental health problems, the relationship between the patient's mental and substance-related disorders, and the patient's current level of mental functioning.

Level I Admission Criteria
Diagnostic and Dimensional Criteria

CRITERIA	LEVEL I — Outpatient Services
DIAGNOSTIC ADMISSION CRITERIA	The patient who is appropriately placed in a Level I program is assessed as meeting the diagnostic criteria for a Substance-Related Disorder (including Substance Use Disorder or Substance-Induced Disorder), as defined in the current *Diagnostic and Statistical Manual of Mental Disorders (DSM)* of the American Psychiatric Association or other standardized and widely accepted criteria, as well as the dimensional criteria for admission. If the patient's presenting alcohol or drug use history is inadequate to substantiate such a diagnosis, the probability of such a diagnosis may be determined from information submitted by collateral parties (such as family members, legal guardians and significant others). **Dual Diagnosis Capable Programs** At Level I, some patients have co-occurring mental disorders that meet the stability criteria for a Dual Diagnosis Capable program. Other patients have difficulties in mood, behavior or cognition as the result of other psychiatric or substance-induced disorders, or the patient's emotional, behavioral or cognitive symptoms are troublesome but not sufficient to meet the criteria for a diagnosed mental disorder. **Dual Diagnosis Enhanced Programs** In contrast to the foregoing criteria, the patient who is identified as in need of Level I Dual Diagnosis Enhanced program services is assessed as meeting the diagnostic criteria for a Mental Disorder as well as a Substance Use Disorder, as defined in the current *Diagnostic and Statistical Manual of Mental Disorders (DSM)* of the American Psychiatric Association or other standardized and widely accepted criteria, as well as the dimensional criteria for admission. If the patient's presenting history is inadequate to substantiate such a diagnosis, the probability of such a diagnosis may be determined from information submitted by collateral parties (such as family members, legal guardians and significant others).
DIMENSIONAL ADMISSION CRITERIA	**All Programs** The patient who is appropriately admitted to a Level I program is assessed as meeting specifications in *all* of the following six dimensions.
DIMENSION 1: **Acute Intoxication and/or Withdrawal**	**All Programs** The patient has no signs or symptoms of withdrawal, or his or her withdrawal needs can be safely managed in a Level I setting (see the separate Dimension 1 criteria).
DIMENSION 2: **Biomedical Conditions and Complications**	**All Programs** The patient's status in Dimension 2 is characterized by biomedical conditions and problems, if any, that are sufficiently stable to permit participation in outpatient treatment. Examples include uncomplicated pregnancy or asymptomatic HIV disease.

Level I Admission Criteria
Diagnostic and Dimensional Criteria

CRITERIA	LEVEL I Outpatient Services
DIMENSION 3: **Emotional,** **Behavioral or** **Cognitive** **Conditions and** **Complications**	**All Programs** The patient's status in Dimension 3 is characterized by (a) *or* (b) *and* (c) *and* (d): (a) The patient has no symptoms of a co-occurring mental disorder, or any symptoms are mild, stable, fully related to substance use, and do not interfere with the patient's ability to focus on addiction treatment issues; *or* (b) The patient's psychiatric symptoms (such as anxiety, guilt, or thought disorders) are mild, mostly stable, and primarily related to substance use or to a co-occurring cognitive, emotional or behavioral condition. Mental health monitoring is needed to maintain stable mood, cognition and behavior; for example, fluctuations in mood only recently stabilized with medication, substance-induced depression that is resolving but still significant, or a patient with schizophrenic disorder recently released from hospital; *and* (c) The patient's mental status does not preclude his or her ability to: (1) understand the information presented and (2) participate in treatment planning and the treatment process; *and* (d) The patient is assessed as not posing a risk of harm to self or others and is not vulnerable to victimization by another. **Dual Diagnosis Enhanced Programs** In addition to the foregoing criteria, the patient's status in Dimension 3 is characterized by *either* (a) *or* (b) *and* (c) *and* (d): (a) The patient has a severe and persistent mental illness that impairs his or her ability to follow through consistently with mental health appointments and psychotropic medication. However, the patient has the ability to access services such as assertive community treatment and intensive case management or supportive living designed to help the patient remain engaged in treatment; *or* (b) The patient has a severe and persistent mental disorder or other emotional, behavioral or cognitive problems, or substance-induced disorder; *and* (c) The patient's mental health functioning is such that he or she has impaired ability to: [1] understand the information presented, and [2] participate in treatment planning and the treatment process. Mental health management is required to stabilize mood, cognition and behavior; *and* (d) The patient is assessed as not posing a risk of harm to self or others and is not vulnerable to victimization by another.

Level I Admission Criteria
Diagnostic and Dimensional Criteria

CRITERIA	LEVEL I Outpatient Services
DIMENSION 4: **Readiness** **to Change**	**All Programs** The patient's status in Dimension 4 is characterized by (a) *and* (b) *or* (c) *or* (d): (a) The patient expresses willingness to participate in treatment planning and to attend all scheduled activities mutually agreed upon in the treatment plan; *and* (b) The patient acknowledges that he or she has a substance-related and/or mental health problem and wants help to change; *or* (c) The patient is ambivalent about a substance-related and/or mental health problem He or she requires monitoring and motivating strategies, but not a structured milieu program. For example, the patient has sufficient awareness and recognition of a substance use and/or mental health problems to allow engagement and follow-through with attendance at intermittent treatment sessions as scheduled; *or* (d) The patient may not recognize that he or she has a substance-related and/or mental health problem. For example, he or she is more invested in avoiding a negative consequence than in the recovery effort. Such a patient may require monitoring and motivating strategies to engage in treatment and to progress through the stages of change.
DIMENSION 5: **Relapse, Continued** **Use or Continued** **Problem Potential**	**All Programs** In Dimension 5, the patient is assessed as able to achieve or maintain abstinence and related recovery goals, or to achieve awareness of a substance problem and related motivational enhancement goals, only with support and scheduled therapeutic contact to assist him or her in dealing with issues that include (but are not limited to) concern or ambivalence about preoccupation with alcohol or other drug use, craving, peer pressure, and lifestyle and attitude changes. **Dual Diagnosis Programs** In addition to the foregoing criteria, the patient is assessed as able to achieve or maintain mental health functioning and related goals only with support and scheduled therapeutic contact to assist him or her in dealing with issues that include (but are not limited to) impulses to harm self or others and difficulty in coping with his or her affects, impulses or cognition. While such impulses and difficulty in coping may apply to patients in both Dual Diagnosis Capable and Dual Diagnosis Enhanced programs, patients in need of Dual Diagnosis Enhanced program services are more unstable and require the outreach and support of assertive community treatment and intensive case management to maintain their mental health function. For example, such a patient may be unable to reliably keep mental health appointments because of instability in cognition, behavior or mood.

Level I Admission Criteria
Diagnostic and Dimensional Criteria

CRITERIA	LEVEL I Outpatient Services
DIMENSION 6: **Recovery Environment**	**All Programs** The patient's status in Dimension 6 is characterized by (a) *or* (b) *or* (c): (a) The patient's psychosocial environment is sufficiently supportive that outpatient treatment is feasible (for example, significant others are in agreement with the recovery effort; there is a supportive work environment or legal coercion; adequate transportation to the program is available; and support meeting locations and non-alcohol/drug-centered work are near the home environment and accessible); *or* (b) The patient does not have an adequate primary or social support system, but he or she has demonstrated motivation and willingness to obtain such a support system; *or* (c) The patient's family, guardian or significant others are supportive but require professional interventions to improve the patient's chance of treatment success and recovery. Such interventions may involve assistance in limit setting, communication skills, a reduction in rescuing behaviors, and the like. **Dual Diagnosis Enhanced Programs** In addition to the foregoing criteria, the patient's status in Dimension 6 is characterized by (a) *or* (b) *or* (c): (a) The patient does not have an adequate primary or social support system and has mild impairment in his or her ability to obtain a support system. For example, mood, cognition and impulse control fluctuate and distract the patient from focusing on treatment tasks; *or* (b) The family, guardian or significant others require active family therapy or systems interventions to improve the patient's chances of treatment success and recovery. These may include family enmeshment issues, significant guilt or anxiety, or passivity or disengaged aloofness or neglect; *or* (c) The patient's status in Dimension 6 is characterized by *all* of the following: (1) the patient has a severe and persistent mental disorder or emotional, behavioral or cognitive problem, *and* (2) the patient does not have an adequate family or social support system, *and* (3) the patient is chronically impaired, but not in imminent danger, and has limited ability to establish a supportive recovery environment. However, he or she does have access to intensive outreach and case management services that can provide structure and allow him or her to work toward stabilizing both the substance-related and mental disorders.

Level II
Intensive Outpatient Treatment/Partial Hospitalization

Level II encompasses intensive outpatient treatment services, which may be delivered in a wide variety of outpatient or partial hospitalization settings. Such treatment may be offered during the day, before or after work or school, in the evening or on a weekend. For appropriately selected patients, Level II programs provide essential education and treatment services while allowing patients to apply their newly acquired skills in "real world" environments.

Level II treatment programs have the capacity to arrange for medical and psychiatric consultation, psychopharmacological consultation, medication management, and 24-hour crisis services. They provide comprehensive biopsychosocial assessments and individualized treatment plans that are developed in consultation with the patient. Such plans include problem formulation, treatment goals and measurable treatment objectives. In addition, the programs have active affiliations with other levels of care and can help the patient access support services such as child care, vocational training and transportation.

Beyond the essential services, many Level II programs provide psychopharmacological assessment and treatment and have the capacity to effectively treat patients who have complex co-occurring mental and substance-related disorders.

Some programs also can provide overnight housing for patients who have problems related to family environment or transportation but who do not need the supervision or 24-hour access to services afforded by a Level III program. Such structured day and evening treatment programs "unbundle" actual clinical treatment from "around-the-clock" supervised living environments that include overnight housing.

Increasingly, distinctions are made among various subtypes of Level II programs. Criteria are offered here for two variations: Intensive Outpatient (Level II.1) and Partial Hospitalization (Level II.5) programs.

Treatment Levels Within Level II

Level II.1: Intensive Outpatient Treatment. Intensive outpatient programs (IOPs) generally provide 9 or more hours of structured programming per week, consisting primarily of counseling and education about substance-related and mental health problems. The patient's needs for psychiatric and medical services are addressed through consultation and referral arrangements if the patient is stable and requires only maintenance monitoring. (Services provided outside the primary program must be tightly coordinated.)

Intensive outpatient treatment differs from partial hospitalization (Level II.5) programs in the intensity of clinical services that are directly available. Specifically, most intensive outpatient programs have less capacity to effectively treat patients who have substantial unstable medical and psychiatric problems than do partial hospitalization programs.

Level II.5: Partial Hospitalization Programs. Partial hospitalization programs generally feature 20 or more hours of clinically intensive programming per week, as specified in the patient's treatment plan. Level II.5 partial hospitalization programs typically have direct access to psychiatric, medical and laboratory services, and thus are better able than Level II.1 programs to meet needs identified in Dimensions 1, 2 and 3, which warrant daily monitoring or management but which can be appropriately addressed in a structured outpatient setting.

Patients who meet Level III criteria in Dimensions 4, 5 or 6 and who otherwise would be placed in a Level III program may be considered for placement in a Level II.5 program if the patient resides in a facility that provides 24-hour support and structure and that limits access to alcohol and other drugs, such as a correctional facility or other licensed health care facility or a supervised living situation.

Length of Service

The duration of treatment varies with the severity of the patient's illness and his or her response to treatment.

Co-Occurring Mental and Substance-Related Disorders

The services of a Level II treatment program are appropriate for patients with co-occurring mental and substance-related disorders if the mental health and addiction treatment services are integrated into the intensive outpatient or partial hospitalization program. Such patients require active mental health services, which should be delivered through Level II.1 Dual Diagnosis Capable or Dual Diagnosis Enhanced programs.

Adult Criteria
Level II: Intensive Outpatient Treatment/Partial Hospitalization

CHARACTERISTIC	LEVEL II.1 Intensive Outpatient	LEVEL II.5 Partial Hospitalization
EXAMPLES	**All Programs** Examples of Level II.1 programs are day or evening outpatient programs.	**All Programs** Examples of Level II.5 programs are day treatment programs.
SETTING	**All Programs** Level II.1 program services may be offered in any appropriate setting that meets state licensure or certification criteria.	**All Programs** Level II.5 program services may be offered in any appropriate setting that meets state licensure or certification criteria.
SUPPORT SYSTEMS	**All Programs** In Level II.1 programs, necessary support systems include: (a) Medical, psychological, psychiatric, laboratory and toxicology services, which are available through consultation or referral. Psychiatric and other medical consultation is available within 24 hours by telephone and within 72 hours in person. (b) Emergency services, which are available by telephone 24 hours a day, 7 days a week when the treatment program is not in session. (c) Direct affiliation with (or close coordination through referral to) more and less intensive levels of care and supportive housing services. **Dual Diagnosis Enhanced Programs** In addition to the foregoing support systems, which encompass Dual Diagnosis Capable programs, Level II.1 Dual Diagnosis Enhanced programs offer psychiatric services appropriate to the patient's mental health condition. Such services are available by telephone and on site, or closely coordinated off site, within a shorter time than in a Dual Diagnosis Capable program.	**All Programs** In Level II.5 programs, necessary support systems include: (a) Medical, psychological, psychiatric, laboratory and toxicology services, which are available through consultation or referral. Psychiatric and other medical consultation is available within 8 hours by telephone and within 48 hours in person. (b) Emergency services, which are available by telephone 24 hours a day, 7 days a week when the treatment program is not in session. (c) Direct affiliation with (or close coordination through referral to) more and less intensive levels of care and supportive housing services. **Dual Diagnosis Enhanced Programs** In addition to the foregoing support systems, which encompass Dual Diagnosis Capable programs, Level II.5 Dual Diagnosis Enhanced programs offer psychiatric services appropriate to the patient's mental health condition. Such services are available by telephone and on site, or closely coordinated off site, within a shorter time than in a Dual Diagnosis Capable program.

Adult Criteria
Level II: Intensive Outpatient Treatment/Partial Hospitalization

CHARACTERISTIC	LEVEL II.1 Intensive Outpatient	LEVEL II.5 Partial Hospitalization
SUPPORT SYSTEMS (continued)		Dual Diagnosis Enhanced programs also provide ongoing intensive case management for highly crisis-prone (and often homeless) dually diagnosed patients. Such case management is delivered by cross-trained, interdisciplinary staff through mobile outreach, and involves engagement-oriented addiction treatment and psychiatric programming.
STAFF	**All Programs** Level II.1 programs are staffed by an interdisciplinary team of appropriately credentialed addiction treatment professionals, including addiction-credentialed physicians, who assess and treat substance-related disorders. Program staff are able to obtain and interpret information regarding the patient's biopsychosocial needs. Some, if not all, program staff have had sufficient cross-training to understand the signs and symptoms of mental disorders and to understand and explain the uses of psychotropic medications and their interactions with substance-related disorders. **Dual Diagnosis Enhanced Programs** In addition to the staff capabilities listed above, which encompass those of Dual Diagnosis Capable programs, Level II.1 Dual Diagnosis Enhanced programs are staffed by appropriately credentialed mental health professionals, who assess and treat co-occurring mental disorders.	**All Programs** Level II.5 programs are staffed by an interdisciplinary team of appropriately credentialed addiction treatment professionals, including addiction-credentialed physicians, who assess and treat substance-related disorders. Program staff are able to obtain and interpret information regarding the patient's biopsychosocial needs. Some, if not all, program staff have had sufficient cross-training to understand the signs and symptoms of mental disorders and to understand and explain the uses of psychotropic medications and their interactions with substance-related disorders. **Dual Diagnosis Enhanced Programs** In addition to the staff capabilities listed above, which encompass those of Dual Diagnosis Capable programs, Level II.5 Dual Diagnosis Enhanced programs are staffed by appropriately credentialed mental health professionals, who assess and treat co-occurring mental disorders.

Adult Criteria
Level II: Intensive Outpatient Treatment/Partial Hospitalization

CHARACTERISTIC	LEVEL II.1 Intensive Outpatient	LEVEL II.5 Partial Hospitalization
THERAPIES	**All Programs** Therapies offered by Level II.1 programs include: (a) A minimum of 9 hours per week of skilled treatment services. Such services may include individual and group counseling, medication management, family therapy, educational groups, occupational and recreational therapy, and other therapies. Services are provided in amounts, frequencies and intensities appropriate to the objectives of the treatment plan. (b) Family therapy, which involves family members, guardians or significant other(s) in the assessment, treatment and continuing care of the patient. (c) A planned format of therapies, delivered on an individual and group basis and adapted to the patient's developmental stage and comprehension level. (d) Motivational enhancement and engagement strategies, which are used in preference to confrontational approaches. **Dual Diagnosis Programs** The therapies described above typically are offered by Dual Diagnosis Capable programs to patients with co-occurring addictive and mental disorders who are able to tolerate and benefit from a planned programs of therapies. Other patients (especially those who are severely and persistently mentally ill) may not be able to benefit from a full program of therapies and thus may require Dual Diagnosis Enhanced program services that constitute the defined intensity of hours in Level II.1. Such services may involve intensive case management, assertive community treatment, medication management and psychotherapy.	**All Programs** Therapies offered by Level II.5 programs include: (a) A minimum of 20 hours per week of skilled treatment services. Services may include individual and group counseling, medication management, family therapy, educational groups, occupational and recreational therapy, and other therapies. These are provided in the amounts, frequencies and intensities appropriate to the objectives of the treatment plan. (b) Family therapy, which involves family members, guardians or significant other(s) in the assessment, treatment and continuing care of the patient. (c) A planned format of therapies, delivered on an individual and group basis and adapted to the patient's developmental stage and comprehension level. (d) Motivational enhancement and engagement strategies, which are used in preference to confrontational approaches. **Dual Diagnosis Programs** The therapies described above typically are offered by Level II.5 Dual Diagnosis Capable programs to patients with co-occurring addictive and mental disorders who are able to tolerate and benefit from a planned programs of therapies. Other patients (especially those who are severely and persistently mentally ill) may not be able to benefit from a full program of therapies and thus may require Dual Diagnosis Enhanced program services that constitute the defined intensity of hours in Level II.5. Such services may involve intensive case management, assertive community treatment, medication management and psychotherapy.

Adult Criteria
Level II: Intensive Outpatient Treatment/Partial Hospitalization

CHARACTERISTIC	LEVEL II.1 Intensive Outpatient	LEVEL II.5 Partial Hospitalization
ASSESSMENT/ TREATMENT PLAN REVIEW	**All Programs** In Level II.1 programs, the assessment and treatment plan review include: (a) A comprehensive substance use history, obtained as part of the initial assessment and reviewed by a physician, if necessary. A physical examination may be performed within a reasonable time, as determined by the patient's medical condition. Such determinations are made according to established protocols, which include reliance on the patient's personal physician whenever possible. They are based on the staff's capabilities and the severity of the patient's symptoms, and are approved by a physician. (In states where physician assistants or nurse practitioners are under physician supervision and are licensed as physician extenders, they may perform the duties designated here for a physician.) (b) An individual biopsychosocial assessment. (c) An individualized treatment plan, including problem formulation and articulation of short-term, measurable treatment goals and activities designed to achieve those goals. The plan is developed in consultation with the patient and reflects the patient's personal goals. Treatment plan reviews are conducted at specified times, as noted in the treatment plan. **Dual Diagnosis Enhanced Programs** In addition to the foregoing activities, which encompass Dual Diagnosis Capable programs, Level II.1 Dual Diagnosis Enhanced programs provide a review of the patient's recent psychiatric history and a mental status examination (which are reviewed by a psychiatrist, if necessary). A comprehensive psychiatric history and examination and a psychodiagnostic	**All Programs** In Level II.5 programs, the assessment and treatment plan review include: (a) A comprehensive substance use history, obtained as part of the initial assessment and reviewed by a physician, if necessary. A physical examination may be performed within a reasonable time, as determined by the patient's medical condition. Such determinations are made according to established protocols, which include reliance on the patient's personal physician whenever possible. They are based on the staff's capabilities and the severity of the patient's symptoms, and are approved by a physician. (In states where physician assistants or nurse practitioners are under physician supervision and are licensed as physician extenders, they may perform the duties designated here for a physician.) (b) An individual biopsychosocial assessment. (c) An individualized treatment plan, including problem formulation and articulation of short-term, measurable treatment goals and activities designed to achieve those goals. The plan is developed in consultation with the patient and reflects the patient's personal goals. Treatment plan reviews are conducted at specified times, as noted in the treatment plan. **Dual Diagnosis Enhanced Programs** In addition to the foregoing activities, which encompass Dual Diagnosis Capable programs, Level II.5 Dual Diagnosis Enhanced programs provide a review of the patient's recent psychiatric history and a mental status examination (which are reviewed by a psychiatrist, if necessary). A comprehensive psychiatric history and examination and a psychodiagnostic

Adult Criteria
Level II: Intensive Outpatient Treatment/Partial Hospitalization

CHARACTERISTIC	LEVEL II.1 Intensive Outpatient	LEVEL II.5 Partial Hospitalization
ASSESSMENT/ TREATMENT PLAN REVIEW (continued)	assessment are performed within a reasonable time frame, as determined by the patient's psychiatric condition.	assessment are performed within a reasonable time frame, as determined by the patient's psychiatric condition.
DOCUMENTATION	**All Programs** Documentation standards for Level II.1 programs include individualized progress notes in the patient's record that clearly reflect implementation of the treatment plan and the patient's response to therapeutic interventions for all disorders treated, as well as subsequent amendments to the plan. **Dual Diagnosis Programs** In addition to the documentation standards described above, Level II.1 Dual Diagnosis Capable and Dual Diagnosis programs document the patient's mental health problems, the relationship between the mental and substance-related disorders, and the patient's current level of mental functioning.	**All Programs** Documentation standards for Level II.5 programs include individualized progress notes in the patient's record that clearly reflect implementation of the treatment plan and the patient's response to therapeutic interventions for all disorders treated, as well as subsequent amendments to the plan. **Dual Diagnosis Programs** In addition to the documentation standards described above, Level II.5 Dual Diagnosis Capable and Dual Diagnosis Enhanced programs document the patient's mental health problems, the relationship between the mental and substance-related disorders, and the patient's current level of mental functioning.

Level II Admission Criteria
Diagnostic and Dimensional Criteria

CRITERIA	LEVEL II.1 Intensive Outpatient	LEVEL II.5 Partial Hospitalization
DIAGNOSTIC ADMISSION CRITERIA	**All Programs** The patient who is appropriately placed in a Level II.1 program is assessed as meeting the diagnostic criteria for a Substance-Related Disorder (including Substance Use Disorder or Substance-Induced Disorder), as defined in the current *Diagnostic and Statistical Manual of Mental Disorders (DSM)* of the American Psychiatric Association or other standardized and widely accepted criteria, as well as the dimensional criteria for admission. If the patient's presenting alcohol or drug use history is inadequate to substantiate such a diagnosis, the probability of such a diagnosis may be determined from information submitted by collateral parties (such as family members, legal guardians and significant others). **Dual Diagnosis Enhanced Programs** The patient in need of Level II.1 Dual Diagnosis Enhanced program services is assessed as meeting the diagnostic criteria for a Mental Disorder as well as a Substance-Related Disorder, as defined in the current *Diagnostic and Statistical Manual of Mental Disorders (DSM)* of the American Psychiatric Association or other standardized and widely accepted criteria, as well as the dimensional criteria for admission. If the patient's presenting history is inadequate to substantiate such a diagnosis, the probability of such a diagnosis may be determined from information submitted by collateral parties (such as family members, legal guardians and significant others).	**All Programs** The patient who is appropriately placed in a Level II.5 program is assessed as meeting the diagnostic criteria for a Substance-Related Disorder (including Substance Use Disorder or Substance-Induced Disorder), as defined in the current *Diagnostic and Statistical Manual of Mental Disorders (DSM)* of the American Psychiatric Association or other standardized and widely accepted criteria, as well as the dimensional criteria for admission. If the patient's presenting alcohol or drug use history is inadequate to substantiate such a diagnosis, the probability of such a diagnosis may be determined from information submitted by collateral parties (such as family members, legal guardians and significant others). **Dual Diagnosis Enhanced Programs** The patient in need of Level II.5 Dual Diagnosis Enhanced program services is assessed as meeting the diagnostic criteria for a Mental Disorder as well as a Substance-Related Disorder, as defined in the current *Diagnostic and Statistical Manual of Mental Disorders (DSM)* of the American Psychiatric Association or other standardized and widely accepted criteria, as well as the dimensional criteria for admission. If the patient's presenting history is inadequate to substantiate such a diagnosis, the probability of such a diagnosis may be determined from information submitted by collateral parties (such as family members, legal guardians and significant others).

Level II Admission Criteria
Diagnostic and Dimensional Criteria

CRITERIA	LEVEL II.1 Intensive Outpatient	LEVEL II.5 Partial Hospitalization
DIMENSIONAL ADMISSION CRITERIA	**All Programs** *Direct admission* to a Level II.1 program is advisable for the patient who meets specifications in Dimension 2 (if any biomedical conditions or problems exist) and in Dimension 3 (if any emotional, behavioral or cognitive conditions or problems exist), as well as in *one* of Dimensions 4, 5 or 6. *Transfer* to a Level II.1 program is advisable for the patient who (a) has met the essential treatment objectives at a more intensive level of care *and* (b) requires the intensity of services provided at Level II.1 in at least one dimension. A patient also may be transferred to Level II.1 from a Level I program when the services provided at Level I have proved insufficient to address the patient's needs or when Level I services have consisted of motivational interventions to prepare the patient for participation in a more intensive level of service, for which he or she now meets the admission criteria.	**All Programs** *Direct admission* to a Level II.5 program is advisable for the patient who meets specifications in Dimension 2 (if any biomedical conditions or problems exist), as well as in *one* of Dimensions 4, 5 or 6. *Transfer* to a Level II.5 program is advisable for the patient who (a) has met essential treatment objectives at a more intensive level of care *and* (b) requires the intensity of services provided at Level II.5 in at least one dimension. A patient also may be transferred to Level II.5 from a Level I or Level II.1 program when the services provided at the lower level have proved insufficient to address the patient's needs or when those services have consisted of motivational interventions to prepare the patient for participation in a more intensive level of service, for which he or she now meets the admission criteria.
DIMENSION 1: Acute Intoxication and/or Withdrawal	**All Programs** The patient has no signs or symptoms of withdrawal, or his or her withdrawal needs can be safely managed in a Level II.1 setting (see the separate Dimension 1 criteria).	**All Programs** The patient has no signs or symptoms of withdrawal, or his or her withdrawal needs can be safely managed in a Level II.5 setting (see the separate Dimension 1 criteria).

ASAM Patient Placement Criteria, Second Edition–Revised

Level II Admission Criteria
Diagnostic and Dimensional Criteria

CRITERIA	LEVEL II.1 Intensive Outpatient	LEVEL II.5 Partial Hospitalization
DIMENSION 2: **Biomedical Conditions and Complications**	**All Programs** In Dimension 2, the patient's biomedical conditions and problems, if any, are stable or are being addressed concurrently and thus will not interfere with treatment. Examples include mild pregnancy-related hypertension.	**All Programs** In Dimension 2, the patient's biomedical conditions and problems, if any, are not sufficient to interfere with treatment but are severe enough to distract from recovery efforts. Examples include unstable hypertension requiring medication adjustment or chronic back pain that distracts from recovery efforts. Such problems require medical monitoring and/or medical management, which can be provided by a Level II.5 program, either directly or through an arrangement with another treatment provider.
DIMENSION 3: **Emotional, Behavioral or Cognitive Conditions and Complications**	**All Programs** Problems in Dimension 3 are not necessary for admission to a Level II.1 program. However, if any of the Dimension 3 conditions are present, the patient must be admitted to either a Dual Diagnosis Capable or Dual Diagnosis Enhanced program, depending on the patient's level of function, stability and degree of impairment in this dimension.	**All Programs** Problems in Dimension 3 are not necessary for admission to a Level II.1 program. However, if any of the Dimension 3 conditions are present, the patient must be admitted to either a Dual Diagnosis Capable or Dual Diagnosis Enhanced program, depending on the patient's level of function, stability and degree of impairment in this dimension. The severity of the patient's problems in Dimension 3 may require partial hospitalization or a similar supportive living environment in conjunction with a Level III.1 program. On the other hand, if the patient receives adequate support from his or her family or significant other(s), a Level II.5 program may suffice.

Level II Admission Criteria
Diagnostic and Dimensional Criteria

CRITERIA	LEVEL II.1 Intensive Outpatient	LEVEL II.5 Partial Hospitalization
DIMENSION 3: Emotional, Behavioral or Cognitive Conditions and Complications (continued)	**Dual Diagnosis Capable Programs** The patient's status in Dimension 3 is characterized by (a) *or* (b): (a) The patient engages in abuse of family members or significant others, and requires intensive outpatient treatment to reduce the risk of further deterioration; *or* (b) The patient has a diagnosed emotional, behavioral or cognitive disorder that requires intensive outpatient monitoring to minimize distractions from his or her treatment or recovery. **Dual Diagnosis Enhanced Programs** The patient's status in Dimension 3 is characterized by (a) *or* (b) *or* (c): (a) The patient has a diagnosed emotional, behavioral or cognitive disorder that requires management because the patient's history suggests a high potential for distracting him or her from treatment; such a disorder requires stabilization concurrent with addiction treatment (for example, an unstable borderline personality disorder, compulsive personality disorder, unstable anxiety or mood disorder); *or* (b) The patient is assessed as at mild risk of behaviors endangering self, others or property (for example, he or she has suicidal or homicidal thoughts but no active plan); *or* (c) The patient is at significant risk of victimization by another. However, the risk is not severe enough to require 24-hour supervision (for example, the patient has sufficient coping skills to maintain safety through attendance at treatment sessions at least 9 hours per week).	**Dual Diagnosis Capable Programs** The patient's status in Dimension 3 is characterized by a history of mild to moderate psychiatric decompensation (marked by paranoia or mild psychotic symptoms) on discontinuation of the drug of abuse. Such decompensation may occur and requires monitoring to permit early intervention. **Dual Diagnosis Enhanced Programs** The patient's status in Dimension 3 is characterized by (a) *or* (b) *or* (c): (a) The patient evidences current inability to maintain behavioral stability over a 48-hour period (as evidenced by distractibility, negative emotions or generalized anxiety that significantly affects his or her daily functioning); *or* (b) The patient has a history of moderate psychiatric decompensation (marked by severe, non-suicidal depression) on discontinuation of the drug of abuse. Such decompensation is currently observable; *or* (c) The patient is at mild to moderate risk of behaviors endangering self, others or property, and is at imminent risk of relapse, with dangerous emotional, behavioral or cognitive consequences, in the absence of Level II.5 structured services. For example, the patient does not have sufficient internal coping skills to maintain safety to self, others or property without the consistent structure achieved through attendance at treatment sessions daily or at least 20 hours per week.

Level II Admission Criteria
Diagnostic and Dimensional Criteria

CRITERIA	LEVEL II.1 Intensive Outpatient	LEVEL II.5 Partial Hospitalization
DIMENSION 4: **Readiness** **to Change**	**All Programs** The patient's status in Dimension 4 is characterized by (a) *or* (b): (a) The patient requires structured therapy and a programmatic milieu to promote treatment progress and recovery because motivational interventions at another level of care have failed. Such interventions are not feasible or are not likely to succeed in a Level I program; *or* (b) The patient's perspective inhibits his or her ability to make behavioral changes without repeated, structured, clinically directed motivational interventions. (For example, the patient attributes his or her alcohol or other drug and mental health problems to other persons or external events rather than to an addictive or mental disorder.) Such interventions are not feasible or are not likely to succeed in a Level I program. However, the patient's willingness to participate in treatment and to explore his or her level of awareness and readiness to change suggest that treatment at Level II.1 can be effective.	**All Programs** The patient's status in Dimension 4 is characterized by (a) *or* (b): (a) The patient requires structured therapy and a programmatic milieu to promote treatment progress and recovery because motivational interventions at another level of care have failed. Such interventions are not feasible or are not likely to succeed in a Level II.1 program; *or* (b) The patient's perspective and lack of impulse control inhibit his or her ability to make behavioral changes without repeated, structured, clinically directed motivational interventions. (For example, the patient has unrealistic expectations that his or her alcohol, drug or mental health problem will resolve quickly, with little or no effort, or the patient experiences frequent impulses to harm himself or herself. He or she is willing to reach out but has poor ability to ask for help.) Such interventions are not feasible or are not likely to succeed in a Level I or Level II.1 program. However, the patient's willingness to participate in treatment and to explore his or her level of awareness and readiness to change suggest that treatment at Level II.5 can be effective.

Level II Admission Criteria
Diagnostic and Dimensional Criteria

CRITERIA	LEVEL II.1 Intensive Outpatient	LEVEL II.5 Partial Hospitalization
DIMENSION 4: **Readiness to Change**	**Dual Diagnosis Enhanced Programs** The patient's status in Dimension 4 is characterized by (a) *or* (b) *or* (c): (a) The patient is reluctant to agree to treatment and is ambivalent about his or her commitment to change a co-occurring mental health problem; *or* (b) The patient's follow-through in treatment is so poor or inconsistent that Level I services are not succeeding or are not feasible; *or* (c) The patient is assessed as requiring intensive services to improve his or her awareness of the need to change. The patient has such limited awareness of or commitment to change that he or she cannot maintain an adequate level of functioning without Level II.1 services (for example, the patient continues to experience mild to moderate depression, anxiety or mood swings, and is inconsistent in taking medication, keeping appointments and completing mental health assignments).	**Dual Diagnosis Enhanced Programs** The patient's status in Dimension 4 is characterized by (a) *or* (b) *or* (c): (a) The patient has little awareness of his or her co-occurring mental disorder; *or* (b) The patient's follow-through in treatment is so poor or inconsistent that Level II.1 services are not succeeding or are not feasible; *or* (c) The patient is assessed as requiring more intensive engagement, community or case management services than are available at Level II.1 in order to maintain an adequate level of functioning (for example, the patient experiences frequent impulses to harm himself or herself, with poor commitment to reach out for help).
DIMENSION 5: **Relapse, Continued Use or Continued Problem Potential**	**All Programs** The patient's status in Dimension 5 is characterized by the following: Although the patient has been an active participant at a less intensive level of care, he or she is experiencing an intensification of symptoms of the substance-related disorder (such as difficulty postponing immediate gratification and related drug-seeking behavior) and his or her level of functioning is deteriorating despite modification of the treatment plan.	**All Programs** The patient's status in Dimension 5 is characterized by (a) *or* (b): (a) Although the patient has been an active participant at a less intensive level of care, he or she is experiencing an intensification of symptoms of the substance-related disorder (such as difficulty postponing immediate gratification and related drug-seeking behavior) and his or her level of functioning is deteriorating despite modification of the treatment plan; *or*

Level II Admission Criteria
Diagnostic and Dimensional Criteria

CRITERIA	LEVEL II.1 Intensive Outpatient	LEVEL II.5 Partial Hospitalization
DIMENSION 5: **Relapse,** **Continued Use** **or Continued** **Problem** **Potential** **(continued)**		(b) There is a high likelihood that the patient will continue to use or relapse to use of alcohol or other drugs without close outpatient monitoring and structured therapeutic services, as indicated by his or her lack of awareness of relapse triggers, difficulty in coping or in postponing immediate gratification or ambivalence toward treatment. The patient has unsuccessfully attempted treatment at a less intensive level of care, or such treatment is adjudged insufficient to stabilize the patient's condition.
	Dual Diagnosis Enhanced Programs The patient's status in Dimension 5 is characterized by psychiatric symptoms that pose a moderate risk of relapse to the alcohol, drug or psychiatric disorder. Such a patient has impaired recognition or understanding of—and difficulty in managing—relapse issues and requires Level II.1 Dual Diagnosis Enhanced program services to maintain an adequate level of functioning.	**Dual Diagnosis Enhanced Programs** The patient's status in Dimension 5 is characterized by psychiatric symptoms that pose a high risk of relapse to the alcohol, drug or psychiatric disorder. Such a patient has impaired recognition or understanding of relapse issues and poor skills in coping with and interrupting mental disorders and/or avoiding or limiting relapse. Such a patient's follow-through in treatment is so poor or inconsistent, and his or her relapse problems are escalating to such a degree, that treatment at Level II.1 is not succeeding or not feasible.
	For example, the patient may have persistent difficulty in controlling his or her anger, with impulses to damage property, or the patient continues to increase his or her medication dose beyond the prescribed level in an attempt to control continued symptoms of anxiety or panic.	For example, the patient may continue to inflict superficial wounds on himself or herself and have continuing suicidal ideation and impulses. However, he or she has no specific suicide plan and agrees to reach out for help if seriously suicidal. Or the patient's continuing substance-induced psychotic symptoms are resolving, but difficulties in controlling his or her substance use exacerbate the psychotic symptoms.

Level II Admission Criteria
Diagnostic and Dimensional Criteria

CRITERIA	LEVEL II.1 Intensive Outpatient	LEVEL II.5 Partial Hospitalization
DIMENSION 6: **Recovery** **Environment**	**All Programs** The patient's status in Dimension 6 is characterized by (a) *or* (b): (a) Continued exposure to the patient's current school, work or living environment will render recovery unlikely. The patient lacks the resources or skills necessary to maintain an adequate level of functioning without the services of a Level II.1 program; *or* (b) The patient lacks social contacts, or has inappropriate social contacts that jeopardize recovery, or has few friends or peers who do not use alcohol or other drugs. He or she also lacks the resources or skills necessary to maintain an adequate level of functioning without Level II.1 services. **Dual Diagnosis Enhanced Programs** The patient's status in Dimension 6 is characterized by a living, working, social and/or community environment that is not supportive of good mental functioning. The patient has insufficient resources and skills to deal with this situation. For example, the patient is unable to cope with continuing stresses caused by hostile and alcoholic family members, and he or she evidences increasing depression and anxiety. The support and intermittent structure of a Level II.1 Dual Diagnosis Enhanced program provide sufficient stability to prevent further deterioration.	**All Programs** The patient's status in Dimension 6 is characterized by (a) *or* (b): (a) Continued exposure to the patient's current school, work or living environment will render recovery unlikely. The patient lacks the resources or skills necessary to maintain an adequate level of functioning without the services of a Level II.5 program; *or* (b) Family members and/or significant other(s) who live with the patient are not supportive of his or her recovery goals, or are passively opposed to his or her treatment. The patient requires the intermittent structure of Level II.5 treatment services and relief from the home environment in order to remain focused on recovery, but may live at home because there is no active opposition to, or sabotaging of, his or her recovery efforts. **Dual Diagnosis Enhanced Programs** The patient's status in Dimension 6 is characterized by a living, working, social and/or community environment that is not supportive of good mental functioning. The patient has such limited resources and skills to deal with this situation that treatment is not succeeding or not feasible. For example, the patient is unable to cope with continuing stresses caused by homelessness, unemployment and isolation, and evidences increasing depression and hopelessness. The support and intermittent structure of a Level II.5 Dual Diagnosis Enhanced program provide sufficient stability to prevent further deterioration.

Level III
Residential/Inpatient Treatment

Level III programs offer organized treatment services that feature a planned regimen of care in a 24-hour residential setting. Treatment services adhere to defined policies, procedures and clinical protocols. They are housed in, or affiliated with, permanent facilities where patients can reside safely. (One of the purposes of these programs is to demonstrate aspects of a positive recovery environment.) They are staffed 24 hours a day. Mutual/self-help group meetings usually are available on-site.

Level III encompasses four types of programs:

- Level III.1: Clinically Managed Low-Intensity Residential Treatment
- Level III.3: Clinically Managed Medium-Intensity Residential Treatment
- Level III.5: Clinically Managed High-Intensity Residential Treatment
- Level III.7: Medically Monitored Inpatient Treatment

The defining characteristic of all Level III programs is that they serve individuals who, because of specific functional deficits, need safe and stable living environments in order to develop their recovery skills. Such living environments may be housed in the same facility as the treatment services, or they may be in separate facilities that are affiliated with the treatment provider. In the latter situation, the relationship between the living environment and the treatment provider must be sufficiently close to allow specific aspects of the individual treatment plan to be addressed in both facilities.

The sublevels within Level III exist on a continuum ranging from the least intensive residential services to the most intensive medically monitored intensive inpatient services. Indeed, Level III always has consisted of a range of intensities of service. The intent never was to create just four discrete sublevels of care within Level III, but rather to create a range of intensities, with each designated sublevel (such as Level III.3) suggesting a particular *point* within that range. When a program provides Level III services that exceed the intensity usually ascribed to that level, or can appropriately treat an individual who has a more severe illness than usually is addressed at that level, it should be considered an *enhanced service*.

The term "clinically managed" is used to describe Level III.1 through III.5 programs. Individuals who are appropriately placed in the clinically managed levels of care have minimal problems with intoxication or withdrawal (Dimension 1) and few biomedical complications (Dimension 2), so on-site physician services are not required. Such individuals may have relatively stable problems in Axis I and/or less stable problems in Axis II (Dimension 3) of the *Diagnostic and Statistical Manual of Mental Disorders (DSM)* of the American Psychiatric Association. Many also have significant deficits in the areas of readiness to change (Dimension 4), relapse, continued use or continued problem potential (Dimension 5) or recovery environment (Dimension 6). Therefore, they are in need of interventions directed by appropriately trained and credentialed addiction treatment staff. Such individuals also need case management services to facilitate their reintegration into the larger community.

Treatment Levels Within Level III

Level III.1: Clinically Managed Low-Intensity Residential Services

Level III.1 programs offer at least 5 hours per week of low-intensity treatment of substance-related disorders (or as specified by state licensure requirements). Treatment is directed toward applying recovery skills, preventing relapse, improving emotional functioning, promoting personal responsibility and reintegrating the individual into the worlds of work, education and family life. The services provided may include individual, group and family therapy; medication management and medication education. Mutual/self-help meetings usually are available on-site.

The kinds of care delivered by Level III.1 programs are best understood in their component parts. The treatment services provided by Level III.1 programs, when considered separately from the residential component and other concurrent services, are low-intensity (Level I) outpatient services that are focused on improving the individual's functioning and coping skills in Dimensions 5 and 6. The other component of care is a structured recovery environment, staffed 24 hours a day, which provides sufficient stability to prevent or minimize relapse or continued use and continued problem potential (Dimension 5). Interpersonal and group living skills generally are promoted through the use of community or house meetings of residents and staff. When these components are provided together, Level III.1 programs often are considered appropriate for individuals who need time and structure to practice and integrate their recovery and coping skills.

Some persons require the structure of a Level III.1 program to achieve engagement in treatment (Dimension 4). Those who are in the early stages of readiness to change may need to be removed from an unsupportive living environment in order to minimize their continued alcohol or other drug use.

The residential component of Level III.1 programs also can be combined with intensive (Level II.1) outpatient services for individuals whose living situations are incompatible with their recovery goals, if they otherwise meet the dimensional admission criteria for intensive outpatient care.

The functional deficits found in populations typically treated at Level III.1 include problems in the application of recovery skills, lack of personal responsibility, or lack of connection to the worlds of work, education or family life. In a setting that provides 24-hour structure and support, residents have an opportunity to develop and practice their interpersonal and group living skills, strengthen their recovery skills, reintegrate into the community and possibly family, and find or return to school or employment.

Level III.1 programs also can meet the needs of individuals who may not yet acknowledge that they have an alcohol or other drug problem. Such individuals may be living in a recovery environment that is too toxic to permit treatment on an outpatient basis. Because these individuals are at an early stage of readiness to change ("Precontemplation" in Prochaska and DiClemente's Transtheoretical Stages of Change), they may need monitoring and motivating strategies to prevent deterioration, engage them in treatment and facilitate their progress through the stages of change to recovery. They are appropriately placed in a Level III.1 supportive environment while receiving "discovery" services as opposed to "recovery" services. (Because continued use of substances in a "discovery" population likely will be more common than in a "recovery" population, consideration should be given to the problems inherent in housing the two populations together.)

Intoxication and withdrawal require separate consideration. Intoxication or withdrawal in an individual who is placed in a Level III.1 program usually represents an isolated relapse associated with problems in applying recovery skills (Dimension 5). If the intoxication or withdrawal is associated with deficits in problem recognition or understanding (Dimension 4), the individual is appropriately placed in a Level III.1 program only if Level I or II motivational and engagement services are being provided concurrently. (Both situations are addressed in the Dimensional Admission Criteria.)

Level III.1 is not intended to describe or include sober houses, boarding houses or group homes where treatment services are not provided.

Level III.3: Clinically Managed Medium-Intensity Residential Services

Frequently referred to as extended or long-term care, Level III.3 programs provide a structured recovery environment in combination with medium-intensity clinical services to support recovery from substance-related disorders.

For the typical resident in a Level III.3 program, the effects of the substance-related disorder on the individual's life are so significant, and the resulting level of impairment so great, that outpatient motivational and/or relapse prevention strategies are not feasible or effective.

The functional deficits seen in individuals who are appropriately placed at Level III.3 are primarily cognitive and can be either temporary or permanent. They may result in problems in interpersonal relationships or emotional coping skills. For example, temporary deficits may be seen in the individual who suffers from an organic brain syndrome as a result of his or her substance use and who requires treatment that is slower paced, more concrete and more repetitive until his or her cognitive impairment subsides.

When assessment indicates that such an individual no longer is cognitively impaired, he or she can be transferred to a more intensive level of care (such as a Level III.5 program) or a less intensive level of care (such as a Level I, II or III.1 program), based on a reassessment of his or her severity of illness and rehabilitative needs. (Transfer to a Level III.7 or higher program would not be considered except in the presence of medical or psychiatric problems that require medical and nursing care.)

By contrast, the individual who suffers from chronic brain syndrome, or the older adult who has age- and substance-related cognitive deficits, or the individual who has experienced a traumatic brain injury, or the mentally retarded resident would continue to receive treatment in a Level III.3 program. For such an individual, the effects of the addictive disorder or co-occurring condition are so significant and the level of his or her impairment so great that outpatient care would not be feasible or effective.

Some individuals have such severe deficits in interpersonal and coping skills that the treatment process is one of "habilitation" rather than "rehabilitation." Treatment of such individuals is directed toward overcoming their lack of awareness of—or ambivalence about—the effects of substance-related problems on their lives, as well as enhancing their readiness to change. Treatment also is focused on preventing relapse, continued problems and/or continued use, and promoting the eventual reintegration of the individual into the community. In every case, the individual should be involved in planning continuing care to support recovery and improve his or her functioning.

Level III.3 programs generally are considered to deliver medium-intensity services. Such services may be provided in a deliberately repetitive fashion to address the special needs of individuals for whom a Level III.3 program is considered medically necessary. Such individuals often are elderly, cognitively impaired or developmentally delayed, or are those in whom the chronicity and intensity of the primary disease process requires a program that allows sufficient time to integrate the lessons and experiences of treatment into their daily lives. Typically, they need a slower pace of treatment because of mental health problems or reduced cognitive functioning (Dimension 3) or because of the chronicity of their illness (Dimensions 4 and 5). They also may be homeless, although homelessness is not, in itself, a sufficient indication for admission to a Level III.3 program.

Where treatment staff have been specially trained and adequate nursing supervision is available, Level III.3 programs are able to address the needs of residents with certain medical problems. These include patients whose biomedical conditions otherwise would meet medical necessity criteria for placement in a nursing home or other medically staffed facility. For such persons, their general medical condition (Dimension 2 comorbidity) provides the justification for admission to a Level III.3 program.

Reintegration of residents in a Level III.3 program into the community requires case management activities directed toward networking residents into community-based ancillary or "wrap-around" services such as housing, vocational services, or transportation assistance so that they are able to attend mutual/self-help meetings or vocational activities after discharge.

Level III.5: Clinically Managed High-Intensity Residential Services

Level III.5 programs are designed to treat persons who have significant social and psychological problems. Such programs are characterized by their reliance on the treatment community as a therapeutic agent. The goals of treatment are to promote abstinence from substance use and antisocial behavior and to effect a global change in participants' lifestyles, attitudes and values. This philosophy views substance-related problems as disorders of the whole person that are reflected in problems with conduct, attitudes, moods, values and emotional management. The defining characteristics of these residents are found in their emotional, behavioral and cognitive conditions (Dimension 3) and their living environments (Dimension 6).

Individuals who are appropriately placed in a Level III.5 program typically have multiple deficits, which may include substance-related disorders, criminal activity, psychological problems, impaired functioning and disaffiliation from mainstream values. Their mental disorders may involve serious and persistent Axis I disorders (such as schizophrenia, bipolar disorders, and major depression) and Axis II disorders (such as borderline, narcissistic and antisocial/personality disorders).

Such individuals generally can be characterized as having chaotic, non-supportive and often abusive interpersonal relationships; extensive treatment or criminal justice histories; limited work histories and educational experiences; and antisocial value systems. These deficits require comprehensive, multi-faceted treatment of relatively long duration that can address all of the patient's interrelated problems. For such patients, standard rehabilitation methods are inadequate. Effective treatment approaches are primarily *habilitative* in focus, addressing the patient's educational and vocational deficits, as well as his or her socially dysfunctional behavior.

Residents may present with the sequelae of physical, sexual or emotional trauma. Chronic use of psychoactive substances also may have impaired their judgment, at least temporarily, leaving them vulnerable to relapse, continued problems or continued use outside of a structured environment.

Other functional deficits in residents appropriately placed at this level of care include a constellation of criminal history or antisocial behaviors, with a risk of continued criminal behavior, an extensive history of treatment and/or criminal justice involvement, limited education, little or no work history and limited vocational skills, poor social skills, inadequate anger management skills, extreme impulsivity, emotional immaturity and/or an antisocial value system.

For all such residents, treatment is directed toward ameliorating their deficits through targeted interventions. For example, treatment may be focused on reducing the risk of relapse, reinforcing prosocial behaviors and assisting with healthy reintegration into the community. This treatment is accomplished by providing specialty modalities and skills training while the resident is in a safe and structured environment, thus providing an opportunity for continued improvement. Because treatment plans are individualized, fixed lengths of stay are inappropriate. The intensity and duration of clinical and habilitative services, rather than medical services, are the defining characteristics of Level III.5 programs.

In addition to residents who might meet *DSM* diagnostic criteria for a co-occurring Axis II disorder (such as antisocial personality disorder) or an Axis I disorder (such as attention deficit/hyperactivity disorder), other residents who do not meet diagnostic criteria may exhibit subthreshold Dimension 3 problems. Examples include impulsivity, deficient anger management skills, hostile and violent acting out, resistance and antagonism to limits, problems with authority, hyperactivity and distractibility. When treatment of these deficits cannot be implemented successfully on an outpatient basis, placement in a Level III.5 program should be considered.

Dimension 6 problems that may lead to placement in a Level III.5 program include a living environment in which substance use, crime and unemployment are endemic. The social influences there may represent a sense of hopelessness or an acceptance of deviance as normative (in such an environment, the threat of incarceration is not a source of motivation because it is a common occurrence). Recovery may be perceived by the resident as providing a lesser return for the effort (for example, the resident may not associate recovery from an addiction with outcomes such as vocational and housing opportunity). Some residents may have had no experience in a living environment that is conducive to healthy psychosocial development. Their entire social network may be composed of others who are involved in addictive disorders and/or criminal behaviors.

Treatment in a Level III.5 program is tailored to the resident's level of readiness to change. For some residents, "discovery" may be an appropriate treatment plan, while others may need to focus on maintaining abstinence and preventing relapse to alcohol or drug use as well as to antisocial behavior. Yet other residents may require treatment to develop a sense of personal responsibility and positive character change.

For some residents, treatment must be considered *habilitative* rather than *rehabilitative*. While most residents do not exhibit Dimension 1, 2 or 3 problems of a type that requires the availability of 24-hour medical or nursing interventions, they are not sufficiently stable to benefit from outpatient treatment, no matter how intensive.

Residents may be appropriately placed in a Level III.5 program as direct admissions or as transfers from a Level III.7 or Level IV program when their problems in Dimensions 1, 2 and 3 no longer warrant the availability of 24-hour medical or nursing interventions, but problems in Dimensions 4, 5 and 6 are sufficiently severe to exclude outpatient treatment as a viable option. Residents also may be transferred to a Level III.5 program from a less intensive level of care.

When offered to residents who are being transferred from a Level III.7 program, the services of a Level III.5 program may be provided by a separate treatment program in the resident's home area or as continued care in the program at which they received their Level III.7 treatment, thus providing continuity of care. Providers of Level III.7 services who decide to offer Level III.5 services should consider the liability and legal issues attendant on this decision.

The duration of treatment always depends on an individual's progress. Nevertheless, the length of service in a clinically managed Level III.5 program tends to be longer than in the more intensive medically monitored and medically managed levels of care. Longer exposure to treatment interventions is necessary for residents to acquire basic living skills and to master the application and demonstration of coping and recovery skills. (Because of the longer duration of treatment in Level III programs, the essential nature of the residential component and the fact that clinically managed programs serve as a temporary recovery environment, participants in Level III.5 programs are referred to as "residents.")

The therapeutic community is widely identified as an example of a Level III.5 program, but other types of programs also fall within Level III.5. For example, a Level III.5 program may represent a "step down" for residents of a Level III.7 program if their complications in Dimensions 1, 2 or 3 no longer require subacute medical services, but their problems in Dimensions 4, 5 and 6 warrant 24-hour structure and clinical services to facilitate initial recovery. (One way of conceptualizing this level of service is as a Level III.7 program without the intensive medical and nursing component.)

Where treatment staff have been specially trained and adequate nursing supervision is available, Level III.5 programs are able to address the needs of individuals who have relatively severe biomedical problems (Dimension 2). For example, some residents may require daily medical monitoring or administration of prescription medications. A number of Level III.5 programs offer a full range of medical services.

Level III.7: Medically Monitored Intensive Inpatient Treatment

Level III.7 programs provide a planned regimen of 24-hour professionally directed evaluation, observation, medical monitoring and addiction treatment in an inpatient setting. They feature permanent facilities, including inpatient beds, and function under a defined set of policies, procedures and clinical protocols. They are appropriate for patients whose subacute biomedical and emotional, behavioral or cognitive problems are so severe that they require inpatient treatment, but who do not need the full resources of an acute care general hospital or a medically managed inpatient treatment program.

The services of a Level III.7 program are designed to meet the needs of patients who have functional deficits in Dimensions 1, 2 and/or 3. For example, a patient may present with moderate to severe Dimension 1 problems, such as withdrawal risk. Dimension 2 problems could include such comorbid medical problems as poorly controlled hypertension or diabetes or a co-occurring chronic pain disorder that interferes with the patient's ability to engage in a recovery program. Dimension 3 problems would include either a diagnosable comorbid *DSM-IV* Axis I disorder or symptoms of such a disorder that are subthreshold and not severe enough to meet diagnostic criteria, but that interfere or distract from recovery efforts (for example, anxiety or hypomanic behavior) and thus require the availability of 24-hour nursing and medical interventions.

Because medical and mental health problems exist on a continuum of severity, problems that exist in Dimensions 2 or 3 may fall short of reaching the threshold to meet diagnostic criteria but still require treatment in a Level III.7 program (for example, a patient's high level of anxiety distracts him or her from recovery efforts but falls short of the *DSM-IV* criteria required to meet the diagnosis for an anxiety disorder).

Although Level III.7 was developed to describe a level of care that responds to problems in Dimensions 1, 2 and 3, the *ASAM PPC-2* admission criteria require only that the patient meet specifications in at least two of the six dimensions (p. 88). Thus, an individual could be admitted to a Level III.7 program even if he or she meets the specifications only in Dimensions 4, 5 or 6. This is inconsistent with the distinctions between inpatient and residential care described earlier, and contradicts the original intent of a medically monitored setting. Therefore, with this revision, the requirements for admission to a Level III.7 program have been clarified to indicate that at least one of the two specifications must be in Dimension 1, 2 or 3. Individuals whose major problems are in Dimensions 4, 5 or 6 are better served by admission to a clinically managed residential program or by combining an intensive outpatient program or partial hospitalization with a housing or domiciliary/supportive living component.

The care provided in Level III.7 programs is delivered by an interdisciplinary staff of appropriately credentialed treatment professionals, including addiction-credentialed physicians. Treatment is specific to substance-related disorders, but the skills of the interdisciplinary team and the availability of support services also can accommodate detoxification and/or intensive inpatient treatment of addiction and/or conjoint treatment of co-occurring subacute biomedical and/or emotional, behavioral or cognitive conditions.

Individuals who have a greater severity of illness in Dimension 1 (withdrawal), Dimension 2 (biomedical conditions) or Dimension 3 (emotional, behavioral or cognitive complications) require use of more intensive staffing patterns and support services. For example, patients undergoing medical detoxification or chemical aversion therapy typically require more intensive medical and nursing care than do other patients in a Level III.7 program.

Level III.7 programs that wish to offer Level III.5 services should give some consideration to liability and licensing issues. Where the resident's primary problems are logistical (for example, he or she lacks public transportation, an automobile or a valid driver's license), a combination of a Level II.5 service with a domiciliary or supportive living component may be the most appropriate intervention.

Length of Service

While the duration of treatment varies with the severity of an individual's illness and his or her response to treatment, the length of service in clinically managed Level III programs tends to be longer than in the more intensive medically monitored and medically managed levels of care.

Some individuals enter Level III programs under a court order that specifies their length of stay. However, treatment professionals have a responsibility to make admission, continued service and discharge decisions based on their own clinical impressions of an individual's assessed needs and treatment progress. Thus, if a patient has improved sufficiently to warrant discharge or transfer, the treatment professional has a responsibility to contact the appropriate court and seek to have the court order amended.

Co-Occurring Mental and Substance-Related Disorders

Level III programs that treat individuals with co-occurring mental and substance-related disorders typically integrate mental health and addiction treatment services and incorporate mental health professionals into the treatment staff. Such programs generally are more flexible, more individualized and less confrontational than the typical Level III program. There is considerable variation in program activities, as well as in the duration of program stages. The intensity of interpersonal encounters is considerably reduced, reliance on educational and skill-building approaches is increased, and the programs are more closely tailored to address the specific mental and substance-related problems of individual patients. The mental health component of treatment is not focused on intensive psychiatric, medical or nursing care, but rather on support for reshaping coping skills and mental functioning.

Adult Criteria
Level III: Residential/Inpatient Treatment

CHARACTERISTIC	LEVEL III.1 Clinically Managed Low-Intensity Residential Treatment	LEVEL III.3 Clinically Managed Medium-Intensity Residential Treatment	LEVEL III.5 Clinically Managed High-Intensity Residential Treatment	LEVEL III.7 Medically Monitored Intensive Inpatient Treatment
EXAMPLES	**All Programs** An example of a Level III.1 program is a Halfway House	**All Programs** An example of a Level III.3 program is a Therapeutic Rehabilitation Facility	**All Programs** Examples of Level III.5 programs are a Therapeutic Community or a Residential Treatment Center	**All Programs** An example of a Level III.7 program in an Inpatient Treatment Center
SETTING	**All Programs** Level III.1 program services may be offered in a (usually) freestanding, appropriately licensed facility located in a community setting or a specialty unit within a licensed health care facility.	**All Programs** Level III.3 program services may be offered in a (usually) freestanding, appropriately licensed facility located in a community setting or a specialty unit within a licensed health care facility.	**All Programs** Level III.5 program services may be offered in a (usually) freestanding, appropriately licensed facility located in a community setting or a specialty unit within a licensed health care facility.	**All Programs** Level III.7 program services may be offered in a (usually) freestanding, appropriately licensed facility located in a community setting or a specialty unit in a general or psychiatric hospital or other licensed health care facility.

Adult Criteria
Level III: Residential/Inpatient Treatment

CHARACTERISTIC	LEVEL III.1 Clinically Managed Low-Intensity Residential Treatment	LEVEL III.3 Clinically Managed Medium-Intensity Residential Treatment	LEVEL III.5 Clinically Managed High-Intensity Residential Treatment	LEVEL III.7 Medically Monitored Intensive Inpatient Treatment
SUPPORT SYSTEMS	**All Programs** In Level III.1 programs, necessary support systems include: (a) Telephone or in-person consultation with a physician and emergency services, available 24 hours a day, 7 days a week.	**All Programs** In Level III.3 programs, necessary support systems include: (a) Telephone or in-person consultation with a physician and emergency services, available 24 hours a day, 7 days a week.	**All Programs** In Level III.5 programs, necessary support systems include: (a) Telephone or in-person consultation with a physician and emergency services, available 24 hours a day, 7 days a week.	**All Programs** In Level III.7 programs, necessary support systems include: (a) Physician monitoring and nursing care and observation are available as needed, based on clinical judgment. A physician is available to assess the patient in person within 24 hours of admission and thereafter as medically necessary. (In states where physician assistants or nurse practitioners are licensed as physician extenders, they may perform the duties designated here for a physician.) A registered nurse conducts an alcohol or other drug-focused nursing assessment at the time of admission. An appropriately credentialed and licensed nurse is responsible for monitoring the patient's progress and for medication administration.

Adult Criteria
Level III: Residential/Inpatient Treatment

CHARACTERISTIC	LEVEL III.1 Clinically Managed Low-Intensity Residential Treatment	LEVEL III.3 Clinically Managed Medium-Intensity Residential Treatment	LEVEL III.5 Clinically Managed High-Intensity Residential Treatment	LEVEL III.7 Medically Monitored Intensive Inpatient Treatment
SUPPORT SYSTEMS (continued)	(b) Direct affiliations with other levels of care, or close coordination through referral to more and less intensive levels of care and other services (such as intensive outpatient treatment, vocational assessment and placement, literacy training and adult education). (c) The program is able to arrange for needed procedures (including indicated laboratory and toxicology tests) as appropriate to the severity and urgency of the resident's condition.	(b) Direct affiliations with other levels of care or close coordination through referral to more and less intensive levels of care and other services (such as sheltered workshops, literacy training and adult education). (c) Medical, psychiatric, psychological, laboratory and toxicology services are available through consultation or referral, as appropriate to the severity and urgency of the resident's condition.	(b) Direct affiliations with other levels of care or close coordination through referral to more and less intensive levels of care and other services (such as vocational assessment and training, literacy training and adult education). (c) The program is able to arrange for needed medical, psychiatric, psychological, laboratory and toxicology services, as appropriate to the severity and urgency of the resident's condition.	(b) Additional medical specialty consultation, psychological, laboratory and toxicology services are available through consultation or referral. (c) Direct affiliation with other levels of care or close coordination through referral to more and less intensive levels of care and other services (such as kidney dialysis, vocational assessment and training, literacy training and adult education). (d) Psychiatric services are available through consultation or referral. Such services are available within 8 hours by telephone or 24 hours in person.

ASAM Patient Placement Criteria, Second Edition–Revised

Adult Criteria
Level III: Residential/Inpatient Treatment

CHARACTERISTIC	LEVEL III.1 Clinically Managed Low-Intensity Residential Treatment	LEVEL III.3 Clinically Managed Medium-Intensity Residential Treatment	LEVEL III.5 Clinically Managed High-Intensity Residential Treatment	LEVEL III.7 Medically Monitored Intensive Inpatient Treatment
SUPPORT SYSTEMS (continued)	**Dual Diagnosis Enhanced Programs** In addition to the foregoing support systems, Level III.1 Dual Diagnosis Enhanced programs offer appropriate psychiatric services, including medication evaluation and laboratory services. Such services are provided on-site or closely coordinated off-site, as appropriate to the severity and urgency of the resident's mental condition.	**Dual Diagnosis Enhanced Programs** In addition to the foregoing support systems, Level III.3 Dual Diagnosis Enhanced programs offer psychiatric services, medication evaluation and laboratory services. Such services are available by telephone within 8 hours and on-site or closely coordinated off-site within 24 hours, as appropriate to the severity and urgency of the resident's mental condition.	**Dual Diagnosis Enhanced Programs** In addition to the foregoing support systems, Level III.5 Dual Diagnosis Enhanced programs offer psychiatric services, medication evaluation and laboratory services. Such services are available by telephone within 8 hours and on-site or closely coordinated off-site within 24 hours, as appropriate to the severity and urgency of the resident's mental condition.	**Dual Diagnosis Enhanced Programs** In addition to the foregoing support systems, Level III.7 Dual Diagnosis Enhanced programs offer appropriate psychiatric services, medication evaluation and laboratory services. A psychiatrist assesses the patient within 4 hours of admission by telephone and within 24 hours of admission in person, or sooner, as appropriate to the patient's mental condition, and thereafter as medically necessary (the services of another physician may be required for biomedical concerns). A registered nurse conducts a mental health focused nursing assessment at the time of admission. A registered nurse is responsible for monitoring the patient's progress and administering psychotropic medications.

Adult Criteria
Level III: Residential/Inpatient Treatment

CHARACTERISTIC	LEVEL III.1 Clinically Managed Low-Intensity Residential Treatment	LEVEL III.3 Clinically Managed Medium-Intensity Residential Treatment	LEVEL III.5 Clinically Managed High-Intensity Residential Treatment	LEVEL III.7 Medically Monitored Intensive Inpatient Treatment
STAFF	**All Programs** Level III.1 programs are staffed by: (a) Allied health professional staff, such as counselor aides or group living workers, who are available on-site 24 hours a day or as required by licensing regulations. (b) Clinical staff who are knowledgeable about the biological and psychosocial dimensions of substance dependence disorders and their treatment, and are able to identify the signs and symptoms of acute psychiatric conditions, including psychiatric decompensation.	**All Programs** Level III.3 programs are staffed by: (a) Allied health professional staff, such as counselor aides or group living workers, are on-site 24 hours a day or as required by licensing regulations. One or more clinicians with competence in the treatment of substance dependence disorders are available on-site or by telephone 24 hours a day. (b) Clinical staff are knowledgeable about the biological and psychosocial dimensions of substance dependence and mental health disorders and their treatment, and are able to identify the signs and symptoms of acute psychiatric conditions, including psychiatric decompensation. Staff have specialized training in behavior management techniques.	**All Programs** Level III.5 programs are staffed by: (a) Allied health professional staff, such as counselor aides or group living workers, are on-site 24 hours a day or as required by licensing regulations. One or more clinicians with competence in the treatment of substance dependence disorders are available on-site or by telephone 24 hours a day. (b) Clinical staff are knowledgeable about the biological and psychosocial dimensions of substance dependence and mental health disorders and their treatment, and are able to identify the signs and symptoms of acute psychiatric conditions, including psychiatric decompensation. Staff have specialized training in behavior management techniques.	**All Programs** Level III.7 programs are staffed by: (a) An interdisciplinary staff (including physicians, nurses, addiction counselors and mental health specialists) are able to assess and treat the patient and to obtain and interpret information regarding the patient's mental and substance dependence disorders. (b) Clinical staff are knowledgeable about the biological and psychosocial dimensions of substance dependence and mental disorders and have specialized training in behavior management techniques. The staff are able to provide a planned regimen of 24-hour professionally directed evaluation, care and treatment services (including administration of prescribed medications).

Adult Criteria
Level III: Residential/Inpatient Treatment

CHARACTERISTIC	LEVEL III.1 Clinically Managed Low-Intensity Residential Treatment	LEVEL III.3 Clinically Managed Medium-Intensity Residential Treatment	LEVEL III.5 Clinically Managed High-Intensity Residential Treatment	LEVEL III.7 Medically Monitored Intensive Inpatient Treatment
STAFF (continued)	**Biomedical Enhanced Services** Biomedical Enhanced services are delivered by appropriately credentialed medical staff, who are available to assess and treat co-occurring biomedical disorders and to monitor the resident's administration of medications in accordance with a physician's prescription. The intensity of nursing care and observation is sufficient to meet the resident's needs.	**Biomedical Enhanced Services** Biomedical Enhanced services are delivered by appropriately credentialed medical staff, who are available to assess and treat co-occurring biomedical disorders and to monitor the resident's administration of medications in accordance with a physician's prescription. The intensity of nursing care and observation is sufficient to meet the patient's needs.	**Biomedical Enhanced Services** Biomedical Enhanced services are delivered by appropriately credentialed medical staff, who are available to assess and treat co-occurring biomedical disorders and to monitor the resident's administration of medications in accordance with a physician's prescription. The intensity of nursing care and observation is sufficient to meet the patient's needs.	**Biomedical Enhanced Services** Biomedical Enhanced services are delivered by appropriately credentialed medical staff, who are available to assess and treat co-occurring biomedical disorders and to monitor the resident's administration of medications in accordance with a physician's prescription. The intensity of nursing care and observation is sufficient to meet the patient's needs.

Adult Criteria
Level III: Residential/Inpatient Treatment

CHARACTERISTIC	LEVEL III.1 Clinically Managed Low-Intensity Residential Treatment	LEVEL III.3 Clinically Managed Medium-Intensity Residential Treatment	LEVEL III.5 Clinically Managed High-Intensity Residential Treatment	LEVEL III.7 Medically Monitored Intensive Inpatient Treatment
STAFF (continued)	**Dual Diagnosis Enhanced Programs** In addition to the staff listed above, Level III.1 Dual Diagnosis Enhanced programs are staffed by appropriately credentialed mental health professionals, who are able to assess and treat co-occurring mental disorders.	**Dual Diagnosis Enhanced Programs** In addition to the staff listed above, Level III.3 Dual Diagnosis Enhanced programs are staffed by appropriately credentialed mental health professionals, who are able to assess and treat co-occurring mental disorders and who have specialized training in behavior management techniques.	**Dual Diagnosis Enhanced Programs** In addition to the staff listed above, Level III.5 Dual Diagnosis Enhanced programs are staffed by appropriately credentialed mental health professionals, who are able to assess and treat co-occurring mental disorders and who have specialized training in behavior management techniques.	**Dual Diagnosis Enhanced Programs** In addition to the staff listed above, Level III.7 Dual Diagnosis Enhanced programs are staffed by appropriately credentialed mental health professionals, who are able to assess and treat co-occurring mental disorders and who have specialized training in behavior management techniques.
	Some (if not all) of the addiction treatment professionals have had sufficient cross-training to understand the signs and symptoms of mental disorders and to understand and explain to the resident the purposes of psychotropic medications and their interactions with substance use.	Some (if not all) of the addiction treatment professionals have had sufficient cross-training to understand the signs and symptoms of mental disorders and to understand and explain to the resident the purposes of psychotropic medications and their interactions with substance use.	Some (if not all) of the addiction treatment professionals have had sufficient cross-training to understand the signs and symptoms of mental disorders and to understand and explain to the resident the purposes of psychotropic medications and their interactions with substance use.	Some (if not all) of the addiction treatment professionals have had sufficient cross-training to understand the signs and symptoms of mental disorders and to understand and explain to the patient the purposes of psychotropic medications and their interactions with substance use.
	The intensity of nursing care and observation is sufficient to meet the resident's needs.	The intensity of nursing care and observation is sufficient to meet the resident's needs.	The intensity of nursing care and observation is sufficient to meet the resident's needs.	The intensity of nursing care and observation is sufficient to meet the patient's needs.

Adult Criteria
Level III: Residential/Inpatient Treatment

CHARACTERISTIC	LEVEL III.1 Clinically Managed Low-Intensity Residential Treatment	LEVEL III.3 Clinically Managed Medium-Intensity Residential Treatment	LEVEL III.5 Clinically Managed High-Intensity Residential Treatment	LEVEL III.7 Medically Monitored Intensive Inpatient Treatment
THERAPIES	**All Programs** Therapies offered by Level III.1 programs include: (a) Services designed to improve the resident's ability to structure and organize the tasks of daily living and recovery, such as personal responsibility, personal appearance and punctuality. (b) Planned clinical program activities (constituting at least 5 hours per week of professionally directed treatment) to stabilize and maintain the stability of the resident's substance dependence symptoms and to help him or her develop and apply recovery skills. Activities may include relapse prevention, interpersonal choices and development of a social network supportive of recovery.	**All Programs** Therapies offered by Level III.3 programs include: (a) Daily clinical services to improve the resident's ability to structure and organize the tasks of daily living and recovery, such as personal responsibility, personal appearance and punctuality. Such services are designed to accommodate the cognitive limitations frequently seen in this population. (b) Planned clinical program activities designed to stabilize and maintain the stability of the resident's substance dependence symptoms and to help him or her develop and apply recovery skills. Activities may include relapse prevention, interpersonal choices and development of a social network supportive of recovery.	**All Programs** Therapies offered by Level III.5 programs include: (a) Daily clinical services to improve the resident's ability to structure and organize the tasks of daily living and recovery, such as personal responsibility, personal appearance and punctuality, and to develop and practice prosocial behaviors. (b) Planned clinical program activities to stabilize and maintain stabilization of the resident's substance dependence symptoms and to help him or her develop and apply recovery skills. Activities may include relapse prevention, interpersonal choices and development of a social network supportive of recovery.	**All Programs** Therapies offered by Level III.7 programs include: (a) Daily clinical services (provided by an interdisciplinary treatment team) to assess and address the patient's individual needs. Clinical services may involve appropriate medical services, and individual, group, family and activity services. (b) Planned clinical program activities to stabilize the acute addictive and/or non-medical or psychiatric symptoms. Activities may include pharmacological, cognitive-behavioral and other therapies administered to the patient on an individual and/or group basis. Such activities are adapted to the resident's developmental stage and level of comprehension.

Adult Criteria
Level III: Residential/Inpatient Treatment

CHARACTERISTIC	LEVEL III.1 Clinically Managed Low-Intensity Residential Treatment	LEVEL III.3 Clinically Managed Medium-Intensity Residential Treatment	LEVEL III.5 Clinically Managed High-Intensity Residential Treatment	LEVEL III.7 Medically Monitored Intensive Inpatient Treatment
THERAPIES (continued)	(c) Counseling and clinical monitoring to promote successful initial involvement or reinvolvement in regular, productive daily activity, such as work or school and, as indicated, successful reintegration into family living.	(c) Counseling and clinical monitoring to promote successful initial involvement or reinvolvement in regular, productive daily activity, such as work or school and, as indicated, successful reintegration into family living.	(c) Counseling and clinical monitoring to promote successful initial involvement or reinvolvement in regular, productive daily activity, such as work or school and, as indicated, successful reintegration into family living.	(c) Counseling and clinical monitoring to promote successful initial involvement or reinvolvement in regular, productive daily activity and, as indicated, successful reintegration into family living.
	(d) Random drug screening to shape behavior and reinforce treatment gains, as appropriate to the resident's individual treatment plan.	(d) Random drug screening to shape behavior and reinforce treatment gains, as appropriate to the resident's individual treatment plan.	(d) Random drug screening to shape behavior and reinforce treatment gains, as appropriate to the resident's individual treatment plan.	(d) Random drug screening to shape behavior and reinforce treatment gains, as appropriate to the patient's individual treatment plan.
	(e) Motivational enhancement and engagement strategies appropriate to the resident's stage of readiness to change, which are used in preference to confrontational approaches.	(e) Services may involve (but are not limited to) a range of cognitive, behavioral and other therapies administered on an individual and group basis, medication education and management, educational groups, and occupational or recreational activities, and are adapted to the resident's developmental stage and level of comprehension.	(e) Services may involve (but are not limited to) a range of cognitive, behavioral and other therapies administered on an individual and group basis, medication education and management, educational groups, and occupational or recreational activities, and are adapted to the resident's developmental stage and level of comprehension.	(e) Counseling and medical monitoring to teach the patient the skills needed for productive daily activity (as at work or school) and, as indicated, successful reintegration into family living.

Adult Criteria
Level III: Residential/Inpatient Treatment

CHARACTERISTIC	LEVEL III.1 Clinically Managed Low-Intensity Residential Treatment	LEVEL III.3 Clinically Managed Medium-Intensity Residential Treatment	LEVEL III.5 Clinically Managed High-Intensity Residential Treatment	LEVEL III.7 Medically Monitored Intensive Inpatient Treatment
THERAPIES (continued)		For residents with significant cognitive deficits (such as chronic brain syndrome, mental retardation or traumatic brain injury), therapies are delivered in a manner that is slower-paced, more concrete and more repetitive.		
	(f) Counseling and clinical monitoring to support successful initial involvement or reinvolvement in regular, productive daily activity (such as work or school) and, as indicated, successful reintegration into family living. Health education services also are provided.	(f) Counseling and clinical monitoring to assist the resident with successful initial involvement or reinvolvement in regular, productive daily activity (such as work or school) and, as indicated, successful reintegration into family living. Health education services are provided.	(f) Motivational enhancement and engagement strategies appropriate to the resident's stage of readiness to change, which are used in preference to confrontational approaches (except for those residents for whom motivational enhancement strategies would be clinically ineffective).	(f) Regular monitoring of the patient's compliance in taking any prescribed medications.
	(g) Regular monitoring of the resident's compliance in taking any prescribed medications.	(g) Regular monitoring of the resident's compliance in taking any prescribed medications.	(g) Counseling and clinical interventions to teach the resident the skills needed for productive daily activity (such as work or school) and, as indicated, successful reintegration into family living. Health education services also are provided.	(g) Planned clinical program activities, designed to enhance the patient's understanding of his or her substance dependence and/or mental disorder.

ASAM Patient Placement Criteria, Second Edition–Revised

Adult Criteria
Level III: Residential/Inpatient Treatment

CHARACTERISTIC	LEVEL III.1 Clinically Managed Low-Intensity Residential Treatment	LEVEL III.3 Clinically Managed Medium-Intensity Residential Treatment	LEVEL III.5 Clinically Managed High-Intensity Residential Treatment	LEVEL III.7 Medically Monitored Intensive Inpatient Treatment
THERAPIES (continued)	(h) Services also are provided to the resident's family and significant others, as appropriate.	(h) Daily scheduled professional addiction and mental health treatment services, designed to develop and apply recovery skills. These may include relapse prevention, interpersonal choices, and development of a social network supportive of recovery from the psychiatric and/or addictive disorder. Such services also may include medical services, nursing services, individual and group counseling, family therapy, educational groups, occupational and recreational therapies, art, music or movement therapies, physical therapy, and vocational rehabilitation activities.	(h) Regular monitoring of the resident's compliance in taking any prescribed medications.	(h) Health education services also are provided.

Adult Criteria
Level III: Residential/Inpatient Treatment

CHARACTERISTIC	LEVEL III.1 Clinically Managed Low-Intensity Residential Treatment	LEVEL III.3 Clinically Managed Medium-Intensity Residential Treatment	LEVEL III.5 Clinically Managed High-Intensity Residential Treatment	LEVEL III.7 Medically Monitored Intensive Inpatient Treatment
THERAPIES (continued)		(i) Clinical and didactic motivational interventions appropriate to the resident's stage of readiness to change, designed to facilitate the resident's understanding of the relationship between his or her substance dependence disorder and attendant life issues.	(i) Planned clinical activities to enhance the resident's understanding of his or her substance dependence and/or mental disorders.	(i) Clinical and didactic motivational enhancement strategies that are appropriate to the patient's stage of readiness to change, and which are designed to facilitate the patient's understanding of the relationship between his or her substance dependence disorder and attendant life issues.
		(j) Services also are provided to the resident's family and significant others.	(j) Daily scheduled professional services, including interdisciplinary assessments and treatment, designed to develop and apply recovery skills. Such services may include relapse prevention, interpersonal choices, and development of a social network supportive of recovery. Such services also may include medical services, nursing services, individual and group counseling, psychotherapy, family therapy, educational groups, occupational and recreational therapies, art, music	(j) Daily treatment services to manage acute symptoms of the patient's biomedical, substance dependence or mental disorder.

ASAM Patient Placement Criteria, Second Edition–Revised

Adult Criteria
Level III: Residential/Inpatient Treatment

CHARACTERISTIC	LEVEL III.1 Clinically Managed Low-Intensity Residential Treatment	LEVEL III.3 Clinically Managed Medium-Intensity Residential Treatment	LEVEL III.5 Clinically Managed High-Intensity Residential Treatment	LEVEL III.7 Medically Monitored Intensive Inpatient Treatment
THERAPIES (continued)			or movement therapies, physical therapy, and vocational rehabilitation activities. (k) Planned community reinforcement designed to foster pro-social values and group living skills. (l) Services also are provided to the resident's family and significant others.	(k) Services also are provided to the patient's family and significant others.
	Dual Diagnosis Enhanced Programs In addition to the therapies described above, Level III.1 Dual Diagnosis Enhanced programs offer planned clinical activities (either directly or through affiliated providers) that are designed to stabilize the resident's mental health problems and psychiatric symptoms and to maintain such stabilization.	**Dual Diagnosis Enhanced Programs** In addition to the therapies described above, Level III.3 Dual Diagnosis Enhanced programs offer planned clinical activities designed to stabilize the resident's mental health problems and psychiatric symptoms and to maintain such stabilization.	**Dual Diagnosis Enhanced Programs** In addition to the therapies described above, Level III.5 Dual Diagnosis Enhanced programs offer planned clinical activities designed to stabilize the resident's mental health problems and psychiatric symptoms and to maintain such stabilization.	**Dual Diagnosis Enhanced Programs** In addition to the therapies described above, Level III.7 Dual Diagnosis Enhanced programs offer planned clinical activities designed to stabilize the patient's mental health problems and psychiatric symptoms and to maintain such stabilization.
	The goals of therapy apply to both the substance dependence	The goals of therapy apply to both the substance dependence	The goals of therapy apply to both the substance dependence	The goals of therapy apply to both the substance dependence

Adult Criteria
Level III: Residential/Inpatient Treatment

CHARACTERISTIC	LEVEL III.1 Clinically Managed Low-Intensity Residential Treatment	LEVEL III.3 Clinically Managed Medium-Intensity Residential Treatment	LEVEL III.5 Clinically Managed High-Intensity Residential Treatment	LEVEL III.7 Medically Monitored Intensive Inpatient Treatment
THERAPIES (continued)	disorder and any co-occurring mental disorder. Specific attention is given to medication education and management and to motivational and engagement strategies, which are used in preference to confrontational approaches. NOTE: The therapies described here encompass Level III.1 Dual Diagnosis Capable program services for residents who are able to tolerate and benefit from a planned program of therapies. Other residents—especially those who are severely and persistently mentally ill—may not be able to benefit from such a program. Once stabilized, such residents will require planning for and integration into intensive case management, medication management and/or psychotherapy.	disorder and any co-occurring mental disorder. Specific attention is given to medication education and management and to motivational and engagement strategies, which are used in preference to confrontational approaches. NOTE: The therapies described above encompass Level III.3 Dual Diagnosis Capable program services for residents who are able to tolerate and benefit from a planned program of therapies. Other residents—especially those who are severely and persistently mentally ill—may not be able to benefit from such a program. Once stabilized, such residents will require planning for and integration into intensive case management, medication management and/or psychotherapy.	disorder and any co-occurring mental disorder. Specific attention is given to medication education and management and to motivational and engagement strategies, which are used in preference to confrontational approaches. NOTE: The therapies described above encompass Level III.5 Dual Diagnosis Capable program services for residents who are able to tolerate and benefit from a planned program of therapies. Other residents—especially those who are severely and persistently mentally ill—may not be able to benefit from such a program. Once stabilized, such residents will require planning for and integration into intensive case management, medication management and/or psychotherapy.	disorder and any co-occurring mental disorder. Specific attention is given to medication education and management and to motivational and engagement strategies, which are used in preference to confrontational approaches. NOTE: The therapies described above encompass Level III.7 Dual Diagnosis Capable program services for patients who are able to tolerate and benefit from a planned program of therapies. Other patients—especially those who are severely and persistently mentally ill—may not be able to benefit from such a program. Once stabilized, such patients will require planning for and integration into intensive case management, medication management and/or psychotherapy.

Adult Criteria
Level III: Residential/Inpatient Treatment

CHARACTERISTIC	LEVEL III.1 Clinically Managed Low-Intensity Residential Treatment	LEVEL III.3 Clinically Managed Medium-Intensity Residential Treatment	LEVEL III.5 Clinically Managed High-Intensity Residential Treatment	LEVEL III.7 Medically Monitored Intensive Inpatient Treatment
ASSESSMENT/ TREATMENT PLAN REVIEW	**All Programs** In Level III.1 programs, the assessment and treatment plan review include: (a) An individualized, comprehensive biopsychosocial assessment of the resident's substance dependence disorder, conducted or updated by staff who are knowledgeable about addiction treatment, to confirm the appropriateness of placement at Level III.1 and to help guide the individualized treatment planning process. (b) An individualized treatment plan, which includes problem formulation and articulation of short-term, measurable treatment goals and activities designed to achieve those goals. The plan is developed in collaboration with the resident and reflects the resident's personal goals.	**All Programs** In Level III.3 programs, the assessment and treatment plan review include: (a) An individualized, comprehensive biopsychosocial assessment of the resident's substance dependence disorder, conducted or updated by staff who are knowledgeable about addiction treatment, to confirm the appropriateness of placement at Level III.3 and to help guide the individualized treatment planning process. (b) An individualized treatment plan, which includes problem formulation and articulation of short-term, measurable treatment goals and activities designed to achieve those goals. The plan is developed in collaboration with the resident and reflects the resident's personal goals.	**All Programs** In Level III.5 programs, the assessment and treatment plan review include: (a) An individualized, comprehensive biopsychosocial assessment of the resident's substance dependence disorder, conducted or updated by staff who are knowledgeable about addiction treatment, to confirm the appropriateness of placement at Level III.5 and to help guide the individualized treatment planning process. (b) An individualized treatment plan, which includes problem formulation and articulation of short-term, measurable treatment goals and activities designed to achieve those goals. The plan is developed in collaboration with the resident and reflects the resident's personal goals.	**All Programs** In Level III.7 programs, the assessment and treatment plan review include: (a) A physical examination, performed by a physician within 24 hours of admission, or a review by a facility physician within 24 hours of admission of the record of a physical examination conducted no more than 7 days prior to admission. (b) A comprehensive nursing assessment, performed at the time of admission.

ASAM Patient Placement Criteria, Second Edition–Revised

Adult Criteria
Level III: Residential/Inpatient Treatment

CHARACTERISTIC	LEVEL III.1 Clinically Managed Low-Intensity Residential Treatment	LEVEL III.3 Clinically Managed Medium-Intensity Residential Treatment	LEVEL III.5 Clinically Managed High-Intensity Residential Treatment	LEVEL III.7 Medically Monitored Intensive Inpatient Treatment
ASSESSMENT/ TREATMENT PLAN REVIEW (continued)	(c) A biopsychosocial assessment, treatment plan and updates that reflect the resident's clinical progress.	(c) A biopsychosocial assessment, treatment plan and updates that reflect the resident's clinical progress, as reviewed by an inter-disciplinary treatment team.	(c) A biopsychosocial assessment, treatment plan and updates that reflect the resident's clinical progress, as reviewed by an inter-disciplinary treatment team.	(c) An individualized, comprehensive biopsychosocial assessment of the patient's substance dependence disorder and mental health problem(s), conducted or updated by staff who are knowledgeable about addiction treatment, to confirm the appropriateness of placement at Level III.7 and to guide the individualized treatment planning process.
	(d) A physical examination, performed within a reasonable time, as determined by the resident's medical condition.	(d) A physical examination, performed within a reasonable time, as determined by the resident's medical condition.	(d) A physical examination, performed within a reasonable time, as determined by the resident's medical condition.	(d) An individualized treatment plan, which includes problem formulation and articulation of short-term, measurable treatment goals and activities designed to achieve those goals. The plan is developed in collaboration with the patient and reflects the patient's personal goals.

Adult Criteria
Level III: Residential/Inpatient Treatment

CHARACTERISTIC	LEVEL III.1 Clinically Managed Low-Intensity Residential Treatment	LEVEL III.3 Clinically Managed Medium-Intensity Residential Treatment	LEVEL III.5 Clinically Managed High-Intensity Residential Treatment	LEVEL III.7 Medically Monitored Intensive Inpatient Treatment
ASSESSMENT/ TREATMENT PLAN REVIEW (continued)	(e) The treatment plan reflects case management conducted by on-site staff; coordination of related addiction treatment, health care, mental health, and social, vocational or housing services (provided concurrently); and the integration of services at this and other levels of care.	(e) The treatment plan reflects case management conducted by on-site staff; coordination of related addiction treatment, health care, mental health, and social, vocational or housing services (provided concurrently); and the integration of services at this and other levels of care.	(e) The treatment plan reflects case management conducted by on-site staff; coordination of related addiction treatment, health care, mental health, and social, vocational or housing services (provided concurrently); and the integration of services at this and other levels of care.	(e) A biopsychosocial assessment, treatment plan and updates that reflect the patient's clinical progress, as reviewed by an interdisciplinary treatment team. (f) The treatment plan reflects case management conducted by on-site staff; coordination of related addiction treatment, health care, mental health, and social, vocational or housing services (provided concurrently); and the integration of services at this and other levels of care.

Adult Criteria
Level III: Residential/Inpatient Treatment

CHARACTERISTIC	LEVEL III.1 Clinically Managed Low-Intensity Residential Treatment	LEVEL III.3 Clinically Managed Medium-Intensity Residential Treatment	LEVEL III.5 Clinically Managed High-Intensity Residential Treatment	LEVEL III.7 Medically Monitored Intensive Inpatient Treatment
ASSESSMENT/ TREATMENT PLAN REVIEW (continued)	**Dual Diagnosis Enhanced Programs** In addition to the assessment and treatment plan review activities described above, Level III.1 Dual Diagnosis Enhanced programs provide a review of the resident's recent psychiatric history and mental status examination. (If necessary, this review is conducted by a psychiatrist.) A comprehensive psychiatric history and examination and psychodiagnostic assessment are performed within a reasonable time, as determined by the resident's needs. Level III.1 Dual Diagnosis Enhanced programs (either directly or through affiliation with another program) also provide active reassessments of the patient's mental status, at a frequency determined by the urgency of the resident's psychiatric problems, and follow-	**Dual Diagnosis Enhanced Programs** In addition to the assessment and treatment plan review activities described above, Level III.3 Dual Diagnosis Enhanced programs provide a review of the resident's recent psychiatric history and mental status examination. (If necessary, this review is conducted by a psychiatrist.) A comprehensive psychiatric history and examination and psychodiagnostic assessment are performed within a reasonable time, as determined by the resident's needs. Level III.3 Dual Diagnosis Enhanced programs also provide active reassessments of the patient's mental status, at a frequency determined by the urgency of the resident's psychiatric problems, and follow-through with mental health treatment and psychotropic medications.	**Dual Diagnosis Enhanced Programs** In addition to the assessment and treatment plan review activities described above, Level III.5 Dual Diagnosis Enhanced programs provide a review of the resident's recent psychiatric history and mental status examination. (If necessary, this review is conducted by a psychiatrist.) A comprehensive psychiatric history and examination and psychodiagnostic assessment are performed within a reasonable time, as determined by the resident's needs. Level III.5 Dual Diagnosis Enhanced programs also provide active reassessments of the patient's mental status, at a frequency determined by the urgency of the resident's psychiatric problems, and follow-through with mental health treatment and psychotropic medications.	**Dual Diagnosis Enhanced Programs** In addition to the assessment and treatment plan review activities described above, Level III.7 Dual Diagnosis Enhanced programs provide a review of the patient's recent psychiatric history and mental status examination. (If necessary, this review is conducted by a psychiatrist.) A comprehensive psychiatric history and examination and psychodiagnostic assessment are performed within a reasonable time, as determined by the patient's needs. Level III.7 Dual Diagnosis Enhanced programs also provide active reassessments of the patient's mental status, at a frequency determined by the urgency of the patient's psychiatric problems, and follow-through with mental health treatment and psychotropic medications.

ASAM Patient Placement Criteria, Second Edition–Revised

Adult Criteria
Level III: Residential/Inpatient Treatment

CHARACTERISTIC	LEVEL III.1 Clinically Managed Low-Intensity Residential Treatment	LEVEL III.3 Clinically Managed Medium-Intensity Residential Treatment	LEVEL III.5 Clinically Managed High-Intensity Residential Treatment	LEVEL III.7 Medically Monitored Intensive Inpatient Treatment
ASSESSMENT/ TREATMENT PLAN REVIEW (continued)	through with mental health treatment and psychotropic medications.			In Level III.7 Dual Diagnosis Enhanced programs, a psychiatric assessment is performed within 24 hours of admission.
	NOTE: Certain residents may need the kinds of assessment and treatment services described here for Dual Diagnosis Enhanced, but at a reduced level of frequency and comprehensiveness to match the greater stability of the resident's mental health problems. For such residents, placement in a Dual Diagnosis Capable program may be appropriate.	NOTE: Certain residents may need the kinds of assessment and treatment services described here for Dual Diagnosis Enhanced, but at a reduced level of frequency and comprehensiveness to match the greater stability of the resident's mental health problems. For such residents, placement in a Dual Diagnosis Capable program may be appropriate.	NOTE: Certain residents may need the kinds of assessment and treatment services described here for Dual Diagnosis Enhanced, but at a reduced level of frequency and comprehensiveness to match the greater stability of the resident's mental health problems. For such residents, placement in a Dual Diagnosis Capable program may be appropriate.	NOTE: Certain patients may need the kinds of assessment and treatment services described here for Dual Diagnosis Enhanced, but at a reduced level of frequency and comprehensiveness to match the greater stability of the patient's mental health problems. For such patients, placement in a Dual Diagnosis Capable program may be appropriate.

ASAM Patient Placement Criteria, Second Edition–Revised

Adult Criteria
Level III: Residential/Inpatient Treatment

CHARACTERISTIC	LEVEL III.1 Clinically Managed Low-Intensity Residential Treatment	LEVEL III.3 Clinically Managed Medium-Intensity Residential Treatment	LEVEL III.5 Clinically Managed High-Intensity Residential Treatment	LEVEL III.7 Medically Monitored Intensive Inpatient Treatment
DOCUMENTATION	**All Programs** Documentation standards for Level III.1 programs include individualized progress notes in the resident's record that clearly reflect implementation of the treatment plan and the resident's response to therapeutic interventions for all disorders treated, as well as subsequent amendments to the plan. Treatment plan reviews are conducted at specified times and recorded in the treatment plan. **Dual Diagnosis Enhanced Programs** In addition to the information described above, Level III.1 Dual Diagnosis Enhanced programs document the resident's mental health problems, the relationship between the mental and substance dependence disorders, and the resident's current level of mental functioning.	**All Programs** Documentation standards for Level III.3 programs include individualized progress notes in the resident's record that clearly reflect implementation of the treatment plan and the resident's response to therapeutic interventions for all disorders treated, as well as subsequent amendments to the plan. Treatment plan reviews are conducted at specified times and recorded in the treatment plan. **Dual Diagnosis Enhanced Programs** In addition to the information described above, Level III.3 Dual Diagnosis Enhanced programs document the resident's mental health problems, the relationship between the mental and substance dependence disorders, and the resident's current level of mental functioning.	**All Programs** Documentation standards for Level III.5 programs include individualized progress notes in the resident's record that clearly reflect implementation of the treatment plan and the resident's response to therapeutic interventions for all disorders treated, as well as subsequent amendments to the plan. Treatment plan reviews are conducted at specified times and recorded in the treatment plan. **Dual Diagnosis Enhanced Programs** In addition to the information described above, Level III.5 Dual Diagnosis Enhanced programs document the resident's mental health problems, the relationship between the mental and substance dependence disorders, and the resident's current level of mental functioning.	**All Programs** Documentation standards for Level III.7 programs include individualized progress notes in the patient's record that clearly reflect implementation of the treatment plan and the patient's response to therapeutic interventions for all disorders treated, as well as subsequent amendments to the plan. Treatment plan reviews are conducted at specified times and recorded in the treatment plan. **Dual Diagnosis Enhanced Programs** In addition to the information described above, Level III.7 Dual Diagnosis Enhanced programs document the patient's mental health problems, the relationship between the mental and substance dependence disorders, and the patient's current level of mental functioning.

ASAM Patient Placement Criteria, Second Edition–Revised

Level III Admission Criteria
Diagnostic and Dimensional Criteria

CRITERIA	LEVEL III.1 Clinically Managed Low-Intensity Residential Treatment	LEVEL III.3 Clinically Managed Medium-Intensity Residential Treatment	LEVEL III.5 Clinically Managed High-Intensity Residential Treatment	LEVEL III.7 Medically Monitored Intensive Inpatient Treatment
DIAGNOSTIC ADMISSION CRITERIA	**All Programs** The resident who is appropriately placed in a Level III.1 program meets the diagnostic criteria for a Substance Dependence Disorder, as defined in the current *Diagnostic and Statistical Manual of Mental Disorders (DSM)* of the American Psychiatric Association or other standardized and widely accepted criteria, as well as the dimensional criteria for admission. If the resident's presenting history is inadequate to substantiate such a diagnosis, the probability of such a diagnosis may be determined from information submitted by collateral parties (such as family members, legal guardians and significant others).	**All Programs** The resident who is appropriately placed in a Level III.3 program meets the diagnostic criteria for a Substance Dependence Disorder, as defined in the current *Diagnostic and Statistical Manual of Mental Disorders (DSM)* of the American Psychiatric Association or other standardized and widely accepted criteria, as well as the dimensional criteria for admission. If the resident's presenting history is inadequate to substantiate such a diagnosis, the probability of such a diagnosis may be determined from information submitted by collateral parties (such as family members, legal guardians and significant others).	**All Programs** The resident who is appropriately placed in a Level III.5 program meets the diagnostic criteria for a Substance Dependence Disorder, as defined in the current *Diagnostic and Statistical Manual of Mental Disorders (DSM)* of the American Psychiatric Association or other standardized and widely accepted criteria, as well as the dimensional criteria for admission. If the resident's presenting history is inadequate to substantiate such a diagnosis, the probability of such a diagnosis may be determined from information submitted by collateral parties (such as family members, legal guardians and significant others).	**All Programs** The patient who is appropriately placed in a Level III.7 program meets the diagnostic criteria for a Substance Dependence Disorder, as defined in the current *Diagnostic and Statistical Manual of Mental Disorders (DSM)* of the American Psychiatric Association or other standardized and widely accepted criteria, as well as the dimensional criteria for admission. If the resident's presenting history is inadequate to substantiate such a diagnosis, the probability of such a diagnosis may be determined from information submitted by collateral parties (such as family members, legal guardians and significant others).

Level III Admission Criteria
Diagnostic and Dimensional Criteria

CRITERIA	LEVEL III.1 Clinically Managed Low-Intensity Residential Treatment	LEVEL III.3 Clinically Managed Medium-Intensity Residential Treatment	LEVEL III.5 Clinically Managed High-Intensity Residential Treatment	LEVEL III.7 Medically Monitored Intensive Inpatient Treatment
DIAGNOSTIC ADMISSION CRITERIA (continued)	NOTE: Residents in Level III.1 Dual Diagnosis Capable programs may have co-occurring Mental Disorders that meet the stability criteria for placement in a Dual Diagnosis Capable program; or difficulties with mood, behavior or cognition related to a substance use or mental disorder; or emotional, behavioral or cognitive symptoms that are troublesome but do not meet the *DSM* criteria for a mental disorder. **Dual Diagnosis Enhanced Programs** The resident who is appropriately admitted to a Level III.1 Dual Diagnosis Enhanced program meets the diagnostic criteria for a Mental Disorder as well as a Substance Dependence Disorder, as defined in the current *Diagnostic and Statistical Manual of Mental Disorders (DSM)* of the American Psychiatric Association or other	NOTE: Residents in Level III.3 Dual Diagnosis Capable programs may have co-occurring Mental Disorders that meet the stability criteria for placement in a Dual Diagnosis Capable program; or difficulties with mood, behavior or cognition related to a substance use or mental disorder; or emotional, behavioral or cognitive symptoms that are troublesome but do not meet the *DSM* criteria for a mental disorder. **Dual Diagnosis Enhanced Programs** The resident who is appropriately admitted to a Level III.3 Dual Diagnosis Enhanced program meets the diagnostic criteria for a Mental Disorder as well as a Substance Dependence Disorder, as defined in the current *Diagnostic and Statistical Manual of Mental Disorders (DSM)* of the American Psychiatric Association or other	NOTE: Residents in Level III.5 Dual Diagnosis Capable programs may have co-occurring Mental Disorders that meet the stability criteria for placement in a Dual Diagnosis Capable program; or difficulties with mood, behavior or cognition related to a substance use or mental disorder; or emotional, behavioral or cognitive symptoms that are troublesome but do not meet the *DSM* criteria for a mental disorder. **Dual Diagnosis Enhanced Programs** The resident who is appropriately admitted to a Level III.5 Dual Diagnosis Enhanced program meets the diagnostic criteria for a Mental Disorder as well as a Substance Dependence Disorder, as defined in the current *Diagnostic and Statistical Manual of Mental Disorders (DSM)* of the American Psychiatric Association or other	NOTE: Patients in Level III.7 Dual Diagnosis Capable programs may have co-occurring Mental Disorders that meet the stability criteria for placement in a Dual Diagnosis Capable program; or difficulties with mood, behavior or cognition related to a substance use or mental disorder; or emotional, behavioral or cognitive symptoms that are troublesome but do not meet the *DSM* criteria for a mental disorder. **Dual Diagnosis Enhanced Programs** The patient who is appropriately admitted to a Level III.7 Dual Diagnosis Enhanced program meets the diagnostic criteria for a Mental Disorder as well as a Substance Dependence Disorder, as defined in the current *Diagnostic and Statistical Manual of Mental Disorders (DSM)* of the American Psychiatric Association or other

ASAM Patient Placement Criteria, Second Edition–Revised

Level III Admission Criteria
Diagnostic and Dimensional Criteria

CRITERIA	LEVEL III.1 Clinically Managed Low-Intensity Residential Treatment	LEVEL III.3 Clinically Managed Medium-Intensity Residential Treatment	LEVEL III.5 Clinically Managed High-Intensity Residential Treatment	LEVEL III.7 Medically Monitored Intensive Inpatient Treatment
DIAGNOSTIC ADMISSION CRITERIA (continued)	standardized and widely accepted criteria, as well as the dimensional criteria for admission. If the resident's presenting history is inadequate to substantiate such a diagnosis, the probability of such a diagnosis may be determined from information submitted by collateral parties (such as family members, legal guardians and significant others).	standardized and widely accepted criteria, as well as the dimensional criteria for admission. If the resident's presenting history is inadequate to substantiate such a diagnosis, the probability of such a diagnosis may be determined from information submitted by collateral parties (such as family members, legal guardians and significant others).	standardized and widely accepted criteria, as well as the dimensional criteria for admission. If the resident's presenting history is inadequate to substantiate such a diagnosis, the probability of such a diagnosis may be determined from information submitted by collateral parties (such as family members, legal guardians and significant others).	standardized and widely accepted criteria, as well as the dimensional criteria for admission. If the resident's presenting history is inadequate to substantiate such a diagnosis, the probability of such a diagnosis may be determined from information submitted by collateral parties (such as family members, legal guardians and significant others).

Level III Admission Criteria
Diagnostic and Dimensional Criteria

CRITERIA	LEVEL III.1 Clinically Managed Low-Intensity Residential Treatment	LEVEL III.3 Clinically Managed Medium-Intensity Residential Treatment	LEVEL III.5 Clinically Managed High-Intensity Residential Treatment	LEVEL III.7 Medically Monitored Intensive Inpatient Treatment
DIMENSIONAL ADMISSION CRITERIA	**All Programs** The resident who is appropriately admitted to a Level III.1 program meets specifications in each of the six dimensions.	**All Programs** The resident who is appropriately admitted to a Level III.3 program meets specifications in each of the six dimensions.	**All Programs** The resident who is appropriately admitted to a Level III.5 program meets specifications in each of the six dimensions.	**All Programs** The patient who is appropriately admitted to a Level III.7 program meets specifications in *two* of the six dimensions, at least *one* of which is in Dimension 1, 2 or 3.
DIMENSION 1: Acute Intoxication and/or Withdrawal	**All Programs** The resident has no signs or symptoms of withdrawal, or his or her withdrawal needs can be safely managed in a Level III.1 setting (see the separate Dimension 1 criteria).	**All Programs** The resident has no signs or symptoms of withdrawal, or his or her withdrawal needs can be safely managed in a Level III.3 setting (see the separate Dimension 1 criteria).	**All Programs** The resident has no signs or symptoms of withdrawal, or his or her withdrawal needs can be safely managed in a Level III.5 setting (see the separate Dimension 1 criteria).

NOTE: A resident who is being transferred from a Level III.7 program should not require medically managed or monitored detoxification services. | **All Programs** See the separate Dimension 1 criteria. |

Level III Admission Criteria
Diagnostic and Dimensional Criteria

CRITERIA	LEVEL III.1 Clinically Managed Low-Intensity Residential Treatment	LEVEL III.3 Clinically Managed Medium-Intensity Residential Treatment	LEVEL III.5 Clinically Managed High-Intensity Residential Treatment	LEVEL III.7 Medically Monitored Intensive Inpatient Treatment
DIMENSION 2: Biomedical Conditions and Complications	**All Programs** The resident's status in Dimension 2 is characterized by *one* of the following: (a) Biomedical problems, if any, are stable and do not require medical or nurse monitoring, and the resident is capable of self-administering any prescribed medications; *or* (b) A current biomedical condition is not severe enough to warrant inpatient treatment but is sufficient to distract from treatment or recovery efforts. The problem requires medical monitoring, which can be provided by the program or through an established arrangement with another provider.	**All Programs** The resident's status in Dimension 2 is characterized by *one* of the following: (a) Biomedical problems, if any, are stable and do not require medical or nurse monitoring, and the resident is capable of self-administering any prescribed medications; *or* (b) A current biomedical condition is not severe enough to warrant inpatient treatment but is sufficient to distract from treatment or recovery efforts. The problem requires medical monitoring, which can be provided by the program or through an established arrangement with another provider.	**All Programs** The resident's status in Dimension 2 is characterized by *one* of the following: (a) Biomedical problems, if any, are stable and do not require 24-hour medical or nurse monitoring, and the resident is capable of self-administering any prescribed medications; *or* (b) A current biomedical condition is not severe enough to warrant inpatient treatment but is sufficient to distract from treatment or recovery efforts. The problem requires medical monitoring, which can be provided by the program or through an established arrangement with another provider.	**All Programs** The patient's status in Dimension 2 is characterized by *one* of the following: (a) The interaction of the patient's biomedical condition and continued alcohol or other drug use places the patient in imminent danger of serious damage to physical health or concomitant biomedical conditions (such as pregnancy with vaginal bleeding or ruptured membranes); *or* (b) A current biomedical condition requires 24-hour nursing and medical monitoring or active treatment, but not the full resources of an acute care hospital.

Level III Admission Criteria
Diagnostic and Dimensional Criteria

CRITERIA	LEVEL III.1 Clinically Managed Low-Intensity Residential Treatment	LEVEL III.3 Clinically Managed Medium-Intensity Residential Treatment	LEVEL III.5 Clinically Managed High-Intensity Residential Treatment	LEVEL III.7 Medically Monitored Intensive Inpatient Treatment
DIMENSION 2: Biomedical Conditions and Complications (continued)	**Biomedical Enhanced Services** The resident who has a biomedical problem that requires a degree of staff attention (such as monitoring of medications or assistance with mobility) that is not available in other Level III.1 programs is in need of Biomedical Enhanced services.	**Biomedical Enhanced Services** The resident who has a biomedical problem that requires a degree of staff attention (such as monitoring of medications or assistance with mobility) that is not available in other Level III.3 programs is in need of Biomedical Enhanced services.	**Biomedical Enhanced Services** The resident who has a biomedical problem that requires a degree of staff attention (such as monitoring of medications or assistance with mobility) that is not available in other Level III.5 programs is in need of Biomedical Enhanced services.	**Biomedical Enhanced Services** The patient who has a biomedical problem that requires a degree of staff attention (such as monitoring of medications or assistance with mobility) that is not available in other Level III.7 programs is in need of Biomedical Enhanced services.
DIMENSION 3: Emotional, Behavioral or Cognitive Conditions and Complications	**All Programs** The resident may not have any significant problems in this dimension. However, if any of the Dimension 3 conditions are present, the resident must be admitted to a Dual Diagnosis Capable or Dual Diagnosis Enhanced program (depending on his or her level of function, stability and degree of impairment). **Dual Diagnosis Capable Programs** The resident's status in Dimension 3 is characterized by (a) *or* (b) *or* (c) *or* (d) *and* (e):	**All Programs** If any of the Dimension 3 conditions are present, the resident must be admitted to a Dual Diagnosis Capable or Dual Diagnosis Enhanced program (depending on his or her level of function, stability and degree of impairment). **Dual Diagnosis Capable Programs** The resident's status in Dimension 3 is characterized by (a) *or* (b) *or* (c) *and* (d):	**All Programs** If any of the Dimension 3 conditions are present, the resident must be admitted to a Dual Diagnosis Capable or Dual Diagnosis Enhanced program (depending on his or her level of function, stability and degree of impairment). **Dual Diagnosis Capable Programs** The resident's status in Dimension 3 is characterized by (a) *or* (b) *or* (c) *or* (d) *or* (e) *and* (f):	**All Programs** Problems in Dimension 3 are not necessary for admission to a Level III.7 program. However, if any of the Dimension 3 conditions are present, the patient must be admitted to a Dual Diagnosis Capable or Dual Diagnosis Enhanced program (depending on his or her level of function, stability and degree of impairment). **Dual Diagnosis Capable Programs** The patient's status in Dimension 3 is characterized by *one* of the following:

ASAM Patient Placement Criteria, Second Edition–Revised

Level III Admission Criteria
Diagnostic and Dimensional Criteria

CRITERIA	LEVEL III.1 Clinically Managed Low-Intensity Residential Treatment	LEVEL III.3 Clinically Managed Medium-Intensity Residential Treatment	LEVEL III.5 Clinically Managed High-Intensity Residential Treatment	LEVEL III.7 Medically Monitored Intensive Inpatient Treatment
DIMENSION 3: Emotional, Behavioral or Cognitive Conditions and Complications (continued)	(a) The resident's psychiatric condition is stable, and he or she is assessed as having minimal problems in this area, as evidenced by *both* of the following: [1] the resident's thought disorder, anxiety, guilt and/or depression may be related to substance use problems or to a stable co-occurring emotional, behavioral or cognitive condition, with imminent likelihood of relapse with dangerous consequences outside of a structured environment; *and* [2] the resident is assessed as not posing a risk to self or others; *or*	(a) The resident's psychiatric condition is stabilizing, but he or she is assessed as in need of a 24-hour structured environment, as evidenced by *one* of the following: [1] depression or other emotional, behavioral or cognitive conditions significantly interfere with activities of daily living and recovery; *or* [2] the resident exhibits violent or disruptive behavior when intoxicated and is assessed as posing a danger to self or others; *or* [3] the resident exhibits stress behaviors related to recent or threatened losses in work, family or social arenas, such that activities of daily living are significantly impaired and the resident requires a secure environment to focus on the substance dependence or mental health problem; *or* [4] concomitant personality disorders are of such severity that the accompanying dysfunctional behaviors require continuing structured interventions; *or*	(a) The resident's psychiatric condition is stabilizing. However, despite his or her best efforts, the resident is unable to control his or her use of alcohol or other drugs and/or antisocial behaviors, with attendant probability of harm to self or others. The resulting level of dysfunction is so severe that it precludes the resident's participation in a less structured and intensive level of care; *or*	(a) The patient's psychiatric condition is unstable. Depression and/or other emotional, behavioral or cognitive symptoms (which may include compulsive behaviors, suicidal or homicidal ideation with a recent history of attempts but no specific plan, or hallucinations and delusions without acute risk to self or others) are interfering with abstinence, recovery and stability to such a degree that the patient needs a structured 24-hour, medically monitored (but not medically managed) environment to address recovery efforts; *or*

Level III Admission Criteria
Diagnostic and Dimensional Criteria

CRITERIA	LEVEL III.1 Clinically Managed Low-Intensity Residential Treatment	LEVEL III.3 Clinically Managed Medium-Intensity Residential Treatment	LEVEL III.5 Clinically Managed High-Intensity Residential Treatment	LEVEL III.7 Medically Monitored Intensive Inpatient Treatment
DIMENSION 3: Emotional, Behavioral or Cognitive Conditions and Complications (continued)	(b) The resident's symptoms and functional deficits, when considered in the context of his or her home environment, are sufficiently severe that he or she is assessed as not likely to maintain mental stability and/or abstinence if treatment is provided in a non-residential setting. Functional deficits may include—but are not limited to—residual psychiatric symptoms, chronic addictive disorder, history of criminality, marginal intellectual ability, limited educational achievement, poor vocational skills, inadequate anger management skills, and the sequelae of physical, sexual or emotional trauma. These deficits may be complicated by problems in Dimensions 2 through 6; *or*	(b) The resident's symptoms and functional deficits, when considered in the context of his or her home environment, are assessed as sufficiently severe that the resident is not likely to maintain mental stability and/or abstinence if treatment is provided in a non-residential setting. Functional deficits may include—but are not limited to—cognitive impairment, developmental disability, manifest chronicity and intensity of the primary addictive disease process, residual psychiatric symptoms, cognitive deficits resulting from traumatic brain injury, limited educational achievement, poor vocational skills, inadequate anger management skills, and other equivalent indications that services need to be presented at a pace that is slower and/or more repetitive and	(b) The resident demonstrates repeated inability to control his or her impulses to use alcohol or other drugs and/or to engage in antisocial behavior, and is in imminent danger of relapse, with attendant likelihood of harm to self, others or property. The resulting level of dysfunction is of such severity that it precludes participation in treatment in the absence of the 24-hour support and structure of a Level III.5 program; *or*	(b) The patient exhibits stress behaviors associated with recent or threatened losses in work, family or social domains, to a degree that his or her ability to manage the activities of daily living are significantly impaired. The patient thus requires a secure, medically monitored environment in which to address self-care problems (such as those associated with eating, weight loss, sleeplessness or personal hygiene) and to focus on his or her substance abuse or mental health problems; *or*

Level III Admission Criteria
Diagnostic and Dimensional Criteria

CRITERIA	LEVEL III.1 Clinically Managed Low-Intensity Residential Treatment	LEVEL III.3 Clinically Managed Medium-Intensity Residential Treatment	LEVEL III.5 Clinically Managed High-Intensity Residential Treatment	LEVEL III.7 Medically Monitored Intensive Inpatient Treatment
DIMENSION 3: Emotional, Behavioral or Cognitive Conditions and Complications (continued)		concrete than is found at other levels of care. These deficits may be complicated by problems in Dimensions 2 through 6; *or*		
	(c) The resident demonstrates (through distractibility, negative emotions, or generalized anxiety) an inability to maintain stable behavior over a 24-hour period without the structure and support of a 24-setting; *or*	(c) The resident is at mild risk of behaviors endangering self, others or property, and is in imminent danger of relapse (with dangerous emotional, behavioral or cognitive consequences) without the 24-hour support and structure of a Level III.3 program; *and*	(c) The resident demonstrates antisocial behavior patterns (as evidenced by criminal activity) that have led or could lead to significant criminal justice problems, lack of concern for others and extreme lack of regard for authority (expressed through distrust, conflict or opposition), and which precludes participation in a less structured and intensive level of care; *or*	(c) The patient has significant functional deficits that require active psychiatric monitoring. They may include—but are not limited to—problems with activities of daily living, problems with self-care, lethality or dangerousness, and problems with social functioning. These deficits may be complicated by problems in Dimensions 2 through 6; *or*

Level III Admission Criteria
Diagnostic and Dimensional Criteria

CRITERIA	LEVEL III.1 Clinically Managed Low-Intensity Residential Treatment	LEVEL III.3 Clinically Managed Medium-Intensity Residential Treatment	LEVEL III.5 Clinically Managed High-Intensity Residential Treatment	LEVEL III.7 Medically Monitored Intensive Inpatient Treatment
DIMENSION 3: Emotional, Behavioral or Cognitive Conditions and Complications (continued)	(d) The resident's co-occurring psychiatric, emotional, behavioral or cognitive conditions are being addressed concurrently through appropriate psychiatric services; *and*	(d) The resident's mental status (including emotional stability and cognitive functioning) is assessed as sufficiently stable to permit the resident to participate in the therapeutic interventions provided at this level of care and to benefit from treatment.	(d) The resident has significant functional deficits, which are likely to respond to staff interventions. These symptoms and deficits, when considered in the context of his or her home environment, are sufficiently severe that the resident is not likely to maintain mental stability and/or abstinence if treatment is provided in a non-residential setting. The functional deficits are of a pervasive nature, requiring treatment that is primarily habilitative in focus; they do not require medical monitoring or management. They may include—but are not limited to—residual psychiatric symptoms, chronic addictive disorder, history of criminality, marginal intellectual ability, limited educational achievement, poor vocational skills, inadequate anger management skills, poor impulse control, and the sequelae of physical, sexual or	(d) The patient is at moderate risk of behaviors endangering self, others or property, and is in imminent danger of relapse (with dangerous emotional, behavioral or cognitive consequences) without the 24-hour support and structure of a Level III.7 program; *or*

ASAM Patient Placement Criteria, Second Edition–Revised

Level III Admission Criteria
Diagnostic and Dimensional Criteria

CRITERIA	LEVEL III.1 Clinically Managed Low-Intensity Residential Treatment	LEVEL III.3 Clinically Managed Medium-Intensity Residential Treatment	LEVEL III.5 Clinically Managed High-Intensity Residential Treatment	LEVEL III.7 Medically Monitored Intensive Inpatient Treatment
DIMENSION 3: Emotional, Behavioral or Cognitive Conditions and Complications (continued)	(e) The resident's mental status (including emotional stability and cognitive functioning) is assessed as sufficiently stable to allow the resident to participate in the therapeutic interventions provided at this level of care and to benefit from treatment.		emotional trauma. These deficits may be complicated by problems in Dimensions 2 through 6; *or* (e) The resident's concomitant personality disorders (e.g., antisocial personality disorder with verbal aggressive behavior requiring consistent limit-setting) are of such severity that the accompanying dysfunctional behaviors require continuous boundary-setting interventions; *and* (f) The resident's mental status (including emotional stability and cognitive functioning) is assessed as sufficiently stable to permit the resident to participate in the therapeutic interventions provided at this level of care and to benefit from treatment.	(e) The patient is actively intoxicated, with resulting violent or disruptive behavior that poses imminent danger to self or others; *or* (f) The patient has a thought disorder or cognitive limitations that require stabilization but not medical management.

Level III Admission Criteria
Diagnostic and Dimensional Criteria

CRITERIA	LEVEL III.1 Clinically Managed Low-Intensity Residential Treatment	LEVEL III.3 Clinically Managed Medium-Intensity Residential Treatment	LEVEL III.5 Clinically Managed High-Intensity Residential Treatment	LEVEL III.7 Medically Monitored Intensive Inpatient Treatment
DIMENSION 3: Emotional, Behavioral or Cognitive Conditions and Complications (continued)	**Dual Diagnosis Enhanced Programs** The resident's status in Dimension 3 is characterized by (a) *or* (b) *and* (c): (a) The resident has a diagnosed emotional, behavioral or cognitive disorder that requires monitoring of medications or assessment of psychiatric symptoms or behavioral management techniques, because the resident's history suggests that these disorders are likely to distract him or her from treatment efforts; *or*	**Dual Diagnosis Enhanced Programs** The resident's status in Dimension 3 is characterized by (a) *or* (b): (a) The resident has a diagnosed emotional, behavioral or cognitive disorder that requires active management (involving monitoring of medications or assessment of psychiatric symptoms or behavioral management techniques, for example). Such disorders complicate treatment of the resident's Substance Dependence or Substance-Induced disorder and require differential diagnosis. The resident thus is in need of stabilization of psychiatric symptoms concurrent with addiction treatment (examples include a patient with unstable borderline or compulsive personality disorder, unstable anxiety or mood disorder, in addition to his or her Substance Dependence or Substance-Induced disorder).	**Dual Diagnosis Enhanced Programs** The resident's status in Dimension 3 is characterized by a range of psychiatric symptoms that require active monitoring, such as poor anger management. These are assessed as posing a risk of harm to self or others if the resident is not contained in a 24-hour structured environment. Although such residents do not require specialized psychiatric nursing and close observation, they do need monitoring and interventions by mental health staff to limit and de-escalate their behaviors. A 24-hour milieu is sufficient to contain such impulses in most cases, but enhanced staff and therapeutic interventions are required to manage unpredictable losses of impulse control.	**Dual Diagnosis Enhanced Programs** The patient's status in Dimension 3 is characterized by *one* of the following: (a) The patient has a history of moderate psychiatric decompensation (involving paranoia, moderate psychotic symptoms or severe, non-suicidal depression) on discontinuation of drugs of abuse, and such decompensation is present; *or*

Level III Admission Criteria
Diagnostic and Dimensional Criteria

CRITERIA	LEVEL III.1 Clinically Managed Low-Intensity Residential Treatment	LEVEL III.3 Clinically Managed Medium-Intensity Residential Treatment	LEVEL III.5 Clinically Managed High-Intensity Residential Treatment	LEVEL III.7 Medically Monitored Intensive Inpatient Treatment
DIMENSION 3: Emotional, Behavioral or Cognitive Conditions and Complications (continued)		Because cognitive deficits are commonly seen in residents treated at Level III.3, such residents may require treatment that is delivered at a slower pace or in a more concrete or repetitive fashion; *or*	The treatment regimen should avoid highly confrontational strategies that are intended to induce submissive behavior or strong affect.	
	(b) The resident needs monitoring of psychiatric symptoms concurrent with addiction treatment (as may occur in a patient with borderline or compulsive personality disorder, anxiety or mood disorder, or persistent schizophrenic disorder in addition to a stabilizing Substance Dependence or Substance-Induced Disorder); *and*	(b) The resident is assessed as at mild to moderate risk of behaviors endangering self, others or property (for example, he or she has suicidal or homicidal thoughts, but lacks an active plan).		(b) The patient is assessed as at moderate to high risk of behaviors endangering self, others or property, and is in imminent danger of relapse (with dangerous emotional, behavioral or cognitive consequences) without 24-hour structure and support and medically monitored treatment. For example, without medically monitored inpatient treatment, the patient does not have sufficient coping skills to avoid harm to self, others or property because of co-occurring mania; *or*

Level III Admission Criteria
Diagnostic and Dimensional Criteria

CRITERIA	LEVEL III.1 Clinically Managed Low-Intensity Residential Treatment	LEVEL III.3 Clinically Managed Medium-Intensity Residential Treatment	LEVEL III.5 Clinically Managed High-Intensity Residential Treatment	LEVEL III.7 Medically Monitored Intensive Inpatient Treatment
DIMENSION 3: Emotional, Behavioral or Cognitive Conditions and Complications (continued)	(c) The resident is assessed as able to safely access the community for work, education and other community resources. NOTE: Such a resident may be receiving specific dual diagnosis services in a Level II.1 or II.5 program, or be receiving Level I outpatient services with intensive case management.	NOTE: The resident who has a severe and persistent mental disorder may manifest inadequate skills to manage the activities of daily living, poor social functioning, disorganized thinking, and/or periods of confusion, disorientation, or impaired reality testing. The resident's dysfunction is so severe that 24-hour structure is required to provide sufficient stabilization so that the resident can safely survive at a less intensive level of care.		(c) The patient is severely depressed, with suicidal impulses and a plan. However, he or she is able to contract to reach out for help as needed and does not require a one-on-one suicide watch; *or* (d) The patient has a co-occurring psychiatric disorder (such as anxiety, distractibility or depression) that is interfering with his or her addiction treatment and thus requires stabilization with psychotropic medications; *or* (e) The patient has a co-occurring psychiatric disorder of moderate to high severity that is marginally and tenuously stable and which requires care to prevent exacerbation.

Level III Admission Criteria
Diagnostic and Dimensional Criteria

CRITERIA	LEVEL III.1 Clinically Managed Low-Intensity Residential Treatment	LEVEL III.3 Clinically Managed Medium-Intensity Residential Treatment	LEVEL III.5 Clinically Managed High-Intensity Residential Treatment	LEVEL III.7 Medically Monitored Intensive Inpatient Treatment
DIMENSION 3: Emotional, Behavioral or Cognitive Conditions and Complications (continued)		During the stabilization period, expectations for the resident's involvement in group, community and activities therapy are limited. A more highly individualized regimen of individual, group and activities involvement may be required.		The patient thus requires the type of close management available only in an addiction treatment program with integrated mental health services, or in a mental health program with integrated addiction treatment services.
DIMENSION 4: Readiness to Change	**All Programs** The resident's status in Dimension 4 is characterized by *one* of the following: (a) The resident acknowledges the existence of a psychiatric condition and/or substance use problem. He or she recognizes specific negative consequences and dysfunctional behaviors and their effect on his or her desire to change. He or she is sufficiently ready to change and cooperative enough to respond to treatment at Level III.1 ; *or*	**All Programs** The resident's status in Dimension 4 is characterized by *one* of the following: (a) Because of the intensity and chronicity of the addictive disorder or the resident's cognitive limitations, he or she has little awareness of the need for continuing care or the existence of his or her substance use or mental health problem and need for treatment, and thus has limited readiness to change; *or*	**All Programs** The resident's status in Dimension 4 is characterized by *one* of the following: (a) Because of the intensity and chronicity of the addictive disorder or the resident's mental health problems, he or she has little awareness of the need for continuing care or the existence of his or her substance use or mental health problem and need for treatment, and thus has limited readiness to change; *or*	**All Programs** The patient's status in Dimension 4 is characterized by *one* of the following: (a) Despite experiencing serious consequences or effects of the addictive disorder or mental health problem, the patient does not accept or relate the addictive disorder to the severity of these problems; *or*

Level III Admission Criteria
Diagnostic and Dimensional Criteria

CRITERIA	LEVEL III.1 Clinically Managed Low-Intensity Residential Treatment	LEVEL III.3 Clinically Managed Medium-Intensity Residential Treatment	LEVEL III.5 Clinically Managed High-Intensity Residential Treatment	LEVEL III.7 Medically Monitored Intensive Inpatient Treatment
DIMENSION 4: Readiness to Change (continued)	(b) The resident is assessed as appropriately placed at Level I or II and is receiving Level III.1 services concurrently. The resident may be at an early stage of readiness to change and thus in need of engagement and motivational strategies; *or*	(b) Despite experiencing serious consequences or effects of the addictive disorder or mental health problem, the resident has marked difficulty in understanding the relationship between his or her substance use, addiction, mental health or life problems, and impaired coping skills and level of functioning; *or*	(b) Despite experiencing serious consequences or effects of the addictive disorder or mental health problem, the resident has marked difficulty in understanding the relationship between his or her substance use, addiction, mental health or life problems and his or her impaired coping skills and level of functioning, often blaming others for his or her substance dependence problems; *or*	(b) The patient is in need of intensive motivating strategies, activities and processes available only in a 24-hour structured, medically monitored setting; *or*
	(c) The resident requires a 24-hour structured milieu to promote treatment progress and recovery, because motivating interventions have failed in the past and are assessed as not likely to succeed in the future in an outpatient setting; *or*	(c) The resident's continued substance use poses a danger of harm to self or others, and he or she demonstrates no awareness of the need to address the severity of his or her addiction or psychiatric problem or does not recognize the need for treatment. However, assessment indicates that treatment interventions available at Level III.3 may increase the resident's degree of readiness to change; *or*	(c) The resident demonstrates passive or active opposition to addressing the severity of his or her mental or addiction problem, or does not recognize the need for treatment. Such continued substance use or inability to follow through with mental health treatment poses a danger of harm to self or others. However, assessment indicates that treatment interventions available at Level III.5 may increase the resident's degree of readiness to change; *or*	(c) The patient needs ongoing 24-hour psychiatric monitoring to assure follow-through with the treatment regimen and to deal with issues such as ambivalence about compliance with psychiatric medications.

ASAM Patient Placement Criteria, Second Edition–Revised

Level III Admission Criteria
Diagnostic and Dimensional Criteria

CRITERIA	LEVEL III.1 Clinically Managed Low-Intensity Residential Treatment	LEVEL III.3 Clinically Managed Medium-Intensity Residential Treatment	LEVEL III.5 Clinically Managed High-Intensity Residential Treatment	LEVEL III.7 Medically Monitored Intensive Inpatient Treatment
DIMENSION 4: Readiness to Change (continued)	(d) The resident's perspective impairs his or her ability to make behavior changes without the support of a structured environment. For example, the resident attributes his or her alcohol, drug or mental health problem to other persons or external events, rather than to a substance dependence or mental disorder. Interventions are assessed as not likely to succeed in an outpatient setting.	(d) The resident's perspective impairs his or her ability to make behavior changes without repeated, structured, clinically directed motivational interventions, delivered in a 24-hour milieu. For example, because of cognitive deficits, the resident attributes his or her alcohol, drug or mental health problem to other persons or external events, rather than to a substance dependence or mental disorder. Interventions are assessed as not feasible or likely to succeed in an outpatient setting.	(d) The resident requires structured therapy and a 24-hour programmatic milieu to promote treatment progress and recovery, because motivational interventions have failed at less intensive levels of care and are assessed as not likely to succeed in the future at a less intensive level of care; *or* (e) The resident's perspective impairs his or her ability to make behavior changes without repeated, structured, clinically directed motivational interventions, delivered in a 24-hour milieu. For example, the resident attributes his or her alcohol, drug or mental health problem to other persons or external events, rather than to a substance dependence or mental disorder. Interventions are adjudged as not feasible or likely to succeed at a less intensive level of care.	

Level III Admission Criteria
Diagnostic and Dimensional Criteria

CRITERIA	LEVEL III.1 Clinically Managed Low-Intensity Residential Treatment	LEVEL III.3 Clinically Managed Medium-Intensity Residential Treatment	LEVEL III.5 Clinically Managed High-Intensity Residential Treatment	LEVEL III.7 Medically Monitored Intensive Inpatient Treatment
DIMENSION 4: Readiness to Change (continued)	Dual Diagnosis Enhanced Programs The resident's status in Dimension 4 is characterized by ambivalence in his or her commitment to change a co-occurring mental health problem.	Dual Diagnosis Enhanced Programs The resident's status in Dimension 4 is characterized by ambivalence in his or her commitment to change and reluctance to engage in activities necessary to address a co-occurring mental health problem. For example, such a resident does not understand the need for antipsychotic medications, so that his or her compliance with the medication regimen is inconsistent.	Dual Diagnosis Enhanced Programs The resident's status in Dimension 4 is characterized by a lack of commitment to change and reluctance to engage in activities necessary to address a co-occurring mental health problem. For example, the resident does not understand the need for antidepressant or antimania medications and so refuses to comply with the medication regimen.	Dual Diagnosis Enhanced Programs The patient's status in Dimension 4 is characterized by a lack of commitment to change and refusal to engage in activities necessary to address a co-occurring mental health problem. For example, the patient with bipolar affective disorder desires his or her manic states and thus refuses to comply with a regimen of mood-stabilizing medications.
	Similarly, the resident who is not consistently able to follow through with treatment, or who demonstrates minimal awareness of a problem, or who is unaware of the need to change requires active interventions with family, significant others and other external systems to create leverage and align incentives so as to promote engage-ment in treatment is appropriately placed in a Level III.1 Dual Diagnosis Enhanced program.	Similarly, the resident who is not consistently able to follow through with treatment, or who demonstrates minimal awareness of a problem, or who is unaware of the need to change, requires active interventions with family, significant others and other external systems to create leverage and align incentives so as to promote engage-ment in treatment is appropriately placed in a Level III.3 Dual Diagnosis Enhanced program.	Similarly, the resident who is not consistently able to follow through with treatment, or who demonstrates minimal awareness of a problem, or who is unaware of the need to change, requires active interventions with family, significant others and other external systems to create leverage and align incentives so as to promote engage-ment in treatment is appropriately placed in a Level III.5 Dual Diagnosis Enhanced program.	Similarly, the patient who is not consistently able to follow through with treatment, or who demonstrates minimal awareness of a problem, or who is unaware of the need to change, requires active interventions with family, significant others and other external systems to create leverage and align incentives so as to promote engage-ment in treatment is appropriately placed in a Level III.7 Dual Diagnosis Enhanced program.

Level III Admission Criteria
Diagnostic and Dimensional Criteria

CRITERIA	LEVEL III.1 Clinically Managed Low-Intensity Residential Treatment	LEVEL III.3 Clinically Managed Medium-Intensity Residential Treatment	LEVEL III.5 Clinically Managed High-Intensity Residential Treatment	LEVEL III.7 Medically Monitored Intensive Inpatient Treatment
DIMENSION 5: Relapse, Continued Use or Continued Problem Potential	**All Programs** The resident's status in Dimension 5 is characterized by *one* of the following: (a) The resident demonstrates limited coping skills to address relapse triggers and urges and/or deteriorating mental functioning. He or she thus is in imminent danger of relapse, with dangerous emotional, behavioral or cognitive consequences, and needs 24-hour structure to help him or her apply recovery and coping skills; *or*	**All Programs** The resident's status in Dimension 5 is characterized by *one* of the following: (a) The resident does not recognize relapse triggers and has little awareness of the need for continuing care. Because of the intensity or chronicity of the resident's addictive disorder or the chronicity of the mental health problem or cognitive limitations, he or she is in imminent danger of continued substance use or mental health problems, with dangerous emotional, behavioral or cognitive consequences. The resident thus needs 24-hour monitoring and structure to assist in the application of recovery and coping skills, as well as active staff interventions to prevent relapse; *or*	**All Programs** The resident's status in Dimension 5 is characterized by *one* of the following: (a) The resident does not recognize relapse triggers and is not committed to continuing care. His or her continued substance use poses an imminent danger of harm to self or others in the absence of 24-hour monitoring and structured support; *or*	**All Programs** The patient's status in Dimension 5 is characterized by *one* of the following: (a) The patient is experiencing an acute psychiatric or substance use crisis, marked by intensification of symptoms of his or her addictive or mental disorder (such as difficulty postponing immediate gratification, drug-seeking behavior, or increasing severity of anxiety or depressive symptoms). This situation poses an imminent danger of harm to self or others in the absence of 24-hour monitoring and structured support; *or*

Level III Admission Criteria
Diagnostic and Dimensional Criteria

CRITERIA	LEVEL III.1 Clinically Managed Low-Intensity Residential Treatment	LEVEL III.3 Clinically Managed Medium-Intensity Residential Treatment	LEVEL III.5 Clinically Managed High-Intensity Residential Treatment	LEVEL III.7 Medically Monitored Intensive Inpatient Treatment
DIMENSION 5: Relapse, Continued Use or Continued Problem Potential (continued)	(b) The resident understands his or her substance dependence and/or mental disorder but is at risk of relapse in a less structured level of care because he or she is unable to consistently address either or both; *or*	(b) The resident is experiencing an intensification of symptoms of his or her substance dependence disorder (such as difficulty in postponing immediate gratification and related drug-seeking behavior) or mental disorder (for example, increasing suicidal thoughts or impulses without a plan), and his or her level of functioning is deteriorating despite amendment of the treatment plan; *or*	(b) The resident's psychiatric condition is stabilizing. However, despite his or her best efforts, the resident is unable to control his or her use of alcohol or other drugs and/or antisocial behaviors, with attendant probability of harm to self or others. The resident has little ability to interrupt the relapse process or to use peer supports when at risk for relapse to his or her substance dependence or mental disorder. His or her continued substance use poses an imminent danger of harm to self or others in the absence of 24-hour monitoring and structured support; *or*	(b) The patient is experiencing an escalation of relapse behaviors and/or reemergence of acute symptoms. This situation poses an imminent danger of harm to self or others in the absence of the type of 24-hour monitoring and structured support found in a medically monitored setting; *or*

ASAM Patient Placement Criteria, Second Edition–Revised

Level III Admission Criteria
Diagnostic and Dimensional Criteria

CRITERIA	LEVEL III.1 Clinically Managed Low-Intensity Residential Treatment	LEVEL III.3 Clinically Managed Medium-Intensity Residential Treatment	LEVEL III.5 Clinically Managed High-Intensity Residential Treatment	LEVEL III.7 Medically Monitored Intensive Inpatient Treatment
DIMENSION 5: Relapse, Continued Use or Continued Problem Potential (continued)	(c) The resident needs staff support to maintain engagement in his or her recovery program while transitioning to life in the community; *or*	(c) The resident's cognitive impairment has limited his or her ability to identify and cope with relapse triggers and high-risk situations. He or she requires relapse prevention activities that are delivered at a slower pace, more concretely and more repetitively, in a setting that provides 24-hour structure and support to prevent imminent dangerous consequences; *or*	(c) The resident is experiencing psychiatric or addiction symptoms such as drug craving, difficulty in postponing immediate gratification and other drug-seeking behaviors. This situation poses an imminent danger of harm to self or others in the absence of close 24-hour monitoring and structured support; *or*	(c) The modality of treatment or protocols to address relapse (such as aversion therapy and similar behavioral therapy techniques) require that the patient receive care in a Level III.7 program.
	(d) The resident is at high risk of substance use or deteriorated mental functioning, with dangerous emotional, behavioral or cognitive consequences, in the absence of close 24-hour structured support (as evidenced, for example, by lack of awareness of relapse triggers, difficulty in postponing immediate gratification or ambivalence toward or resistance to treatment), and these issues are being addressed concurrently in a Level II program.	(d) Despite recent, active participation in treatment at a less intensive level of care, the resident continues to use alcohol or other drugs or to deteriorate psychiatrically, with imminent serious consequences, and is at high risk of continued substance use or mental deterioration without close 24-hour monitoring and structured treatment.	(d) The resident is in imminent danger of relapse, with dangerous emotional, behavioral or cognitive consequences, because of a crisis situation.	

ASAM Patient Placement Criteria, Second Edition–Revised

Level III Admission Criteria
Diagnostic and Dimensional Criteria

CRITERIA	LEVEL III.1 Clinically Managed Low-Intensity Residential Treatment	LEVEL III.3 Clinically Managed Medium-Intensity Residential Treatment	LEVEL III.5 Clinically Managed High-Intensity Residential Treatment	LEVEL III.7 Medically Monitored Intensive Inpatient Treatment
DIMENSION 5: Relapse, Continued Use or Continued Problem Potential (continued)			(e) Despite recent, active participation in treatment at a less intensive level of care, the resident continues to use alcohol or other drugs or to deteriorate psychiatrically, with imminent serious consequences, and is at high risk of continued substance use or mental deterioration in the absence of close 24-hour monitoring and structured treatment.	
	Dual Diagnosis Enhanced Programs The resident's status in Dimension 5 is characterized by psychiatric symptoms that pose a moderate risk of relapse to a substance dependence or mental disorder. Such a resident demonstrates limited ability to apply relapse prevention skills, as well as deteriorating psychiatric functioning, which increases his or her risk of serious consequences and requires the types of services and 24-hour	**Dual Diagnosis Enhanced Programs** The resident's status in Dimension 5 is characterized by psychiatric symptoms that pose a moderate risk of relapse to a substance dependence or mental disorder. Such a resident demonstrates limited ability to apply relapse prevention skills, as well as poor skills in coping with mental disorders and/or avoiding or limiting relapse, with imminent serious consequences.	**Dual Diagnosis Enhanced Programs** The resident's status in Dimension 5 is characterized by psychiatric symptoms that pose a moderate to high risk of relapse to a substance dependence or mental disorder. Such a resident demonstrates limited ability to apply relapse prevention skills, as well as poor skills in coping with mental disorders and/or avoiding or limiting relapse, with imminent serious consequences.	**Dual Diagnosis Enhanced Programs** The patient's status in Dimension 5 is characterized by psychiatric symptoms that pose a moderate to high risk of relapse to a substance dependence or mental disorder. Such a patient demonstrates limited ability to apply relapse prevention skills, as well as poor skills in coping with mental disorders and/or avoiding or limiting relapse, with imminent serious consequences.

Level III Admission Criteria
Diagnostic and Dimensional Criteria

CRITERIA	LEVEL III.1 Clinically Managed Low-Intensity Residential Treatment	LEVEL III.3 Clinically Managed Medium-Intensity Residential Treatment	LEVEL III.5 Clinically Managed High-Intensity Residential Treatment	LEVEL III.7 Medically Monitored Intensive Inpatient Treatment
DIMENSION 5: Relapse, Continued Use or Continued Problem Potential (continued)	structure of a Level III.1 Dual Diagnosis Enhanced program in order to maintain an adequate level of functioning. For example, the resident demonstrates deteriorating functioning during outpatient treatment or while in a Halfway House that does not provide Dual Diagnosis Enhanced services. The resident who is receiving concurrent Level II and Level III.1 services requires case management to coordinate the services across levels of care.	For example, the resident continues to engage in behaviors that pose a risk of relapse (such as non-compliance with the medication regimen or spending time in places where drugs are being sold or used) because he or she has cognitive deficits that prevent understanding of the relationship between those behaviors and relapse to substance-dependence or mental disorders. The presence of these relapse issues requires the types of services and 24-hour structure of a Level III.3 Dual Diagnosis Enhanced program.	For example, the resident continues to engage repetitively and compulsively in behaviors that pose a risk of relapse (such as antisocial behavior or criminal activity, or spending time in places where antisocial behavior is the attraction) because of an inability to understand the relationship between those behaviors and relapse to substance dependence or mental disorders or criminal activity. The presence of these relapse issues requires the intensity and types of services and 24-hour structure of a Level III.5 Dual Diagnosis Enhanced program.	The patient's follow-through in treatment is poor or inconsistent, and his or her relapse problems are escalating to such a degree that treatment at a lower level of care is not succeeding or not feasible. For example, the patient continues to evidence self-harm behaviors, such as superficially cutting himself or herself, or suicidal ideation or impulses with a plan to commit suicide, but agrees to reach out if seriously suicidal and is assessed as capable of enough internal control to do so. Or the patient's continuing substance-induced psychotic symptoms are resolving, but his or her difficulties in controlling substance use and craving for use are exacerbating his or her psychotic symptoms.

Level III Admission Criteria
Diagnostic and Dimensional Criteria

CRITERIA	LEVEL III.1 Clinically Managed Low-Intensity Residential Treatment	LEVEL III.3 Clinically Managed Medium-Intensity Residential Treatment	LEVEL III.5 Clinically Managed High-Intensity Residential Treatment	LEVEL III.7 Medically Monitored Intensive Inpatient Treatment
DIMENSION 5: Relapse, Continued Use or Continued Problem Potential (continued)	Case management and collaboration across levels of care may be needed to manage anti-craving, psychotropic or opioid maintenance medications. For example, the resident may have only recently developed the ability to control his or her anger and impulses to damage property. Or the resident may have only recently become compliant in taking psychotropic medications as prescribed and is not increasing the dose to control continuing symptoms of anxiety or panic.	Case management and collaboration across levels of care may be needed to manage anti-craving, psychotropic or opioid maintenance medications. For example, because of significant cognitive deficits, the resident may have difficulty in managing the activities of daily living without 24-hour interventions and thus require preparation for placement in a group home in order to support his or her continued recovery from a substance use or mental health problem. (Such a group home may involve supervised living for persons with cognitive deficits such as mental retardation or those who are severely and persistently mentally ill.)	Case management and collaboration across levels of care may be needed to manage anti-craving, psychotropic or opioid maintenance medications. For example, because of an external locus of control, the resident may have difficulty in resisting pressures to use psychoactive substances. He or she may continue involvement or become re-involved with peers who are engaged in antisocial and/or criminal behaviors, and thus requires some type of group living situation that provides ongoing structure and support. (Such a group home may be a supervised living arrangement for ex-offenders.)	

ASAM Patient Placement Criteria, Second Edition–Revised

Level III Admission Criteria
Diagnostic and Dimensional Criteria

CRITERIA	LEVEL III.1 Clinically Managed Low-Intensity Residential Treatment	LEVEL III.3 Clinically Managed Medium-Intensity Residential Treatment	LEVEL III.5 Clinically Managed High-Intensity Residential Treatment	LEVEL III.7 Medically Monitored Intensive Inpatient Treatment
DIMENSION 5: Relapse, Continued Use or Continued Problem Potential (continued)	Preparation for transfer of the resident to a less intensive level of care and/or reentry into the community requires case management and staff exploration of supportive living environments, separately from their therapeutic work with the resident.	Preparation for transfer of the resident to a less intensive level of care, a different type of service in the community, and/or reentry into the community requires case management and staff exploration of supportive living environments, separately from their therapeutic work with the resident.	Preparation for transfer of the resident to a less intensive level of care, a different type of service in the community, and/or reentry into the community requires case management and staff exploration of supportive living environments, separately from their therapeutic work with the resident.	
DIMENSION 6: Recovery Environment	**All Programs** The resident's status in Dimension 6 is characterized by *one* of (a) *or* (b) *or* (c) *or* (d) *or* (e) *and* (f): (a) The resident has been living in an environment that is characterized by a moderately high risk of initiation or repetition of physical, sexual or emotional abuse, or substance use so endemic that the resident is assessed as being unable to achieve or maintain recovery at a less intensive level of care; *or*	**All Programs** The resident's status in Dimension 6 is characterized by *one* of the following: (a) The resident has been living in an environment that is characterized by a moderately high risk of initiation or repetition of physical, sexual or emotional abuse, or substance use so endemic that the resident is assessed as being unable to achieve or maintain recovery at a less intensive level of care; *or*	**All Programs** The resident's status in Dimension 6 is characterized by *one* of the following: (a) The resident has been living in an environment that is characterized by a moderately high risk of initiation or repetition of physical, sexual or emotional abuse, or substance use so endemic that the resident is assessed as being unable to achieve or maintain recovery at a less intensive level of care; *or*	**All Programs** The patient's status in Dimension 6 is characterized by *one* of the following: (a) The patient requires continuous medical monitoring while addressing his or her substance use and/or psychiatric problems, because his or her current living situation is characterized by a high risk of initiation or repetition of physical, sexual or emotional abuse, or substance use so endemic that the patient is assessed as

Level III Admission Criteria
Diagnostic and Dimensional Criteria

CRITERIA	LEVEL III.1 Clinically Managed Low-Intensity Residential Treatment	LEVEL III.3 Clinically Managed Medium-Intensity Residential Treatment	LEVEL III.5 Clinically Managed High-Intensity Residential Treatment	LEVEL III.7 Medically Monitored Intensive Inpatient Treatment
DIMENSION 6: Recovery Environment (continued)				being unable to achieve or maintain recovery at a less intensive level of care. For example, because of mania (which is treated with mood-stabilizing medications), the patient is believes he or she is able to control the people in his or her environment who pose the risk; *or*
	(b) The resident lacks social contacts or has inappropriate social contacts that jeopardize his or her recovery, or the resident's social network is characterized by significant social isolation and withdrawal. The resident's social network includes few friends who are not regular users of alcohol or other drugs, leading recovery goals to be assessed as unachievable outside of a 24-hour supportive setting; *or*	(b) The resident is in significant danger of victimization and thus requires 24-hour supervision. For example, the resident has sustained a traumatic brain injury, as a result of which he or she is vulnerable to victimization when using psychoactive substances; *or*	(b) The resident's social network includes regular users of alcohol or other drugs, such that recovery goals are assessed as unachievable at a less intensive level of care; *or*	(b) Family members or significant others living with the patient are not supportive of his or her recovery goals and are actively sabotaging treatment. This situation requires structured treatment services and relief from the home environment in order for the patient to focus on recovery; *or*

Level III Admission Criteria
Diagnostic and Dimensional Criteria

CRITERIA	LEVEL III.1 Clinically Managed Low-Intensity Residential Treatment	LEVEL III.3 Clinically Managed Medium-Intensity Residential Treatment	LEVEL III.5 Clinically Managed High-Intensity Residential Treatment	LEVEL III.7 Medically Monitored Intensive Inpatient Treatment
DIMENSION 6: Recovery Environment (continued)	(c) The resident's social network involves living in an environment that is so highly invested in alcohol or other drug use that the resident's recovery goals are assessed as unachievable; *or*	(c) The resident's social network includes regular users of alcohol or other drugs, such that recovery goals are assessed as unachievable at a less intensive level of care; *or*	(c) The resident's social network is characterized by significant social isolation or withdrawal, such that recovery goals are assessed as unachievable at a less intensive level of care; *or*	(c) The patient is unable to cope, for even limited periods of time, outside of 24-hour care. The patient needs staff monitoring to learn to cope with Dimension 6 problems before he or she can be transferred safely to a less intensive setting.
	(d) Continued exposure to the resident's school, work or living environment makes recovery unlikely, and the resident has insufficient resources and skills to maintain an adequate level of functioning outside of a 24-hour supportive environment; *or*	(d) The resident's social network involves living with an individual who is a regular user, abuser or dealer of alcohol or other drugs, or the resident's living environment is so highly invested in alcohol or other drug use that his or her recovery goals are assessed as unachievable; *or*	(d) The resident's social network involves living with an individual who is a regular user, abuser or dealer of alcohol or other drugs, or the resident's living environment is so highly invested in alcohol or other drug use that his or her recovery goals are assessed as unachievable; *or*	
	(e) The resident is in danger of victimization by another and thus requires 24-hour supervision; *and*	(e) Because of cognitive limitations, the resident is in danger of victimization by another and thus requires 24-hour supervision; *or*	(e) The resident is unable to cope, for even limited periods of time, outside of 24-hour care. He or she needs staff monitoring to learn to cope with Dimension 6 problems before being transferred safely to a less intensive setting; *or*	

Level III Admission Criteria
Diagnostic and Dimensional Criteria

CRITERIA	LEVEL III.1 Clinically Managed Low-Intensity Residential Treatment	LEVEL III.3 Clinically Managed Medium-Intensity Residential Treatment	LEVEL III.5 Clinically Managed High-Intensity Residential Treatment	LEVEL III.7 Medically Monitored Intensive Inpatient Treatment
DIMENSION 6: Recovery Environment (continued)	(f) The resident is able to cope, for limited periods of time, outside the 24-hour structure of a Level III.1 program in order to pursue clinical, vocational, educational and community activities.	(f) The resident is unable to cope, for even limited periods of time, outside the 24-hour structure of a Level III.3 program. He or she needs staff monitoring to assure his or her safety and well-being.	(f) The resident's living environment is characterized by criminal behavior, victimization, and other antisocial norms and values.	
	Dual Diagnosis Enhanced Programs The resident's status in Dimension 6 is characterized by severe and persistent mental illness. He or she may be too ill to benefit from skills training to learn to cope with problems in the recovery environment. Such a resident requires planning for assertive community treatment, intensive case management or other community outreach and support services.	**Dual Diagnosis Enhanced Programs** The resident's status in Dimension 6 is characterized by severe and persistent mental illness. He or she may be too ill to benefit from skills training to learn to cope with problems in the recovery environment. Such a resident requires planning for assertive community treatment, intensive case management or other community outreach and support services.	**Dual Diagnosis Enhanced Programs** The resident's status in Dimension 6 is characterized by severe and persistent mental illness. He or she may be too ill to benefit from skills training to learn to cope with problems in the recovery environment. Such a resident requires planning for assertive community treatment, intensive case management or other community outreach and support services.	**Dual Diagnosis Enhanced Programs** The patient's status in Dimension 6 is characterized by severe and persistent mental illness. He or she may be too ill to benefit from skills training to learn to cope with problems in the recovery environment. Such a resident requires planning for assertive community treatment, intensive case management or other community outreach and support services.

Level III Admission Criteria
Diagnostic and Dimensional Criteria

CRITERIA	LEVEL III.1 Clinically Managed Low-Intensity Residential Treatment	LEVEL III.3 Clinically Managed Medium-Intensity Residential Treatment	LEVEL III.5 Clinically Managed High-Intensity Residential Treatment	LEVEL III.7 Medically Monitored Intensive Inpatient Treatment
DIMENSION 6: Recovery Environment (continued)	The resident's living, working, social and/or community environment is not supportive of good mental health functioning. He or she has insufficient resources and skills to deal with this situation. For example, the resident may be unable to cope with the continuing stress of homelessness, or hostile or alcoholic family members, and thus exhibits increasing anxiety and depression. Such a resident needs the support and structure of a Level III.1 Dual Diagnosis Enhanced program to achieve stabilization and prevent further deterioration.	The resident's living, working, social and/or community environment is not supportive of good mental health functioning. He or she has insufficient resources and skills to deal with this situation. For example, the resident may be unable to cope with the continuing stress of decreased cognitive functioning, or hostile or alcoholic family members, and thus exhibits increasing anxiety and depression. Such a resident needs the support and structure of a Level III.3 Dual Diagnosis Enhanced program to achieve stabilization and prevent further deterioration.	Such a resident's living, working, social and/or community environment is not supportive of good mental health functioning. He or she has insufficient resources and skills to deal with this situation. For example, the resident may be unable to cope with the continuing stress of peer pressure to be involved in criminal behavior, or threats by former criminal associates, or hostile or alcoholic family members, and thus exhibits increasing anxiety and depression. Such a resident needs the support and structure of a Level III.5 Dual Diagnosis Enhanced program to achieve stabilization and prevent further deterioration.	Such a resident's living, working, social and/or community environment is not supportive of good mental health functioning. He or she has insufficient resources and skills to deal with this situation. For example, the resident may be unable to cope with a hostile or alcoholic family member and thus exhibits increasing anxiety and depression. Such a resident needs the support and structure of a Level III.7 Dual Diagnosis Enhanced program to achieve stabilization and prevent further deterioration.

Level IV
Medically Managed Intensive Inpatient Treatment

Level IV medically managed intensive inpatient treatment is an organized service, delivered in an acute care inpatient setting. It is appropriate for patients whose acute biomedical, emotional, behavioral and cognitive problems are so severe that they require primary medical and nursing care.

Level IV program services are delivered by an interdisciplinary staff of addiction-credentialed physicians and other appropriately credentialed treatment professionals. Such a program encompasses a planned regimen of 24-hour medically directed evaluation and treatment services, provided under a defined set of policies, procedures and clinical protocols.

Treatment is provided 24 hours a day in a permanent facility with inpatient beds. The full resources of a general acute care or psychiatric hospital are available. Although treatment is specific to substance dependence disorders, the skills of the interdisciplinary team and the availability of support services allow the conjoint treatment of any co-occurring biomedical conditions and mental disorders that need to be addressed.

Length of Service

The duration of treatment varies with the severity of the patient's illness and his or her response to treatment.

Co-Occurring Mental and Substance-Related Disorders

The services of a Level IV program are appropriate for patients who have severe, unstable mental and substance dependence disorders. Such disorders typically require a range of medical, nursing and other clinical interventions that can be delivered safely only in a 24-hour medically managed setting. They may involve:

- Co-occurring severe substance-related and mental disorders, such as an acutely suicidal patient who also is acutely in need of medical detoxification.

- Severe intoxication or withdrawal problems or other severe biomedical conditions that occur simultaneously with more stabilized mental health problems.

- Severe mental health problems that co-occur with more stabilized substance dependence problems.

Because Level IV program services are the most intensive in the continuum of care, their principal focus is the stabilization of the patient and preparation for his or her transfer to a less intensive setting for continuing care.

Adult Criteria
Level IV: Medically Managed Intensive Inpatient Services

CHARACTERISTIC	ESSENTIAL FEATURES
EXAMPLES	**All Programs** Level IV programs typically are housed in three types of settings: (a) an acute care general hospital, (b) an acute psychiatric hospital or psychiatric unit within an acute care general hospital, and (c) a licensed chemical dependency specialty hospital with acute care medical and nursing staff.
SETTING	**All Programs** Level IV program services may be offered in any appropriately licensed acute care setting that offers addiction treatment services in concert with intensive biomedical and/or psychiatric services. Such a program must offer medically directed acute detoxification and related treatment directed at alleviating acute emotional, behavioral or cognitive and/or biomedical distress resulting from, or co-occurring with, a patient's use of alcohol or other drugs. The program may provide life support care and treatment—either directly, or through transfer of the patient to another service within the facility, or to another medical facility equipped to provide such care. Patients who meet the criteria for Dimension 1 may be admitted to a Level IV program in an acute care general hospital, a psychiatric hospital or a chemical dependency specialty hospital. Those who meet criteria in Dimension 2 would be admitted to a Level IV program in an acute care general hospital or a chemical dependency specialty hospital. Those who meet the criteria in Dimension 3 may be admitted to a Level IV program in a psychiatric specialty hospital or a psychiatric specialty unit in a general hospital.
SUPPORT SYSTEMS	**All Programs** In Level IV programs, necessary support systems include a full range of acute care services, specialty consultation and intensive care.
STAFF	**All Programs** Level IV programs are staffed by: (a) An interdisciplinary team of appropriately credentialed clinical staff (including addiction-credentialed physicians, nurses, counselors, psychologists and social workers) who assess and treat patients with substance dependence disorders or addicted patients with concomitant acute biomedical, emotional or behavioral disorders. Staff are knowledgeable about the biopsychosocial dimensions of addiction as well as biomedical, emotional, behavioral and cognitive disorders. (b) A team of appropriately trained and credentialed professionals who provide medical management by physicians 24 hours a day, primary nursing care and observation 24 hours a day, and professional counseling services 16 hours a day.

Adult Criteria
Level IV: Medically Managed Intensive Inpatient Services

CHARACTERISTIC	ESSENTIAL FEATURES
STAFF (continued)	(c) Facility-approved addiction counselors or licensed, certified or registered addiction clinicians who administer planned interventions according to the assessed needs of the patient. Some, if not all, program staff have had sufficient cross-training to understand the signs and symptoms of mental disorders and to understand and explain the uses of psychotropic medications and their interactions with substance-related disorders. **Dual Diagnosis Programs** In addition to the staff listed above, which encompass Dual Diagnosis Capable programs, Level IV Dual Diagnosis Enhanced programs are staffed by appropriately credentialed mental health professionals, who assess and treat the patient's co-occurring mental disorders. Such staff are knowledgeable about the biological and psychosocial dimensions of psychiatric disorders and their treatment. The staff includes cross-trained and appropriately credentialed addiction and mental health professionals.
THERAPIES	**All Programs** Therapies offered by Level IV programs include: (a) A highly individualized program of treatment for substance-related disorders, as well as any concurrent biomedical, emotional, behavioral or cognitive problems, delivered by an interdisciplinary treatment team. (b) Cognitive, behavioral, medication and other therapies, provided on an individual or group basis, depending on the patient's needs. For the patient who has a severe biomedical disorder, biomedical interventions are available to supplement addiction treatment. For the patient who has stable psychiatric symptoms, Level IV Dual Diagnosis Capable programs offer individualized treatment activities designed to monitor the patient's mental health and to address the interaction of the mental health problems and substance use disorders. (c) Health education services. (d) Planned clinical interventions that are designed to enhance the patient's acceptance of his or her substance dependence problem. (e) Services for the patient's family, guardian or significant other(s). Because the length of stay in a Level IV program typically is sufficient only to stabilize the patient's acute signs and symptoms, a primary focus of the treatment plan is case management and coordination of care to ensure a smooth transition to continuing treatment at another level of care.

Adult Criteria
Level IV: Medically Managed Intensive Inpatient Services

CHARACTERISTIC	ESSENTIAL FEATURES
THERAPIES (continued)	**Dual Diagnosis Enhanced Programs** In addition to the therapies described above, Level IV Dual Diagnosis Enhanced programs offer individualized treatment activities designed to stabilize the patient's active psychiatric symptoms. Specific attention is given to medication evaluation and management. Treatment features motivational and engagement strategies, which are used in preference to confrontational approaches.
ASSESSMENT/ TREATMENT PLAN REVIEW	**All Programs** In Level IV programs, the assessment and treatment plan review include: (a) A comprehensive nursing assessment, conducted at the time of admission. (b) Physician approval of the admission. (c) A comprehensive history and physical examination, performed by a physician within 24 hours of admission. (d) A comprehensive biopsychosocial assessment, begun at the time of admission. (e) An individualized treatment plan, which includes problem formulation and articulation of short-term, measurable treatment goals and activities designed to achieve those goals. The plan is developed in collaboration with the patient and reflects the patient's personal goals. Treatment plan reviews are conducted at specified times, as noted in the treatment plan. **Dual Diagnosis Capable Programs** In addition to the assessment and treatment plan activities described above, Level IV Dual Diagnosis Capable programs offer skilled assessment and monitoring of the patient's co-occurring mental disorder. However, the primary focus of these programs is the assessment, stabilization and treatment of the patient's substance-induced intoxication, withdrawal or biomedical problem(s), rather than the more stable co-occurring mental health problem(s). **Dual Diagnosis Enhanced Programs** In addition to the assessment and treatment plan activities described above, staff of Level IV Dual Diagnosis Enhanced programs give equal attention to the patient's co-occurring mental disorder. Because acute stabilization usually occurs in a Level IV program that is focused on the patient's most acute problem, any acute substance-induced psychiatric disorder or co-occurring mental disorder is appropriately addressed at this level of care. Level IV Dual Diagnosis Enhanced programs offer assessment and treatment planning for all aspects of a patient's substance dependence and mental health problems.

Adult Criteria
Level IV: Medically Managed Intensive Inpatient Services

CHARACTERISTIC	ESSENTIAL FEATURES
DOCUMENTATION	**All Programs** Documentation standards for Level IV programs include individualized progress notes in each patient's record for every shift. Such notes clearly reflect implementation of the treatment plan and the patient's response to therapeutic interventions for all disorders treated, as well as subsequent amendments to the plan. The focus of documentation is the degree of stabilization of the patient's substance-related disorder and any concurrent biomedical, emotional, behavioral or cognitive problem(s). Documentation also focuses on the elements of the treatment plan that are related to case management and coordination of care to ensure a smooth transition to continuing service or another level of care.

Level IV Admission Criteria
Diagnostic and Dimensional Criteria

CRITERIA	LEVEL IV Medically Managed Intensive Inpatient Services
DIAGNOSTIC ADMISSION CRITERIA	**All Programs** The patient who is appropriately placed in a Level IV program is assessed as meeting the diagnostic criteria for a Substance-Related Disorder (including Substance-Use Disorder or Substance-Induced Disorder), as defined in the current *Diagnostic and Statistical Manual of Mental Disorders (DSM)* of the American Psychiatric Association or other standardized and widely accepted criteria, as well as the dimensional criteria for admission. If the patient's presenting alcohol or drug use history is inadequate to substantiate such a diagnosis, the probability of such a diagnosis may be determined from information submitted by collateral parties (such as family members, legal guardian and significant others). **Dual Diagnosis Capable Programs** Some patients have co-occurring mental disorders that meet stability criteria for admission to a Dual Diagnosis Capable program. Other patients may have difficulties with mood, behavior or cognition as the result of other psychiatric or substance-induced disorders, or the patient's emotional, behavioral or cognitive symptoms may be troublesome but not sufficient to meet the criteria for a diagnosed mental disorder. **Dual Diagnosis Enhanced Programs** In contrast to the foregoing criteria, the patient who is appropriately placed in a Level IV Dual Diagnosis Enhanced program is assessed as meeting the diagnostic criteria for a Mental Disorder as well as a Substance-Related Disorder, as defined in the current *Diagnostic and Statistical Manual of Mental Disorders (DSM)* of the American Psychiatric Association or other standardized and widely accepted criteria, as well as the dimensional criteria for admission. If the patient's presenting history is inadequate to substantiate such a diagnosis, the probability of such a diagnosis may be determined from information submitted by collateral parties (such as family members, legal guardians and significant others).
DIMENSIONAL ADMISSION CRITERIA	**All Programs** The patient who is appropriately admitted to a Level IV program meets specifications in at least *one* of Dimensions 1, 2 or 3.
DIMENSION 1: **Acute Intoxication and/or Withdrawal**	**All Programs** See the separate Dimension 1 criteria.

Level IV Admission Criteria
Diagnostic and Dimensional Criteria

CRITERIA	LEVEL IV Medically Managed Intensive Inpatient Services
DIMENSION 2: **Biomedical Conditions and Complications**	**All Programs** The patient's status in Dimension 2 is characterized by *one* of the following: (a) Biomedical complications of the addictive disorder require medical management and skilled nursing care; *or* (b) A concurrent biomedical illness or pregnancy requires stabilization and daily medical management, with daily primary nursing interventions; *or* (c) The patient has a concurrent biomedical condition(s) in which continued alcohol or other drug use presents an imminent danger to life or severe danger to health (including pregnancy); *or* (d) The patient is experiencing recurrent or multiple seizures; *or* (e) The patient is experiencing a disulfiram-alcohol reaction; *or* (f) The patient has life-threatening symptoms (such as stupor, convulsions, and the like) that are related to use of alcohol or other drugs; *or* (g) The patient's alcohol or other drug use are gravely complicating or exacerbating a previously diagnosed medical condition; *or* (h) Changes in the patient's medical status, such as significant worsening of a medical condition, make abstinence imperative; *or* (i) Significant improvement in a previously unstable medical condition allows the patient to respond to addiction treatment; *or* (j) The patient has another biomedical problem(s) that requires 24-hour observation and evaluation.
DIMENSION 3: **Emotional, Behavioral or Cognitive Conditions and Complications**	**All Programs** The patient whose status in Dimension 3 is characterized by stabilized emotional, behavioral or cognitive conditions is appropriately assessed as in need of Level IV Dual Diagnosis Capable program services. On the other hand, if the patient's symptoms in Dimension 3 are so severe as to require admission to a Level IV program, then only placement in a Dual Diagnosis Enhanced program is sufficient to meet the patient's needs.

Level IV Admission Criteria
Diagnostic and Dimensional Criteria

CRITERIA	LEVEL IV Medically Managed Intensive Inpatient Services
DIMENSION 3: **Emotional, Behavioral or Cognitive Conditions and Complications (continued)**	**Dual Diagnosis Enhanced Programs** For admission to a Level IV Dual Diagnosis Enhanced program, the patient's status in Dimension 3 is characterized by *one* of the following: (a) Emotional, behavioral or cognitive complications of the patient's addictive disorder require psychiatric management and skilled nursing care; *or* (b) A concurrent emotional, behavioral or cognitive illness requires stabilization, daily psychiatric management and primary nursing interventions; *or* (c) The patient's uncontrolled behavior poses an imminent danger to self or others; *or* (d) The patient's mental confusion or fluctuating orientation poses an imminent danger to self or others (for example, severe self-care problems, violence or suicide); *or* (e) A coexisting serious emotional, behavioral or cognitive disorder complicates the treatment of addiction and requires differential diagnosis and treatment; *or* (f) The patient's extreme depression poses an imminent risk to his or her safety; *or* (g) Impairment of the patient's thought processes or abstract thinking, limitations in his or her ability to conceptualize, and impairment in the patient's ability to manage the activities of daily living pose an imminent risk to his or her safety; *or* (h) The patient's continued alcohol or drug use is causing grave complications or exacerbation of a previously diagnosed psychiatric or emotional or behavioral condition; *or* (i) The patient is experiencing altered mental status, with or without delirium, as manifested by: [1] disorientation to self, or [2] alcoholic hallucinosis, or [3] toxic psychosis.
DIMENSION 4: **Readiness to Change**	**All Programs** Only a patient who meets criteria in Dimensions 1, 2 or 3 is appropriately placed in a Level IV program. Problems in Dimensions 4, 5 or 6 alone are not sufficient for placement at Level IV.

Level IV Admission Criteria
Diagnostic and Dimensional Criteria

CRITERIA	LEVEL IV Medically Managed Intensive Inpatient Services
DIMENSION 5: **Relapse, Continued Use or Continued Problem Potential**	**All Programs** Only a patient who meets criteria in Dimensions 1, 2 or 3 is appropriately placed in a Level IV program. Problems in Dimensions 4, 5 or 6 alone are not sufficient for placement at Level IV.
DIMENSION 6: **Recovery Environment**	**All Programs** Only a patient who meets criteria in Dimensions 1, 2 or 3 is appropriately placed in a Level IV program. Problems in Dimensions 4, 5 or 6 alone are not sufficient for placement at Level IV.

Opioid Maintenance Therapy

"Opioid maintenance therapy" is an umbrella term that encompasses a variety of pharmacologic and nonpharmacologic treatment modalities, including the therapeutic use of specialized opioid compounds such as methadone and LAAM (levo-alpha-acetylmethadol) to psychopharmacologically occupy opiate receptors in the brain, extinguish drug craving and establish a maintenance state. The result is a continuously maintained state of drug tolerance in which the therapeutic agent does not produce euphoria, intoxication or withdrawal symptoms.

Opioid maintenance therapy is best conceptualized as a separate service that can be provided at many levels of care, depending on the patient's status in Dimensions 1 through 6. Adjunctive nonpharmacologic interventions are essential and may be provided in the clinic or through coordination with another addiction treatment provider.

Opioid maintenance therapy is presented here as a Level I service because that is the context in which it is most commonly offered. Identical elements must be present in any program that offers opioid maintenance therapy, regardless of the level of care.

Brief Description of Treatment Level

Opioid maintenance therapy is an organized, usually ambulatory, addiction treatment service for opiate-addicted patients. It is delivered by addiction-trained personnel or addiction-credentialed clinicians, who provide individualized treatment, case management, and health education (including education about human immunodeficiency virus [HIV], tuberculosis [TB], and sexually transmitted diseases [STD]). The nature of the services provided (such as dose, level of care, length of service or frequency of visits) is determined by the patient's clinical needs, but such services always include regularly scheduled psychosocial treatment sessions and daily or other scheduled medication visits within a structured program (for patients who are doing well enough to have take-home doses of methadone or who are taking LAAM).

Opioid maintenance therapy is provided under a defined set of policies and procedures, including admission, discharge and continued service criteria stipulated by state law and regulation and the federal regulations at *FDA 21 CFR Part 291*.

Treatment with methadone or LAAM is designed to address the patient's need to achieve changes in his or her level of functioning, including elimination of illicit opiate and other alcohol or drug use. To accomplish such change, the patient's treatment plan must address major lifestyle, attitudinal and behavioral issues that have the potential to undermine the goals of recovery and inhibit the individual's ability to cope with major life tasks.

Note: At the time this edition was completed, the U.S. Food and Drug Administration had not yet approved buprenorphine, alone or in combination with naloxone, for the treatment of opiate addiction. Therefore, the use of buprenorphine is not addressed in the *ASAM PPC-2R*. It is anticipated that it will be included in a future edition.

Length of Service

Duration of treatment varies with the severity of the patient's illness and his or her response to treatment and desire to continue treatment.

Adult Criteria
Opioid Maintenance Therapy

CHARACTERISTIC	OPIOID MAINTENANCE THERAPY
EXAMPLES	Examples of opioid maintenance therapy (OMT) include methadone and LAAM therapy.
SETTING	OMT may be offered in any licensed program with the necessary and appropriate licenses and certifications. Opioid maintenance therapy typically is provided in permanent freestanding clinics, community mental health centers, community health centers, hospital medication units, satellite clinics and mobile units attached to a permanent clinic site.
SUPPORT SYSTEMS	In OMT programs, necessary support systems include: (a) Linkage with or access to psychological, medical and psychiatric consultation. (b) Linkage with or access to emergency medical and psychiatric care through affiliations with more intensive levels of care. (c) Linkage with or access to evaluation and ongoing primary medical care. (d) Ability to conduct or arrange for appropriate laboratory and toxicology tests. (e) Availability of physicians to evaluate, prescribe and monitor use of methadone or LAAM, and of nurses and pharmacists to dispense and administer methadone or LAAM. (f) Ability to provide or assist in arrangements for transportation services for patients who are unable to drive safely or who lack transportation.
STAFF	Staff of OMT programs include: (a) An interdisciplinary team of appropriately trained and credentialed addiction professionals, including a medical director, counselors and the medical staff delineated in (b) below. The team will include social workers and licensed psychologists, as needed. Team members must be knowledgeable in the assessment, interpretation, and treatment of the biopsychosocial dimensions of alcohol or other drug dependence. They would receive supervision appropriate to their level of training and experience. (b) Licensed medical, nursing or pharmacy staff, who are available to administer medications in accordance with the physician's prescriptions or orders. The intensity of nursing care is appropriate to the services provided by an outpatient treatment program that uses methadone or LAAM. (c) A physician, who is available during medication dispensing and clinic operating hours, either in person or by telephone.

Adult Criteria
Opioid Maintenance Therapy

CHARACTERISTIC	OPIOID MAINTENANCE THERAPY
THERAPIES	Therapies offered in OMT programs include: (a) Individualized assessment and treatment. (b) Medication: Assessing, prescribing, administering, reassessing and regulating dose levels appropriate to the individual; supervising detoxification from opiates, methadone or LAAM; overseeing and facilitating access to appropriate treatment, including medication for other physical and mental health disorders, provided as needed. (c) Monitored urine testing. (d) Counseling: A range of cognitive, behavioral and other addiction-focused therapies, reflecting a variety of treatment approaches, provided to the patient on an individual, group or family basis. (e) Case management: Case management, including medical monitoring and coordination of on- and off-site treatment services, provided as needed. Case managers also assure the provision of, or referral to, educational and vocational counseling, treatment of psychiatric illness, child care, parenting skills development, primary health care and other adjunct services, as needed. (f) Psychoeducation, including HIV/AIDS and other health education services.
ASSESSMENT/ TREATMENT PLAN REVIEW	In OMT programs, the assessment and treatment plan review include: (a) A comprehensive medical history, physical examination and laboratory tests, provided or obtained in accordance with federal regulations. The tests must be done at the time of admission and reviewed by a physician as soon as possible, but no later than 14 days after admission [*FDA 21 CFR Part 291*]. (b) An individual biopsychosocial assessment. (c) An appropriate regimen of methadone or LAAM (as required by FDA regulation), at a dose established by a physician at the time of admission and monitored carefully until the patient is stable and an adequate dose has been established. The dose then is reviewed as indicated by the patient's course of treatment. (d) Continuing evaluation and referral for care of any serious biomedical problems. (e) An individualized treatment plan, including problem formulation and articulation of short-term, measurable treatment goals and activities designed to achieve those goals. The plan is developed in collaboration with the patient and reflects the patient's personal goals. Treatment plan reviews are conducted at specified times, as noted in the plan.

Adult Criteria
Opioid Maintenance Therapy

CHARACTERISTIC	OPIOID MAINTENANCE THERAPY
DOCUMENTATION	Documentation standards of OMT programs include individualized progress notes in each patient's record for every shift. Such notes clearly reflect implementation of the treatment plan and the patient's response to therapeutic interventions for all disorders treated, as well as subsequent amendments to the plan. Because of special recordkeeping requirements for OMT programs, records also should include documentation of each dose of methadone or LAAM administered, with a copy of the physician's order for methadone or LAAM.
DIAGNOSTIC ADMISSION CRITERIA	The patient who is appropriately placed in opioid maintenance therapy is assessed as meeting the diagnostic criteria for Opioid Dependence Disorder, as defined in the current *Diagnostic and Statistical Manual of Mental Disorders (DSM)* or other standardized and widely accepted criteria, aside from those exceptions listed in the *Federal Register* of the U.S. Department of Health and Human Services, Food and Drug Administration, *21 CFR Part 291*. If the patient's drug use history is inadequate to substantiate such a diagnosis, the probability of such a diagnosis may be determined from information submitted by other health care professionals and programs and collateral parties (such as family members, legal guardian or significant others). Individuals who are admitted to treatment with methadone or LAAM must demonstrate specific objective and subjective signs of opiate dependence, as defined in *FDA 21 CFR Part 291*.
DIMENSIONAL ADMISSION CRITERIA	The patient who is appropriately placed in opioid maintenance therapy is assessed as meeting the required specifications in Dimensions 1 through 6.

Adult Criteria
Diagnostic and Dimensional Criteria

CRITERIA	OPIOID MAINTENANCE THERAPY
DIMENSION 1: Acute Intoxication and/or Withdrawal	In Dimension 1, the patient meets specifications in (a) *and* (b), *or one of* (c), (d) *or* (e): (a) A physician determines that the patient is "physiologically dependent upon an opiate drug and became physiologically dependent at least one year before admission to methadone maintenance." This means that the patient was addicted "continuously or episodically for most of the year immediately before admission" *[FDA 21 CFR Part 291]; and* (b) The patient's current physiological dependence (in addition to a history of addiction) is confirmed by vital signs, early physical signs of narcotic withdrawal, a urine screen that is positive for opiates, the presence of old or fresh needle marks, and documented reports from medical professionals, the patient or family, treatment history, or (if necessary) a positive reaction to a naloxone test; *or* (c) A patient can be admitted from a criminal justice or chronic care setting within 14 days of release, or up to 6 months after release without documented evidence of physiological dependence if the patient was eligible for admission prior to incarceration *[FDA 21 CFR Part 291]; or* (d) A pregnant women who has a documented history of opiate dependence without physiological dependence can be admitted if the program physician certifies that the woman is pregnant and finds that treatment is medically justified *[FDA 21 CFR Part 291]; or* (e) A previously treated patient who has been voluntarily detoxified from methadone within two years of discharge can be admitted, in the absence of current physiological dependence, if the program can document prior methadone treatment of 6 months' or more duration and, in the judgment of the program physician, readmission to opioid maintenance therapy is medically indicated *[FDA 21 CFR Part 291]*.
DIMENSION 2: Biomedical Conditions and Complications	In Dimension 2, the patient meets specifications in *one* of the following: (a) The patient meets the biomedical criteria for opiate dependence, with or without the complications of opiate addiction, and requires outpatient medical monitoring and skilled care; *or* (b) The patient has a concurrent biomedical illness or pregnancy, which can be treated on an outpatient basis with minimal daily medical monitoring; *or* (c) The patient has biomedical problems that can be managed on an outpatient basis, such as: [1] liver disease or problems with potential hepatic decompensation, [2] pancreatitis, [3] gastrointestinal problems, [4] cardiovascular disorders, [5] HIV and AIDS, [6] sexually transmitted diseases, and [7] tuberculosis.

Adult Criteria
Diagnostic and Dimensional Criteria

CRITERIA	OPIOID MAINTENANCE THERAPY
DIMENSION 3: Emotional, Behavioral or Cognitive Conditions and Complications	In Dimension 3, the patient meets specifications in *one* of the following: (a) The patient's emotional, behavioral or cognitive problems, if present, are manageable in an outpatient structured environment; *or* (b) The patient's substance-related abuse or neglect of his or her spouse, children or significant others require intensive outpatient treatment to reduce the risk of further deterioration; *or* (c) The patient has a diagnosed and stable emotional, behavioral or cognitive problem or thought disorder (such as stable borderline personality disorder or obsessive-compulsive disorder) that requires monitoring, management or medication because of the risk that the problem(s) will distract the patient from his or her focus on treatment; *or* (d) The patient poses a mild risk of harm to self or others, with or without a history of severe depression, suicidal or homicidal behavior, but can be managed safely in a structured outpatient environment; *or* (e) The patient demonstrates emotional and behavioral stability but requires continued pharmacotherapy to prevent relapse to opiate use.
DIMENSION 4: Readiness to Change	In Dimension 4, the patient meets specifications in *one* of the following: (a) The patient requires structured therapy, pharmacotherapy and programmatic milieu to promote treatment progress and recovery; *or* (b) The patient attributes his or her problems to persons or external events rather than to the substance-related disorder. He or she thus is unable to make behavioral changes in the absence of clinically directed and repeated structured motivational interventions. However, the patient's resistance is not so high as to render treatment ineffective.
DIMENSION 5: Relapse, Continued Use or Continued Problem Potential	In Dimension 5, the patient meets specifications in *one* of the following: (a) The patient requires structured therapy, pharmacotherapy and programmatic milieu to promote treatment progress because he or she attributes continued relapse to physiologic craving or the need for opiates; *or* (b) Despite active participation in other treatment interventions without provision for opioid maintenance therapy, the patient is experiencing an intensification of addiction symptoms (such as difficulty in postponing immediate gratification and related drug-seeking behavior) or continued high-risk behaviors (such as shared needle use), and his or her level of functioning is deteriorating, despite revisions of the treatment plan; *or* (c) The patient is at high risk of relapse to opiate use without opioid maintenance therapy, close outpatient monitoring and structured support, as indicated by his or her lack of awareness of relapse triggers, difficulty in postponing immediate gratification or ambivalence toward or resistance to treatment.

Adult Criteria
Diagnostic and Dimensional Criteria

CRITERIA	OPIOID MAINTENANCE THERAPY
DIMENSION 6: Recovery Environment	In Dimension 6, the patient meets specifications in *one* of the following: (a) The patient has a sufficiently supportive psychosocial environment to render opioid maintenance therapy feasible (for example, significant others are supportive of recovery efforts, the patient's workplace is supportive, the patient is subject to legal coercion, the patient has adequate transportation to the program, and the like); *or* (b) The patient's family members or significant others are supportive, but require professional intervention to improve the patient's likelihood of treatment success (such as assistance with limit-setting, communication skills, avoiding rescuing behaviors, education about methadone treatment and HIV risk avoidance, and the like); *or* (c) The patient does not have a positive social support system to assist with immediate recovery efforts, but he or she has demonstrated motivation to obtain such a support system or to pursue (with assistance) an appropriate alternative living environment; *or* (d) The patient has experienced traumatic events in his or her recovery environment (such as physical, emotional, sexual or domestic abuse) or has manifested the effects of emotional, behavioral or cognitive problems in the environment (such as criminal activity), but these are manageable on an outpatient basis.

Dimension 1:
Adult Detoxification

Dimension 1, Acute Intoxication and/or Withdrawal Potential, is the first of the six primary assessment areas to be evaluated in making treatment and placement decisions. The range of clinical severity seen in this dimension has given rise to multiple levels of intensity in the management of detoxification.

In this context, detoxification refers not only to the attenuation of the physiological and psychological features of withdrawal syndromes, but also to the process of interrupting the momentum of compulsive use in persons diagnosed with substance *dependence*. Because of the force of this momentum and the inherent difficulties in overcoming it even when there is no clear withdrawal syndrome, this phase of treatment frequently requires a greater intensity of services initially in order to establish treatment engagement and patient role induction. This is, of course, critical to the course of treatment because of the impossibility of engaging a patient in treatment while that patient is caught up in the cycle of frequent intoxication and withdrawal.

Treatment Levels Within Dimension 1

Level I-D: Ambulatory Detoxification Without Extended On-Site Monitoring

Level I-D detoxification is an organized outpatient service, which may be delivered in an office setting, health care or addiction treatment facility, or in a patient's home by trained clinicians who provide medically supervised evaluation, detoxification and referral services according to a pre-determined schedule. Such services are provided in regularly scheduled sessions. Level I-D services should be delivered under a defined set of policies and procedures or medical protocols.

Outpatient detoxification services should be designed to treat the patient's level of clinical severity and to achieve safe and comfortable withdrawal from mood-altering drugs (including alcohol) and to effectively facilitate the patient's transition into ongoing treatment and recovery.

Level II-D: Ambulatory Detoxification With Extended On-Site Monitoring

Level II-D detoxification is an organized outpatient service, which may be delivered in an office setting, health care or addiction treatment facility by trained clinicians who provide medically supervised evaluation, detoxification and referral services. Level II-D services are provided in regularly scheduled sessions. They are delivered under a defined set of policies and procedures or medical protocols. Outpatient services are designed to treat the patient's level of clinical severity and to achieve safe and comfortable withdrawal from mood-altering drugs (including alcohol) and to effectively facilitate the patient's entry into ongoing treatment and recovery.

Essential to this level of care is the availability of appropriately credentialed and licensed nurses (such as registered nurses or licensed practical nurses), who monitor patients over a period of several hours each day of service.

Level III-D: Residential/Inpatient Detoxification

Criteria are provided for two types of Level III detoxification programs: Level III.2-D (Clinically Managed Residential Detoxification) and Level III.7-D (Medically Monitored Inpatient Detoxification). The "residential" level of care has, in the past, been synonymous with rehabilitation services, whereas detoxification services and the "inpatient" level of care have been synonymous with acute inpatient hospital care. With the increased availability and utilization of Medically Monitored Inpatient Detoxification services, the terms "residential" and "inpatient" are being used more broadly to contrast ambulatory ("outpatient") detoxification with non-ambulatory ("residential" or "inpatient") detoxification services. The difference between these two levels of detoxification is the intensity of clinical services, particularly as demonstrated by the degree of involvement of medical and nursing professionals.

Level III.2-D: Clinically Managed Residential Detoxification (sometimes referred to as "social setting detoxification") is an organized service that may be delivered by appropriately trained staff, who provide 24-hour supervision, observation and support for patients who are intoxicated or experiencing withdrawal. Clinically managed residential detoxification is characterized by its emphasis on peer and social support.

This level provides care for patients whose intoxication/withdrawal signs and symptoms are sufficiently severe to require 24-hour structure and support. However, the full resources of a Level III.7-D, medically monitored inpatient detoxification service, are not necessary.

Some clinically managed residential detoxification programs are staffed to supervise self-administered medications for the management of withdrawal. All programs at this level rely on established clinical protocols to identify patients who are in need of medical services beyond the capacity of the facility and to transfer such patients to more appropriate levels of care.

Level III.7-D: Medically Monitored Inpatient Detoxification is an organized service delivered by medical and nursing professionals, which provides for 24-hour medically supervised evaluation and withdrawal management in a permanent facility with inpatient beds. Services are delivered under a defined set of physician-approved policies and physician-monitored procedures or clinical protocols.

This level provides care to patients whose withdrawal signs and symptoms are sufficiently severe to require 24-hour inpatient care. It sometimes is provided by overlapping with Level IV-D services (as a "step-down" service) in a specialty unit of an acute care general or psychiatric hospital. Twenty-four hour observation, monitoring and treatment are available. However, the full resources of an acute care general hospital or a medically managed intensive inpatient treatment program are not necessary.

Level III.7-D detoxification also can be provided by overlapping with Level IV-D detoxification as a step-down service in a specialty unit of a general or psychiatric hospital.

Level IV-D: Medically Managed Intensive Inpatient Detoxification

Level IV-D detoxification is an organized service delivered by medical and nursing professionals that provides for 24-hour medically directed evaluation and withdrawal management in an acute care inpatient setting. Services are delivered under a defined set of physician-approved policies and physician-managed procedures or medical protocols.

Level IV-D provides care to patients whose withdrawal signs and symptoms are sufficiently severe to require primary medical and nursing care services. Twenty-four hour observation, monitoring and treatment are available. Although Level IV-D is specifically designed for acute medical detoxification, it also is important to assess the patient and develop a care plan for any treatment priorities identified in Dimensions 2 through 6.

Adult Criteria
Comparison of Detoxification Services Across Treatment Levels

CHARACTERISTIC	LEVEL I-D Ambulatory Detoxification without Extended On-Site Monitoring	LEVEL II-D Ambulatory Detoxification with Extended On-Site Monitoring	LEVEL III.2-D Clinically Managed Residential Detoxification	LEVEL III.7-D Medically Monitored Inpatient Detoxification	LEVEL IV-D Medically Managed Intensive Inpatient Detoxification
EXAMPLES	Physician's office or home health care agency	Day hospital service	Social setting detoxification program	Freestanding detoxification center	Psychiatric hospital inpatient unit
SETTING	Level I-D detoxification may be conducted in a general health care facility, such as a physician's office, a freestanding urgent care center or hospital emergency department, an addiction or mental health treatment facility, a hospital outpatient department, or the patient's home, supervised by a licensed home health care agency.	Level II-D detoxification may be conducted in a general health care facility, such as a physician's office, a freestanding urgent care center or hospital emergency department, an addiction or mental health treatment facility, or a hospital outpatient department. When the focus of care initially is on evaluation to determine the need for more or less intensive detoxification services,	Level III.2-D detoxification may be conducted in an appropriately licensed health care or addiction treatment facility.	Level III.7-D detoxification may be conducted in a freestanding or other appropriately licensed health care or addiction treatment facility.	Level IV-D detoxification may be conducted in an appropriately licensed acute care setting that can provide medically directed acute detoxification and related treatment aimed at alleviating acute emotional, behavioral, cognitive or biomedical distress resulting from the patient's use of alcohol or other drugs. At least three types of settings provide this level of care:

ASAM Patient Placement Criteria, Second Edition–Revised

Adult Criteria
Comparison of Detoxification Services Across Treatment Levels

CHARACTERISTIC	LEVEL I-D Ambulatory Detoxification without Extended On-Site Monitoring	LEVEL II-D Ambulatory Detoxification with Extended On-Site Monitoring	LEVEL III.2-D Clinically Managed Residential Detoxification	LEVEL III.7-D Medically Monitored Inpatient Detoxification	LEVEL IV-D Medically Managed Intensive Inpatient Detoxification
SETTING (continued)		Level II-D services may be provided in a "23-hour bed." More often, however, this level of detoxification is conducted in addiction specialty treatment facilities and is fully integrated with Level II addiction services that address Dimensions 2 through 6 of the patient's condition. Thus, intensive outpatient and partial hospitalization facilities, or settings where such services are offered, are appropriate for Level II-D detoxification.			(a) An acute care general hospital; or (b) An acute care psychiatric hospital with ready access to the full resources of an acute care general hospital, or a psychiatric unit in an acute care general hospital; or (c) An appropriately licensed chemical dependency specialty hospital with acute care medical and nursing staff and life support equipment, or an acute care addiction treatment unit in an acute care general hospital.

Adult Criteria
Comparison of Detoxification Services Across Treatment Levels

CHARACTERISTIC	LEVEL I-D Ambulatory Detoxification without Extended On-Site Monitoring	LEVEL II-D Ambulatory Detoxification with Extended On-Site Monitoring	LEVEL III.2-D Clinically Managed Residential Detoxification	LEVEL III.7-D Medically Monitored Inpatient Detoxification	LEVEL IV-D Medically Managed Intensive Inpatient Detoxification
SUPPORT SYSTEMS	In Level I-D detoxification, support systems feature: (a) Availability of specialized clinical consultation and supervision for biomedical, emotional, behavioral and cognitive problems. (b) Ability to obtain a comprehensive medical history and physical examination of the patient at admission.	In Level II-D detoxification, support systems feature: (a) Availability of specialized clinical consultation and supervision for biomedical, emotional, behavioral and cognitive problems. (b) Ability to obtain a comprehensive medical history and physical examination of the patient at admission.	In Level III.2-D detoxification, support systems feature: (a) Availability of specialized clinical consultation and supervision for biomedical, emotional, behavioral and cognitive problems. (b) Protocols used to determine the nature of the medical interventions required (including nursing and physician care and/or transfer to a medically monitored facility or an acute care hospital) are developed and supported by a physician knowledgeable in addiction medicine.	In Level III.7-D detoxification, support systems feature: (a) Availability of specialized clinical consultation and supervision for biomedical, emotional, behavioral and cognitive problems. (b) Availability of medical and nursing care and observation as warranted, based on clinical judgment.	In Level IV-D detoxification, support systems feature: (a) Availability of specialized medical consultation. (b) Full medical acute care services.

ASAM Patient Placement Criteria, Second Edition–Revised

Adult Criteria
Comparison of Detoxification Services
Across Treatment Levels

CHARACTERISTIC	LEVEL I-D Ambulatory Detoxification without Extended On-Site Monitoring	LEVEL II-D Ambulatory Detoxification with Extended On-Site Monitoring	LEVEL III.2-D Clinically Managed Residential Detoxification	LEVEL III.7-D Medically Monitored Inpatient Detoxification	LEVEL IV-D Medically Managed Intensive Inpatient Detoxification
SUPPORT SYSTEMS (continued)	(c) Access to psychological and psychiatric consultation. (d) Direct affiliation with other levels of care, including other levels of specialty addiction treatment, as well as general and psychiatric services for additional problems identified through a comprehensive biopsychosocial assessment. (e) Ability to conduct and/or arrange for appropriate laboratory and toxicology tests. (f) 24-hour access to emergency medical services.	(c) Access to psychological and psychiatric consultation. (d) Direct affiliation with other levels of care, including other levels of specialty addiction treatment, as well as general and psychiatric services for additional problems identified through a comprehensive biopsychosocial assessment. (e) Ability to conduct and/or arrange for appropriate laboratory and toxicology tests. (f) 24-hour access to emergency medical services.	(c) Direct affiliation with other levels of care. (d) Ability to arrange for appropriate laboratory and toxicology tests.	(c) Direct affiliation with other levels of care. (d) Ability to conduct or arrange for appropriate laboratory and toxicology tests.	(c) Intensive care, as needed.

Adult Criteria
Comparison of Detoxification Services
Across Treatment Levels

CHARACTERISTIC	LEVEL I-D Ambulatory Detoxification without Extended On-Site Monitoring	LEVEL II-D Ambulatory Detoxification with Extended On-Site Monitoring	LEVEL III.2-D Clinically Managed Residential Detoxification	LEVEL III.7-D Medically Monitored Inpatient Detoxification	LEVEL IV-D Medically Managed Intensive Inpatient Detoxification
SUPPORT SYSTEMS (continued)	(g) Ability to provide or assist in accessing transportation services for patients who are unable to drive safely for legal or medical reasons, or who otherwise lack transportation.	(g) Ability to provide or assist in accessing transportation services for patients who are unable to drive safely for legal or medical reasons, or who otherwise lack transportation.			
STAFF	Level I-D detoxification programs are staffed by physicians and nurses, who are essential to this type of service, although they need not be present in the treatment setting at all times. (In states where physician assistants or nurse practitioners are licensed as physician extenders, they	Level II-D detoxification programs are staffed by physicians and nurses, who are essential to this type of service, although they need not be present at all times. (In states where physician assistants or nurse practitioners are licensed as physician extenders, they may perform the duties designated for a physician.)	Level III.2-D social detoxification programs are staffed by appropriately credentialed personnel who are trained and competent to implement physician-approved protocols for patient observation and supervision, determination of appropriate level of care,	Level III.7-D detoxification programs are staffed by physicians, who are available 24 hours a day by telephone. (In states where physician assistants or nurse practitioners are licensed as physician extenders, they may perform the duties designated for a physician.)

A physician is available to assess the patient | Level IV-D detoxification programs are staffed by physicians, who are available 24 hours a day as an active member of an interdisciplinary team of appropriately trained professionals, and who medically manage the care of the patient. (In states where physician assistants or nurse practitioners are |

ASAM Patient Placement Criteria, Second Edition–Revised

Adult Criteria
Comparison of Detoxification Services
Across Treatment Levels

CHARACTERISTIC	LEVEL I-D Ambulatory Detoxification without Extended On-Site Monitoring	LEVEL II-D Ambulatory Detoxification with Extended On-Site Monitoring	LEVEL III.2-D Clinically Managed Residential Detoxification	LEVEL III.7-D Medically Monitored Inpatient Detoxification	LEVEL IV-D Medically Managed Intensive Inpatient Detoxification
STAFF (continued)	may perform the duties designated for a physician.) Because Level I-D detoxification is conducted on an outpatient basis, it is important for medical and nursing personnel to be readily available to evaluate and confirm that detoxification in the less supervised setting is relatively safe. (These services are distinguished from Level III.2-D services.) The services of counselors, psychologists and social workers may be available through the detoxification program, or may be accessed through affiliation with	Because Level II-D detoxification is conducted on an outpatient basis, it is important for medical and nursing personnel to be readily available to evaluate and confirm that detoxification in the less supervised setting is relatively safe. The services of counselors, psychologists and social workers may be available through the detoxification program or may be accessed through affiliation with entities providing other Level II services. All clinicians who assess and treat patients are able to obtain	and facilitation of the patient's transition to continuing care. Level III.2-D social detoxification is a clinically managed detoxification service designed explicitly to safely detoxify patients without the need for ready on-site access to medical and nursing personnel. Medical evaluation and consultation is available 24 hours a day, in accordance with treatment/transfer practice guidelines. All clinicians who assess and treat patients are able to obtain and interpret	within 24 hours of admission (or earlier, if medically necessary), and is available to provide on-site monitoring of care and further evaluation on a daily basis. A registered nurse or other licensed and credentialed nurse is available to conduct a nursing assessment on admission. A nurse is responsible for overseeing the monitoring of the patient's progress and medication administration on an hourly basis, if needed. Appropriately licensed and credentialed staff	licensed as physician extenders, they may perform the duties designated for a physician.) A registered nurse or other licensed and credentialed nurse is available for primary nursing care and observation 24 hours a day. Facility-approved addiction counselors or licensed, certified or registered addiction clinicians are available 8 hours a day to administer planned interventions according to the assessed needs of the patient. An interdisciplinary team of

ASAM Patient Placement Criteria, Second Edition–Revised

Adult Criteria
Comparison of Detoxification Services
Across Treatment Levels

CHARACTERISTIC	LEVEL I-D Ambulatory Detoxification without Extended On-Site Monitoring	LEVEL II-D Ambulatory Detoxification with Extended On-Site Monitoring	LEVEL III.2-D Clinically Managed Residential Detoxification	LEVEL III.7-D Medically Monitored Inpatient Detoxification	LEVEL IV-D Medically Managed Intensive Inpatient Detoxification
STAFF (continued)	other entities providing Level I services. All clinicians who assess and treat patients are able to obtain and interpret information regarding the needs of these persons, and are knowledgeable about the biopsychosocial dimensions of alcohol and other drug dependence. Such knowledge includes the signs and symptoms of alcohol and other drug intoxication and withdrawal, as well as the appropriate treatment and monitoring of those conditions and how to facilitate the individual's entry into ongoing care.	and interpret information regarding the needs of these persons, and are knowledgeable about the biopsychosocial dimensions of alcohol and other drug dependence. Such knowledge includes the signs and symptoms of alcohol and other drug intoxication and withdrawal, as well as the appropriate treatment and monitoring of those conditions and how to facilitate entry into ongoing care.	information regarding the needs of these patients. Such knowledge includes the signs and symptoms of alcohol and other drug intoxication and withdrawal, as well as the appropriate treatment and monitoring of those conditions and how to facilitate entry into ongoing care. Facilities that supervise self-administered medications have appropriately licensed or credentialed staff and policies and procedures in accordance with state and federal law.	are available to administer medications in accordance with physician orders. The level of nursing care is appropriate to the severity of patient needs. Licensed, certified or registered clinicians provide a planned regimen of 24-hour, professionally directed evaluation, care and treatment services for patients and their families. An interdisciplinary team of appropriately trained clinicians (such as physicians, nurses, counselors, social workers and	appropriately trained clinicians (such as physicians, nurses, counselors, social workers and psychologists) is available to assess and treat the patient with a substance-related disorder, or an addicted patient with a concomitant acute biomedical, emotional or behavioral disorder.

Adult Criteria
Comparison of Detoxification Services Across Treatment Levels

CHARACTERISTIC	LEVEL I-D Ambulatory Detoxification without Extended On-Site Monitoring	LEVEL II-D Ambulatory Detoxification with Extended On-Site Monitoring	LEVEL III.2-D Clinically Managed Residential Detoxification	LEVEL III.7-D Medically Monitored Inpatient Detoxification	LEVEL IV-D Medically Managed Intensive Inpatient Detoxification
STAFF (continued)	Medical consultation is readily available in emergencies.	Medical consultation is readily available in emergencies.	Staff assure that patients are taking medications according to physician prescription and legal requirements.	psychologists) is available to assess and treat the patient and to obtain and interpret information regarding the patient's needs. The number and disciplines of team members are appropriate to the range and severity of the patient's problems.	
THERAPIES	Therapies offered by Level I-D detoxification programs include individual assessment, medication or non-medication methods of detoxification, involvement of family members or significant other in the detoxification process, and discharge or transfer planning.	Therapies offered by Level II-D detoxification programs include individual assessment, medication or non-medication methods of detoxification, involvement of family members or significant other in the detoxification process, and discharge or transfer planning.	Therapies offered by Level III.2-D detoxification programs include daily clinical services to assess and address the needs of each patient. Such clinical services may include appropriate medical services, individual and group therapies, and withdrawal support.	Therapies offered by Level III.7-D detoxification programs include daily clinical services to assess and address the needs of each patient. Such clinical services may include appropriate medical services, individual and group therapies, and withdrawal support.	Therapies offered by Level IV-D detoxification programs include highly individualized biomedical, emotional, behavioral and addiction treatment. This includes the management of all concomitant biomedical, emotional, behavioral and cognitive

ASAM Patient Placement Criteria, Second Edition–Revised

Adult Criteria
Comparison of Detoxification Services Across Treatment Levels

CHARACTERISTIC	LEVEL I-D Ambulatory Detoxification without Extended On-Site Monitoring	LEVEL II-D Ambulatory Detoxification with Extended On-Site Monitoring	LEVEL III.2-D Clinically Managed Residential Detoxification	LEVEL III.7-D Medically Monitored Inpatient Detoxification	LEVEL IV-D Medically Managed Intensive Inpatient Detoxification
THERAPIES (continued)	Therapies also may include physician and/or nurse monitoring, assessment and management of signs and symptoms of intoxication and withdrawal.	Therapies also may include physician and/or nurse monitoring, assessment and management of signs and symptoms of intoxication and withdrawal.	The following therapies are provided as clinically necessary, depending on the patient's progress through detoxification and his or her assessed needs in Dimensions 2 through 6:	Hourly nurse monitoring of the patient's progress and medication administration are available, if needed.

The following therapies are provided as clinically necessary, depending on the patient's progress through detoxification and the assessed needs in Dimensions 2 through 6: | conditions in the context of addiction treatment. (The extent to which concomitant conditions can be treated depends on the capabilities of the particular Level IV-D setting.)

Hourly or more frequent nurse monitoring is available, if needed.

The following therapies are provided as clinically necessary, depending on the patient's progress through detoxification and the assessed needs in Dimensions 2 through 6: |

Adult Criteria
Comparison of Detoxification Services Across Treatment Levels

CHARACTERISTIC	LEVEL I-D Ambulatory Detoxification without Extended On-Site Monitoring	LEVEL II-D Ambulatory Detoxification with Extended On-Site Monitoring	LEVEL III.2-D Clinically Managed Residential Detoxification	LEVEL III.7-D Medically Monitored Inpatient Detoxification	LEVEL IV-D Medically Managed Intensive Inpatient Detoxification
THERAPIES (continued)			(a) A range of cognitive, behavioral, medical, mental health and other therapies are administered to the patient on an individual or group basis. These are designed to enhance the patient's understanding of addiction, the completion of the detoxification process and referral to an appropriate level of care for continuing treatment.	(a) A range of cognitive, behavioral, medical, mental health and other therapies are administered to the patient on an individual or group basis. These are designed to enhance the patient's understanding of addiction, the completion of the detoxification process and referral to an appropriate level of care for continuing treatment.	(a) A range of cognitive, behavioral, medical, mental health and other therapies. These are designed to enhance the patient's understanding of addiction, the completion of the detoxification process and referral to an appropriate level of care for continuing treatment. For the patient with a severe comorbid psychiatric disorder, psychiatric interventions complement addiction treatment. For the patient with a severe comorbid biomedical disorder, biomedical interventions complement addiction treatment.

Adult Criteria
Comparison of Detoxification Services Across Treatment Levels

CHARACTERISTIC	LEVEL I-D Ambulatory Detoxification without Extended On-Site Monitoring	LEVEL II-D Ambulatory Detoxification with Extended On-Site Monitoring	LEVEL III.2-D Clinically Managed Residential Detoxification	LEVEL III.7-D Medically Monitored Inpatient Detoxification	LEVEL IV-D Medically Managed Intensive Inpatient Detoxification
THERAPIES (continued)			(b) Multidisciplinary individualized assessment and treatment. (c) Health education services. (d) Services to families and significant others.	(b) Multidisciplinary individualized assessment and treatment. (c) Health education services. (d) Services to families and significant others.	(b) Health education services. (c) Services to families and significant others.
ASSESSMENTS/ TREATMENT PLAN REVIEW	In Level I-D detoxification programs, elements of the assessment and treatment plan review include: (a) An addiction-focused history, obtained as part of the initial assessment and reviewed by a physician during the admission process.	In Level II-D detoxification programs, elements of the assessment and treatment plan review include: (a) An addiction-focused history, obtained as part of the initial assessment and reviewed by a physician during the admission process.	In Level III.2-D detoxification programs, elements of the assessment and treatment plan review include: (a) An addiction-focused history, obtained as part of the initial assessment and reviewed with a physician during the admission process if physician-developed protocols indicate concern.	In Level III.7-D detoxification programs, elements of the assessment and treatment plan review include: (a) An addiction-focused history, obtained as part of the initial assessment and reviewed by a physician during the admission process.	In Level IV-D detoxification programs, elements of the assessment and treatment plan review include: (a) A comprehensive nursing assessment, performed at admission.

Adult Criteria
Comparison of Detoxification Services Across Treatment Levels

CHARACTERISTIC	LEVEL I-D Ambulatory Detoxification without Extended On-Site Monitoring	LEVEL II-D Ambulatory Detoxification with Extended On-Site Monitoring	LEVEL III.2-D Clinically Managed Residential Detoxification	LEVEL III.7-D Medically Monitored Inpatient Detoxification	LEVEL IV-D Medically Managed Intensive Inpatient Detoxification
ASSESSMENTS/ TREATMENT PLAN REVIEW (continued)	(b) A physical examination by a physician, physician assistant or nurse practitioner, performed within a reasonable time frame as part of the initial assessment.	(b) A physical examination by a physician, physician assistant, or nurse practitioner within a reasonable time frame as part of the initial assessment.	(b) A physical examination by a physician, physician assistant, or nurse practitioner as part of the initial assessment if self-administered detoxification medications are to be used.	(b) A physical examination by a physician, physician assistant, or nurse practitioner within 24 hours of admission, and appropriate laboratory and toxicology tests. If Level III.7-D detoxification services are step-down services from Level IV-D, records of a physical examination within the preceding 7 days are evaluated by a physician within 24 hours of admission.	(b) Approval of the admission by a physician.
	(c) Sufficient biopsychosocial screening assessments to determine the level of care in which the person should be placed and for the individualized care plan to	(c) Sufficient biopsychosocial screening assessments to determine the level of care in which the patient should be placed for the individualized care plan to	(c) Sufficient biopsychosocial screening assessments to determine the level of care in which the patient should be placed and for the individualized care plan to	(c) Sufficient biopsychosocial screening assessments to determine the level of care in which the patient should be placed and for the individualized care plan to	(c) A comprehensive history and physical examination performed within 24 hours of admission, accompanied by appropriate laboratory and toxicology tests.

Adult Criteria
Comparison of Detoxification Services Across Treatment Levels

CHARACTERISTIC	LEVEL I-D Ambulatory Detoxification without Extended On-Site Monitoring	LEVEL II-D Ambulatory Detoxification with Extended On-Site Monitoring	LEVEL III.2-D Clinically Managed Residential Detoxification	LEVEL III.7-D Medically Monitored Inpatient Detoxification	LEVEL IV-D Medically Managed Intensive Inpatient Detoxification
ASSESSMENTS/ TREATMENT PLAN REVIEW (continued)	address treatment priorities identified in Dimensions 2 through 6. (d) An individualized treatment plan, including problem identification in Dimensions 2 through 6 and development of treatment goals and measurable treatment objectives, as well as activities designed to meet those objectives. (e) Daily assessment of progress during detoxification and any treatment changes (or less frequently, if the severity of withdrawal is sufficiently mild or stable).	address treatment priorities identified in Dimensions 2 through 6. (d) An individualized treatment plan, including problem identification in Dimensions 2 through 6 and development of treatment goals and measurable treatment objectives and activities designed to meet those objectives. (e) Daily assessment of progress during detoxification and any treatment changes.	address treatment priorities identified in Dimensions 2 through 6. (d) An individualized treatment plan, including problem identification in Dimensions 2 through 6 and development of treatment goals and measurable treatment objectives and activities designed to meet those objectives. (e) Daily assessment of patient progress through detoxification and any treatment changes.	address treatment priorities identified in Dimensions 2 through 6. (d) An individualized treatment plan, including problem identification in Dimensions 2 through 6 and development of treatment goals and measurable treatment objectives and activities designed to meet those objectives. (e) Daily assessment of patient progress through detoxification and any treatment changes.	(d) An addiction-focused history, obtained as part of the initial assessment and reviewed by a physician during the admission process. (e) Sufficient biopsychosocial screening assessments to determine placement, and for the individualized care plan to address treatment priorities identified in Dimensions 2 through 6.

Adult Criteria
Comparison of Detoxification Services Across Treatment Levels

CHARACTERISTIC	LEVEL I-D Ambulatory Detoxification without Extended On-Site Monitoring	LEVEL II-D Ambulatory Detoxification with Extended On-Site Monitoring	LEVEL III.2-D Clinically Managed Residential Detoxification	LEVEL III.7-D Medically Monitored Inpatient Detoxification	LEVEL IV-D Medically Managed Intensive Inpatient Detoxification
ASSESSMENTS/ TREATMENT PLAN REVIEW (continued)	(f) Discharge/transfer planning, beginning at admission. (g) Referral arrangements, made as needed.	(f) Discharge/transfer planning, beginning at admission. (g) Referral arrangements, made as needed. (h) Serial nursing assessments, using appropriate measures of withdrawal.	(f) Discharge/transfer planning, beginning at admission. (g) Referral arrangements, made as needed.	(f) Discharge/transfer planning, beginning at admission. (g) Referral arrangements, made as needed.	(f) Discharge/transfer planning, beginning at admission. (g) Referral arrangements, made as needed. (h) An individualized treatment plan, including problem identification in Dimensions 2 through 6 and development of treatment goals and measurable treatment objectives and activities designed to meet those objectives. (i) Daily assessment of patient progress through detoxification and any treatment changes.

Adult Criteria
Comparison of Detoxification Services Across Treatment Levels

CHARACTERISTIC	LEVEL I-D Ambulatory Detoxification without Extended On-Site Monitoring	LEVEL II-D Ambulatory Detoxification with Extended On-Site Monitoring	LEVEL III.2-D Clinically Managed Residential Detoxification	LEVEL III.7-D Medically Monitored Inpatient Detoxification	LEVEL IV-D Medically Managed Intensive Inpatient Detoxification
DOCUMENTATION	Documentation standards of Level I-D programs include progress notes in the patient record that clearly reflect implementation of the treatment plan and the patient's response to treatment, as well as subsequent amendments to the plan. Detoxification rating scale tables and flow sheets (which may include tabulation of vital signs) are used as needed.	Documentation standards of Level I-D programs include progress notes in the patient record that clearly reflect implementation of the treatment plan and the patient's response to treatment, as well as subsequent amendments to the plan. Detoxification rating scale tables and flow sheets (which may include tabulation of vital signs) are used as needed.	Documentation standards of Level I-D programs include progress notes in the patient record that clearly reflect implementation of the treatment plan and the patient's response to treatment, as well as subsequent amendments to the plan. Detoxification rating scale tables and flow sheets (which may include tabulation of vital signs) are used as needed.	Documentation standards of Level I-D programs include progress notes in the patient record that clearly reflect implementation of the treatment plan and the patient's response to treatment, as well as subsequent amendments to the plan. Detoxification rating scale tables and flow sheets (which may include tabulation of vital signs) are used as needed.	Documentation standards of Level I-D programs include progress notes in the patient record that clearly reflect implementation of the treatment plan and the patient's response to treatment, as well as subsequent amendments to the plan. Detoxification rating scale tables and flow sheets (which may include tabulation of vital signs) are used as needed.
DIAGNOSTIC ADMISSION CRITERIA	The patient who is appropriately placed in a Level I-D detoxification program meets the diagnostic criteria for Substance-Induced Disorder of the current	The patient who is appropriately placed in a Level II-D detoxification program meets the diagnostic criteria for Substance-Induced Disorder of the current	The patient who is appropriately placed in a Level III.2-D detoxification program meets the diagnostic criteria for Substance-Induced Disorder	The patient who is appropriately placed in a Level III.7-D detoxification program meets the diagnostic criteria for Substance-Induced Disorder	The patient who is appropriately placed in a Level IV-D detoxification program meets the diagnostic criteria for Substance-Induced Disorder

Adult Criteria
Comparison of Detoxification Services Across Treatment Levels

CHARACTERISTIC	LEVEL I-D Ambulatory Detoxification without Extended On-Site Monitoring	LEVEL II-D Ambulatory Detoxification with Extended On-Site Monitoring	LEVEL III.2-D Clinically Managed Residential Detoxification	LEVEL III.7-D Medically Monitored Inpatient Detoxification	LEVEL IV-D Medically Managed Intensive Inpatient Detoxification
DIAGNOSTIC ADMISSION CRITERIA (continued)	*Diagnostic and Statistical Manual of Mental Disorders* of the American Psychiatric Association or other standardized and widely accepted criteria, as well as the dimensional criteria for admission. In patients whose presenting alcohol or other drug history is inadequate to substantiate such a diagnosis, information provided by collateral parties (such as family members or legal guardian) indicates a high probability of such a diagnosis, subject to confirmation by further evaluation.	*Diagnostic and Statistical Manual of Mental Disorders* of the American Psychiatric Association or other standardized and widely accepted criteria, as well as the dimensional criteria for admission. In patients whose presenting alcohol or other drug history is inadequate to substantiate such a diagnosis, information provided by collateral parties (such as family members or legal guardian) indicates a high probability of such a diagnosis, subject to confirmation by further evaluation.	of the *Diagnostic and Statistical Manual of Mental Disorders* of the American Psychiatric Association or other standardized and widely accepted criteria, as well as the dimensional criteria for admission.	of the *Diagnostic and Statistical Manual of Mental Disorders* of the American Psychiatric Association or other standardized and widely accepted criteria, as well as the dimensional criteria for admission.	of the *Diagnostic and Statistical Manual of Mental Disorders* of the American Psychiatric Association or other standardized and widely accepted criteria, as well as the dimensional criteria for admission.

Adult Criteria
Comparison of Detoxification Services Across Treatment Levels

CHARACTERISTIC	LEVEL I-D Ambulatory Detoxification without Extended On-Site Monitoring	LEVEL II-D Ambulatory Detoxification with Extended On-Site Monitoring	LEVEL III.2-D Clinically Managed Residential Detoxification	LEVEL III.7-D Medically Monitored Inpatient Detoxification	LEVEL IV-D Medically Managed Intensive Inpatient Detoxification
DIMENSIONAL ADMISSION CRITERIA	The patient who is appropriately placed in a Level I-D detoxification program meets specifications in (a) *and* (b) *and* (c): (a) The patient is experiencing at least mild signs and symptoms of withdrawal, or there is evidence (based on history of substance intake, age, gender, previous withdrawal history, present symptoms, physical condition, and/or emotional, behavioral or cognitive condition) that withdrawal is imminent.	The patient who is appropriately placed in a Level II-D detoxification program meets specifications in (a) *and* (b): (a) The patient is experiencing signs and symptoms of withdrawal, or there is evidence (based on history of substance intake, age, gender, previous withdrawal history, present symptoms, physical condition, and/or emotional, behavioral or cognitive condition) that withdrawal is imminent.	The patient who is appropriately placed in a Level III.2-D detoxification program meets specifications in (a) *and* (b): (a) The patient is experiencing signs and symptoms of withdrawal, or there is evidence (based on history of substance intake, age, gender, previous withdrawal history, present symptoms, physical condition, and/or emotional, behavioral or cognitive condition) that withdrawal is imminent.	The patient who is appropriately placed in a Level III.7-D detoxification program meets specifications in (a) *or* (b): (a) The patient is experiencing signs and symptoms of severe withdrawal, or there is evidence (based on history of substance intake, age, gender, previous withdrawal history, present symptoms, physical condition, and/or emotional, behavioral or cognitive condition) that a severe withdrawal syndrome is imminent.	The patient who is appropriately placed in a Level IV-D detoxification program meets specifications in (a) *or* (b): (a) The patient is experiencing signs and symptoms of severe withdrawal, or there is evidence (based on history of substance intake, age, gender, previous withdrawal history, present symptoms, physical condition, and/or emotional, behavioral or cognitive condition) that a severe withdrawal syndrome is imminent.

ASAM Patient Placement Criteria, Second Edition–Revised

Adult Criteria
Comparison of Detoxification Services Across Treatment Levels

CHARACTERISTIC	LEVEL I-D Ambulatory Detoxification without Extended On-Site Monitoring	LEVEL II-D Ambulatory Detoxification with Extended On-Site Monitoring	LEVEL III.2-D Clinically Managed Residential Detoxification	LEVEL III.7-D Medically Monitored Inpatient Detoxification	LEVEL IV-D Medically Managed Intensive Inpatient Detoxification
DIMENSIONAL ADMISSION CRITERIA (continued)	The patient is assessed as being at minimal risk of severe withdrawal syndrome and can be safely managed at this level.	The patient is assessed as being at moderate risk of severe withdrawal syndrome outside the program setting, is free of severe physical and psychiatric complications, and would safely respond to several hours of monitoring, medication and treatment.	The patient is assessed as not being at risk of severe withdrawal syndrome, and moderate withdrawal is safely manageable at this level of service.	The severe withdrawal syndrome is assessed as manageable at this level of service.	
	Examples include, but are not limited to:	Examples include, but are not limited to:	Examples include, but are not limited to:	Examples include, but are not limited to:	Examples include, but are not limited to:
	[1] *Alcohol*: The presence of mild symptoms of withdrawal, with a CIWA-Ar (Clinical Institute Withdrawal Assessment-Alcohol, Revised) score of less than 8, or the equivalent for a comparable standardized scoring system.	[1] *Alcohol*: A CIWA-Ar (Clinical Institute Withdrawal Assessment-Alcohol, Revised) score of 8 to 15, or the equivalent for a comparable standardized scoring system.	[1] *Alcohol*: The patient is intoxicated or is withdrawing from alcohol and the CIWA-Ar (Clinical Institute Withdrawal Assessment-Alcohol, Revised) score is less than 8 at admission, and monitoring is available to assure that it remains less than 8, or the	[1] *Alcohol*: The patient is withdrawing from alcohol, the CIWA-Ar (Clinical Institute Withdrawal Assessment-Alcohol, Revised) score is 10 or greater (or the equivalent for a standardized scoring system) by the end of the period of	[1] *Alcohol*: The patient is withdrawing from alcohol, and the CIWA-Ar score is 10 or greater (or the equivalent for a comparable standardized scoring system), and the patient requires monitoring more often than hourly, requires intravenous

Adult Criteria
Comparison of Detoxification Services Across Treatment Levels

CHARACTERISTIC	LEVEL I-D Ambulatory Detoxification without Extended On-Site Monitoring	LEVEL II-D Ambulatory Detoxification with Extended On-Site Monitoring	LEVEL III.2-D Clinically Managed Residential Detoxification	LEVEL III.7-D Medically Monitored Inpatient Detoxification	LEVEL IV-D Medically Managed Intensive Inpatient Detoxification
DIMENSIONAL ADMISSION CRITERIA (continued)			equivalent for a comparable standardized scoring system.	outpatient monitoring available in Level II-D.	medication or infusions, or requires close behavioral monitoring because of high levels of agitation, confusion or extremes of vital signs.
	[2] *Sedative-hypnotics*: Any recent use is confined to therapeutic levels and is not complicated by daily use of alcohol or other mind-altering drugs known to produce a significant withdrawal syndrome.	[2] *Sedative-hypnotics*: There is a reliable history that the patient is withdrawing from sedative-hypnotics, but there is no evidence of other drug dependence, and withdrawal symptoms have responded to, or are likely to respond to, substitute doses of sedative-hypnotics in the therapeutic range within the observable hours of the program.	[2] *Opiates*: Withdrawal signs and symptoms are distressing but do not require medication for reasonable withdrawal discomfort, and the patient is impulsive and lacks skills needed to prevent immediate continued drug use.	[2] *Sedative-hypnotics*: The patient has ingested sedative-hypnotics at more than therapeutic levels daily for more than 4 weeks and is not responsive to appropriate recent efforts to maintain the dose at therapeutic levels.	[2] *Alcohol and sedative-hypnotics*: The patient is experiencing seizures, *delirium tremens* or severe, persistent hallucinations.

Adult Criteria
Comparison of Detoxification Services Across Treatment Levels

CHARACTERISTIC	LEVEL I-D Ambulatory Detoxification without Extended On-Site Monitoring	LEVEL II-D Ambulatory Detoxification with Extended On-Site Monitoring	LEVEL III.2-D Clinically Managed Residential Detoxification	LEVEL III.7-D Medically Monitored Inpatient Detoxification	LEVEL IV-D Medically Managed Intensive Inpatient Detoxification
DIMENSIONAL ADMISSION CRITERIA (continued)	[3] *Sedative-hypnotics*: There is a reliable history that the patient is withdrawing from therapeutic doses of sedative-hypnotics, but there is no evidence of other alcohol or drug dependence. Withdrawal symptoms have responded to, or are likely to respond to, substitute doses of sedative-hypnotics in the therapeutic range within 2 hours.	[3] *Sedative-hypnotics*: The patient has ingested sedative-hypnotics in excess of therapeutic levels daily for at least 4 weeks, but the risk of seizures, hallucinations, dissociation or severe affective disorder during unobserved periods outside the program is assessed as minimal. Close hourly monitoring is available, if needed. There is no accompanying chronic mental or physical disorder that poses a danger to the patient during withdrawal.	[3] *Stimulants*: The patient has marked lethargy, hypersomnolence, paranoia or mild psychotic symptoms due to stimulant withdrawal, and these are still present beyond a period of outpatient monitoring available in Level II-D services.	[3] *Sedative-hypnotics*: The patient has ingested sedative-hypnotics at more than therapeutic levels daily for more than 4 weeks, in combination with daily alcohol use or regular use of another mind-altering drug known to pose a severe risk of withdrawal. Signs and symptoms of withdrawal are of moderate severity, and the patient cannot be stabilized by the end of the period of outpatient monitoring available at Level II-D.	[3] *Sedative-hypnotics*: The patient has ingested sedative-hypnotics at more than therapeutic levels daily for more than 4 weeks, and the patient has an accompanying acute mental or physical disorder that is complicating withdrawal.
	[4] *Opiates* (for withdrawal management not using opiate substitution methods of detoxification):	[4] *Sedative-hypnotics*: The patient has ingested sedative-hypnotics at not more than therapeutic levels		[4] *Alcohol and sedative-hypnotics*: The patient has marked lethargy or hypersomnolence due to intoxication with	[4] *Sedative-hypnotics*: The patient has ingested sedative-hypnotics daily for at least 6 months, in

Adult Criteria
Comparison of Detoxification Services Across Treatment Levels

CHARACTERISTIC	LEVEL I-D Ambulatory Detoxification without Extended On-Site Monitoring	LEVEL II-D Ambulatory Detoxification with Extended On-Site Monitoring	LEVEL III.2-D Clinically Managed Residential Detoxification	LEVEL III.7-D Medically Monitored Inpatient Detoxification	LEVEL IV-D Medically Managed Intensive Inpatient Detoxification
DIMENSIONAL ADMISSION CRITERIA (continued)	Either the patient's use of high-potency opiates (such as injectable or smoked forms) has not been daily for more than 2 weeks preceding admission or the use of opiates is near the therapeutically recommended level.	daily for at least 6 months, in combination with daily alcohol use or regular use of another mind-altering drug known to have its own dangerous withdrawal syndrome. Nonetheless, the risk of seizures, hallucinations, dissociation or severe affective symptoms outside the program is minimal.		alcohol or other drugs, and a history of severe withdrawal syndrome, or the patient's altered level of consciousness has not stabilized at the end of the period of outpatient monitoring available at Level II-D.	combination with daily alcohol use or regular use of another mind-altering drug known to pose a severe withdrawal syndrome, and the patient has accompanying acute mental or physical disorder that is complicating withdrawal.
	[5] *Opiates* (for withdrawal management using opiate substitution methods of detoxification, such as methadone or other appropriate opiate): Either the patient is being detoxified gradually from opiate maintenance or the patient is	[5] *Opiates* (for withdrawal management not using opiate substitution methods of detoxification): The abstinence syndrome—as indicated by vital signs and evidence of physical discomfort or craving—can be stabilized by the end of each day's		[5] *Opiates* (for withdrawal management not using opiate substitution methods of detoxification): The patient has used injectable opiates daily for more than two weeks and has a history of inability to complete withdrawal as an outpatient or	[5] *Opiates*: The patient is experiencing a severe opiate withdrawal syndrome that has not been stabilized or managed at a less intensive level of service.

ASAM Patient Placement Criteria, Second Edition–Revised

Adult Criteria
Comparison of Detoxification Services Across Treatment Levels

CHARACTERISTIC	LEVEL I-D Ambulatory Detoxification without Extended On-Site Monitoring	LEVEL II-D Ambulatory Detoxification with Extended On-Site Monitoring	LEVEL III.2-D Clinically Managed Residential Detoxification	LEVEL III.7-D Medically Monitored Inpatient Detoxification	LEVEL IV-D Medically Managed Intensive Inpatient Detoxification
DIMENSIONAL ADMISSION CRITERIA (continued)	being treated for mild opiate withdrawal symptoms.	monitoring, so that the patient can manage such symptoms at home with appropriate supervision.		without medication in a Level III.2-D service.	
	[6] *Stimulants*: The patient is withdrawing from stimulants and is experiencing some lethargy, agitation, paranoia, mild psychotic symptoms or depression, but he or she has good impulse control.	[6] *Opiates* (for withdrawal management using opiate substitution methods of detoxification, such as methadone or other appropriate opiate): The withdrawal signs and symptoms are of such severity or instability that extended monitoring is required to determine the appropriate dosage.		[6] *Opiates*: Antagonist medication is to be used in withdrawal in a brief but intensive detoxification (as in multiday pharmacological induction onto naltrexone).	[6] *Opiates*: Antagonist medication is to be used in rapid withdrawal (as in pharmacological induction and resolution of opiate withdrawal with naloxone in 6 hours).

ASAM Patient Placement Criteria, Second Edition–Revised

Adult Criteria
Comparison of Detoxification Services Across Treatment Levels

CHARACTERISTIC	LEVEL I-D Ambulatory Detoxification without Extended On-Site Monitoring	LEVEL II-D Ambulatory Detoxification with Extended On-Site Monitoring	LEVEL III.2-D Clinically Managed Residential Detoxification	LEVEL III.7-D Medically Monitored Inpatient Detoxification	LEVEL IV-D Medically Managed Intensive Inpatient Detoxification
DIMENSIONAL ADMISSION CRITERIA (continued)	[7] *Nicotine*: The patient is withdrawing from nicotine and is experiencing withdrawal symptoms that require either nicotine replacement therapies or non-nicotine agents for symptomatic treatment.	[7] *Stimulants*: The patient is withdrawing from stimulants and is experiencing significant lethargy, agitation, paranoia, psychotic symptoms or depression, and requires extended outpatient monitoring to determine impulse control and readiness for Level I-D ambulatory detoxification services or the need for Level III.2-D detoxification services.		[7] *Stimulants*: The patient has marked lethargy, hypersomnolence, agitation, paranoia, depression or mild psychotic symptoms due to stimulant withdrawal, and has poor impulse control and/or coping skills to prevent immediate continued drug use.	[7] *Stimulants*: Intoxication or withdrawal signs and symptoms require psychiatric or medical monitoring more frequently than hourly (because of psychotic impulsive behavior or depressive suicidality). [8] *All substances*: There is recent (within 24 hours) serious head trauma or loss of consciousness, with persistent mental status or neurological changes resulting in the need to closely observe the patient at least hourly.

ASAM Patient Placement Criteria, Second Edition–Revised

Adult Criteria
Comparison of Detoxification Services Across Treatment Levels

CHARACTERISTIC	LEVEL I-D Ambulatory Detoxification without Extended On-Site Monitoring	LEVEL II-D Ambulatory Detoxification with Extended On-Site Monitoring	LEVEL III.2-D Clinically Managed Residential Detoxification	LEVEL III.7-D Medically Monitored Inpatient Detoxification	LEVEL IV-D Medically Managed Intensive Inpatient Detoxification
DIMENSIONAL ADMISSION CRITERIA (continued)					[9] *All substances*: Drug overdose or intoxication has compromised the patient's mental status, cardiac function or other vital signs or functions. [10] *All substances*: The patient has a significant acute biomedical disorder that poses substantial risk of serious or life-threatening consequences during withdrawal (such as significant hypertension or esophageal varices).
	(b) The patient has withdrawal symptoms but is at minimal risk of severe withdrawal syndrome and is assessed as likely to complete needed	(b) The patient is assessed as likely to complete detoxification and to enter into continued treatment or self-help recovery, as evidenced by	(b) The patient is assessed as not requiring medication, but requires this level of service to complete detoxification and enter into	(b) There is a strong likelihood that the patient (who requires medication) will not complete detoxification at another level of care and enter	(b) Level IV is the only available level of care that can provide the medical support and comfort care needed by the patient, as evidenced by:

ASAM Patient Placement Criteria, Second Edition–Revised

Adult Criteria
Comparison of Detoxification Services Across Treatment Levels

CHARACTERISTIC	LEVEL I-D Ambulatory Detoxification without Extended On-Site Monitoring	LEVEL II-D Ambulatory Detoxification with Extended On-Site Monitoring	LEVEL III.2-D Clinically Managed Residential Detoxification	LEVEL III.7-D Medically Monitored Inpatient Detoxification	LEVEL IV-D Medically Managed Intensive Inpatient Detoxification
DIMENSIONAL ADMISSION CRITERIA (continued)	detoxification and to enter into continued treatment or self-help recovery, as evidenced by meeting [1] or [2] or [3]:	meeting [1] and either [2] or [3] or [4]:	continued treatment or self-help recovery because of inadequate home supervision or support structure, as evidenced by meeting [1] or [2] or [3]:	into continuing treatment or self-help recovery, as evidenced (for example), by any of the following:	
	[1] The patient has an adequate understanding of ambulatory detoxification and has expressed commitment to enter such a program; *or*	[1] The patient or support persons clearly understand instructions for care and are able to follow instructions; *and*	[1] The patient's recovery environment is not supportive of detoxification and entry into treatment, and the patient does not have sufficient coping skills to safely deal with the problems in the recovery environment; *or*	[1] The patient requires medication and has a recent history of detoxification at a less intensive level of care, marked by past and current inability to complete detoxification and enter into continuing addiction treatment. The patient continues to have insufficient skills or supports to complete detoxification; *or*	[1] A detoxification regimen or a patient's response to that regimen that requires monitoring or intervention more frequently than hourly; *or*

ASAM Patient Placement Criteria, Second Edition–Revised

Adult Criteria
Comparison of Detoxification Services Across Treatment Levels

CHARACTERISTIC	LEVEL I-D Ambulatory Detoxification without Extended On-Site Monitoring	LEVEL II-D Ambulatory Detoxification with Extended On-Site Monitoring	LEVEL III.2-D Clinically Managed Residential Detoxification	LEVEL III.7-D Medically Monitored Inpatient Detoxification	LEVEL IV-D Medically Managed Intensive Inpatient Detoxification
DIMENSIONAL ADMISSION CRITERIA (continued)	[2] The patient has adequate support services to ensure commitment to completion of detoxification and entry into ongoing treatment or recovery; *or*	[2] The patient has an adequate understanding of ambulatory detoxification and has expressed commitment to enter such a program; *or*	[2] The patient has a recent history of detoxification at less intensive levels of service that is marked by inability to complete detoxification or to enter into continuing addiction treatment, and the patient continues to have insufficient skills to complete detoxification; *or*	[2] The patient has a recent history of detoxification at less intensive levels of service that is marked by inability to complete detoxification or to enter into continuing addiction treatment, and the patient continues to have insufficient skills to complete detoxification; *or*	[2] The patient's need for detoxification or stabilization while pregnant, until she can be safely treated in a less intensive level of care. For example, the patient does not require medical management (as in the case of a patient who is soon to have the pregnancy terminated), or she no longer is bleeding or leaking amniotic fluid, or an unstable fetal heartbeat has improved.
	[3] The patient is willing to accept a recommendation for treatment (for example, to begin disulfiram, naltrexone or other medication once withdrawal has been	[3] The patient has adequate support services to ensure commitment to completion of detoxification and entry into ongoing treatment or recovery; *or*	[3] The patient recently has demonstrated an inability to complete detoxification at a less intensive level of service, as by continued use of other-than-prescribed drugs	[3] The patient has a comorbid physical, emotional, behavioral or cognitive condition (such as chronic pain with active exacerbation or post-traumatic	

ASAM Patient Placement Criteria, Second Edition–Revised

Adult Criteria
Comparison of Detoxification Services Across Treatment Levels

CHARACTERISTIC	LEVEL I-D Ambulatory Detoxification without Extended On-Site Monitoring	LEVEL II-D Ambulatory Detoxification with Extended On-Site Monitoring	LEVEL III.2-D Clinically Managed Residential Detoxification	LEVEL III.7-D Medically Monitored Inpatient Detoxification	LEVEL IV-D Medically Managed Intensive Inpatient Detoxification
DIMENSIONAL ADMISSION CRITERIA (continued)	managed, or to attend outpatient sessions or self-help groups). (c) For patients whose withdrawal symptoms are no more severe than those noted in section (a), the patient has, and responds positively to, emotional support and comfort, as evidenced by: [1] Decreased emotional symptoms at the close of the initial treatment session; *and* [2] The patient's or support person's ability to clearly understand instructions for care, and the presence of both the ability and resources to follow instructions.	[4] The patient evidences willingness to accept a recommendation for treatment once withdrawal has been managed (for example, to attend outpatient sessions or self-help groups).	or other mind-altering substances.	stress disorder with brief dissociative episodes) that is manageable in a Level III.7-D setting but which increases the clinical severity of the withdrawal and complicates detoxification.	

Adult Criteria
Comparison of Detoxification Services
Across Treatment Levels

CHARACTERISTIC	LEVEL I-D Ambulatory Detoxification without Extended On-Site Monitoring	LEVEL II-D Ambulatory Detoxification with Extended On-Site Monitoring	LEVEL III.2-D Clinically Managed Residential Detoxification	LEVEL III.7-D Medically Monitored Inpatient Detoxification	LEVEL IV-D Medically Managed Intensive Inpatient Detoxification
LENGTH OF SERVICE/ CONTINUED SERVICE AND DISCHARGE CRITERIA	The patient continues in a Level I-D detoxification program until withdrawal signs and symptoms are sufficiently resolved that he or she can participate in self-directed recovery or ongoing treatment without the need for further medical or nursing detoxification monitoring; *or*	The patient continues in a Level II-D detoxification program until withdrawal signs and symptoms are sufficiently resolved that he or she can be safely managed at a less intensive level of care; *or*	The patient continues in a Level III.2-D detoxification program until withdrawal signs and symptoms are sufficiently resolved that he or she can be safely managed at a less intensive level of care; *or*	The patient continues in a Level III.7-D detoxification program until withdrawal signs and symptoms are sufficiently resolved that he or she can be safely managed at a less intensive level of care; *or*	The patient continues in a Level IV-D detoxification program until withdrawal signs and symptoms are sufficiently resolved that he or she can be safely managed at a less intensive level of care.
	Alternatively, the patient's signs and symptoms of withdrawal have failed to respond to treatment and have intensified (as confirmed by higher scores on the CIWA-Ar or other comparable standardized scoring system), such that transfer to a more	Alternatively, the patient's signs and symptoms of withdrawal have failed to respond to treatment and have intensified (as confirmed by higher scores on the CIWA-Ar or other comparable standardized scoring system), such that transfer to a more	Alternatively, the patient's signs and symptoms of withdrawal have failed to respond to treatment and have intensified (as confirmed by higher scores on the CIWA-Ar or other comparable standardized scoring system), such that transfer to a more	Alternatively, the patient's signs and symptoms of withdrawal have failed to respond to treatment and have intensified (as confirmed by higher scores on the CIWA-Ar or other comparable standardized scoring system), such that transfer to a Level IV-D	

Adult Criteria
Comparison of Detoxification Services Across Treatment Levels

CHARACTERISTIC	LEVEL I-D Ambulatory Detoxification without Extended On-Site Monitoring	LEVEL II-D Ambulatory Detoxification with Extended On-Site Monitoring	LEVEL III.2-D Clinically Managed Residential Detoxification	LEVEL III.7-D Medically Monitored Inpatient Detoxification	LEVEL IV-D Medically Managed Intensive Inpatient Detoxification
LENGTH OF SERVICE/ CONTINUED SERVICE AND DISCHARGE CRITERIA (continued)	intensive level of detoxification service is indicated; *or* The patient is unable to complete detoxification at Level I-D, despite an adequate trial. For example, he or she is experiencing intense craving and evidences insufficient coping skills to prevent continued alcohol or other drug use concurrent with the detoxification medication, indicating a need for more intensive services (such as addition of a supportive living environment).	intensive level of detoxification service is indicated; *or* The patient is unable to complete detoxification at Level II-D, despite an adequate trial. For example, he or she is experiencing intense craving and has insufficient coping skills to prevent continued alcohol or other drug use, indicating a need for more intensive services.	intensive level of detoxification service is indicated; *or* The patient is unable to complete detoxification at Level III.2-D, despite an adequate trial. For example, he or she is experiencing increasing depression and suicidal impulses, complicating cocaine withdrawal and indicating the need for transfer to a more intensive level of care or the addition of other clinical services (such as intensive counseling).	detoxification service is indicated.	

Adolescent Patient Placement Criteria

Preface to the Adolescent Criteria

This revision of the adolescent criteria is an incremental one. As with the adult criteria, experience with the first and second editions of the *ASAM Patient Placement Criteria* identified areas in which the adolescent criteria required expansion or revision. Some of these changes involved updating the adolescent criteria in parallel to the adult criteria (where applicable) to match some of the advances achieved from the first (1991) and second (1996) editions. In other areas, the changes cause the adolescent criteria to diverge even more sharply from the adult criteria than in the past; these changes reflect recent scholarship affirming fundamental differences in adolescents' treatment needs and appropriate differences in treatment delivery.

What's New in the Second Edition-Revised?

Major areas of revision in the *ASAM PPC-2R* adolescent criteria include:

- Expansion of the levels of care to include several sublevels, reflecting gradations of intensity along the continuum of care.

- Expansion of Dimension 3 to include cognitive conditions and complications as well as new subdomains of assessment to address psychiatric comorbidity or "dual diagnosis" issues in more detail.

- Expansion of the Dimension 1 assessment elements to include additional detail and some breakdown by specific drug classes.

- Broadened applicability of the criteria to encompass adolescents involved in the public sector and juvenile justice systems, with more explicit consideration of specifically relevant scenarios and examples.

- Replacement of specific separate continued service and discharge criteria for each level of care, with general guidelines for continued service and transfer/discharge.

- Presentation of an experimental needs-based format (as opposed to a placement-based format) that suggests what future editions of the criteria may be.

The goal of the adolescent criteria (like the adult criteria) is to facilitate the process of matching patients in need of treatment with treatment services and settings in order to maximize treatment accessibility, effectiveness and efficiency. The principle of matching on which the criteria are based is that of *clinical appropriateness*. In considering appropriateness, quality and efficiency are emphasized over cost. The concept of "clinical appropriateness" contrasts with the more familiar "medical necessity," which has become a term associated with restrictions on utilization and thus has come to be defined narrowly, often related only to the first three ASAM assessment dimension. In fact, all six dimensions identified in the *ASAM PPC-2R* are needed to accurately assess the severity of the adolescent's problem, his or her level of functioning, and the clinically appropriate placement.

The ASAM criteria are intended to evolve in response to ongoing advances in the field of adolescent addiction medicine. At present, the criteria are based predominantly on consensus best practices. As the results of additional adolescent treatment outcome studies become available, future editions of the criteria will incorporate empirically tested hypotheses of treatment effectiveness and placement.

Levels of Care Expanded

In keeping with ongoing expansions of the continuum of care, this revision includes gradations of intensity within the original levels of care. These gradations, or sublevels, are designated by decimals following a Roman numeral. The gradations describe discrete sublevels of care, which depict specific types of treatment placement settings. They also are meant to imply a continuum of care, which could encompass a variety of potential treatment placement settings, not every gradation of which is depicted specifically in the criteria.

The reality of limited availability of services continues to be a major problem for a variety of reasons. An indicated level of care may not exist or be accessible in a given community. While accessibility is a common problem in rural areas, it is an issue in many urban areas as well. Funding limitations and other resource constraints also are barriers to the availability of a level of care. Even logistical issues such as waiting lists can render a level of care unavailable. Moreover, the variations in programs within a given level of care sometimes mean that specific treatment services are not available even if an available setting meets the broader criteria.

In general, when the criteria designate a treatment placement that is not available, a strategy must be crafted that gives the patient the needed services in another placement or combination of placements. The paramount objective should be safety and effectiveness, which usually requires opting for a program of greater intensity than the placement criteria indicate.

The following levels of care for adolescents are described in this edition:

    Level 0.5   Early Intervention
    Level I   Outpatient Treatment
    Level II   Intensive Outpatient Treatment/Partial Hospitalization
        II.1   *Intensive Outpatient Treatment*
        II.5   *Partial Hospitalization*
    Level III   Residential/Intensive Inpatient Treatment
        III.1   *Clinically Managed Low-Intensity Residential Treatment*
        III.5   *Clinically Managed Medium-Intensity Residential Treatment*
        III.7   *Medically Monitored High-Intensity Residential/Inpatient Treatment*
    Level IV   Medically Managed Intensive Inpatient Treatment

The sublevels described in the adolescent criteria are somewhat different from those in the adult criteria. Moreover, there are differences in what is intended by certain sublevel designations. For example, sublevel III.1 for adolescents (a group home or halfway house) is intended to convey a somewhat greater intensity of services and staffing than would a similar sublevel III.1 program for adults. This difference reflects adolescents' greater need for supervision. Similarly, the definition of Intensive Outpatient Treatment refers to a minimum of 6 hours of treatment per week for adolescents, as compared to 9 hours a week for adults. This difference reflects the developmental and attentional capacities of adolescents, for whom 6 hours of treatment (generally delivered in two sessions of 3 hours each, or three sessions of 2 hours each) falls more closely within the spectrum of Level II intensive outpatient treatment than of Level I outpatient treatment. (This change by no means implies that 6 hours is automatically sufficient or that 9 (or more) hours is excessive. Rather, it implies a range and continuum. Some programs, for example, offer 3-hour sessions two to five times per week, depending on need.)

The new Level III.5 (clinically managed medium-intensity residential treatment) is intended to describe a variety of settings that provide 24-hour active monitoring and treatment, but relatively limited medical or nursing services. The adult Level III.3 is not included here because Level III.5 encompasses the range of adolescent treatment settings commonly employed, and the distinction between Levels III.3 and III.5 does not have sufficient specificity in adolescent treatment to merit the added complexity of an additional level.

Level III.5 settings include subacute or step-down programs that follow stabilization at a more intensive residential setting, medium- to long-term therapeutic community (TC) model programs, therapeutic group homes, and programs that emphasize a psychoeducational or psychosocial rehabilitation/habilitation model (in contrast to a medical model) for refractory Dimension 3 conditions such as conduct disorder, developmental difficulties, or personality vulnerabilities. While many Level III.5 programs are freestanding, many are provided as an internal step-down or lesser intensity track within a Level III.7 program.

The new Level III.7 (medically monitored high-intensity residential/inpatient treatment) describes a variety of settings that offer 24-hour active monitoring and treatment, with available medical or nursing services. Level III.7 also is distinguished by and often indicated for the overall high intensity of the program and treatment milieu. A patient may need Level III.7 services for the intensity that draws on the overall staffing pattern, including the availability of various professional services to the program as a whole, and not only for specific medical or nursing services provided directly to the patient. The terms "residential" and "inpatient" are used to describe Level III.7 programs because they often are used interchangeably in the field, whereas for Level IV the term "inpatient" is used exclusively to denote the intensity associated with an acute hospital setting.

Dimension 1 Expanded

The *PPC-2R* features an expansion of the Dimension 1 assessment elements, include some detailed information for specific drug classes. It also contains outlines of extra program elements that are required as enhancements for several levels of care in order to support detoxification treatment. While not all programs provide detoxification treatment, programs that offer these enhanced services are considered capable of providing detoxification treatments appropriate to their particular level of care. Such enhancements are designated by the suffix "D" and are listed under the categories of support systems, staff, therapies, and assessment/treatment plan review, following the listing of the routine program elements. For example, the therapies required for detoxification treatment in a Level III.7 program are described at the end of the "Therapies" section for Level III.7 under the heading "III.7-D."

The approach to management of intoxication and withdrawal in the adolescent criteria is different from that of the adult criteria, in which detoxification services have been separated into a separate section. An integrated approach was judged better for the adolescent criteria, because severe physiological withdrawal is seen less often in adolescents than in adults. Therefore, the provision of adolescent detoxification as an unbundled or stand-alone service is less common and less needed. Nevertheless, withdrawal does occur in adolescents and should not be overlooked. In cases where physiological withdrawal is present and its management is necessary, services in a setting separate from other treatment or even their articulation as something separate is clinically undesirable because of the developmental issues involved in the care of adolescents.

The process of detoxification includes not only attenuation of the physiological and psychological features of withdrawal, but also interrupting the momentum of habitual compulsive use in persons with substance dependence. Because of the force of this momentum and the difficulties inherent in overcoming it (even when there is no clear physiological withdrawal syndrome *per se*), this phase of treatment often requires a greater intensity of services to establish initial treatment engagement and patient role induction. This step is critical to the success of treatment because it is difficult for an adolescent to engage or participate in treatment while he or she is caught up in a cycle of intoxication and recovery from intoxication.

Dimension 3 Expanded

In the *PPC-2R*, Dimension 3 has been retitled "Emotional, Behavioral and Cognitive Conditions and Complications" to signify the importance attached to cognition by adolescents' developmental status. The new title is intended to convey the importance of cognitive considerations in assessment and treatment. Cognitive abilities, as well as global or focal cognitive impairments, play a large role in an adolescent's functional capacity. Regardless of whether cognitive problems are expressions of pre-existing conditions (such as borderline intellectual functioning, fetal alcohol effects or learning disorders) or complications of substance use (such as marijuana-induced amnestic disorders), they can interfere significantly with treatment and recovery. To be most effective, treatment providers must adapt their methods and strategies to respond to adolescents' cognitive vulnerabilities and strengths, as well as a developmental perspective that evolves dynamically.

Dimension 3 has been expanded to include new subdomains that address psychiatric comorbidity or "dual diagnosis" issues. These subdomains are:

(a) Dangerousness/Lethality
(b) Interference with Addiction Recovery Efforts
(c) Social Functioning
(d) Ability for Self-Care
(e) Course of Illness

The subdomains are designed to guide the assessment of severity and treatment needs. They are defined in the Glossary (Appendix E). The use of Dimension 3 to assess problems in the emotional, behavioral or cognitive realms does not require that the adolescent have an additional co-occurring psychiatric diagnosis or a formal psychiatric evaluation (although it may suggest that he or she should). Rather, the subdomains emphasize the broad functional impairments that are associated with both substance-related disorders and mental health problems.

Broadened Applicability

A criticism leveled against earlier editions of the criteria is that they were insensitive to the circumstances of publicly funded treatment programs and the special needs of the juvenile justice system. It is true that the continuum of services described and the range of benefits implied often are not available to disadvantaged or public sector populations. In an effort to address this criticism, the *PPC-2R* describes the full range of treatment services that should be available to all drug-involved adolescents, regardless of whether they are privately insured, publicly insured, underinsured or uninsured. In fact, many indigent adolescents need an even broader continuum and a greater intensity of services than do adolescents who are in better economic circumstances. These needs persist, whether or not the world has yet met them, and it is the intention of the *PPC-2R* to explicitly highlight this dichotomy.

This revision aims to broaden the scope of the criteria to encompass more explicitly the circumstances of adolescents in the public sector and the juvenile justice system. While adolescents who are confined in juvenile justice settings (such as detention centers) may have extended periods of enforced abstinence, they usually have not had active treatment. In this context, their treatment needs should not be assessed on a narrow standard that relies solely on the recency of their alcohol or drug use. Rather, assessment should be multidimensional, incorporating the adolescent's recovery skills and capacity for re-integration into the community. The *PPC-2R* anticipates that active treatment, including the full continuum of services, will become the rule rather than the exception for all adolescents.

The *ASAM PPC-2R* also anticipates that families and their needs and involvement will be interpreted broadly and encompass a wide variety of arrangements, including extended families, surrogate families and other caretakers. The importance of cultural diversity and the role of cultural competence in treatment engagement also should be emphasized in the implementation of these criteria.

Continued Service and Discharge Criteria

To simplify the adolescent criteria, the separate continued service and discharge criteria for each level of care have been eliminated as redundant. They have been replaced by more general continued service and transfer/discharge criteria that are applicable to any level of care. These criteria speak to the general issues of identification of, progress toward and resolution of treatment problems and goals. The more specific content is intended to come from the treatment problems, needs and goals identified in the application of the initial admission criteria, or new problems, needs and goals that emerge over time.

Special Considerations in the Care of Adolescents

Adolescents who use alcohol and other drugs differ from adults in significant ways. While substance use disorders in adolescents and adults may have common biopsychosocial elements of etiology, they are different in many aspects of their expression and treatment. Adolescence affords a unique opportunity to modify risk factors that are still active and not yet complete in their influence on development. Adolescents must be approached differently from adults because of differences in their stages of emotional, cognitive, physical, social and moral development. Examples of these fundamental developmental issues include the extremely potent influences of the adolescent's interactions with family and peers, the expected immaturity of adolescents' independent living skills, and the fact that some amount of testing limits is a normative developmental task of adolescence.

Most adolescents do not develop classic physical dependence or well-defined withdrawal symptoms, nor do they exhibit the physiological deterioration seen in many adults suffering from substance-related disorders, because of the shorter duration of their exposure to alcohol or drugs. Nevertheless, they are vulnerable to the full range of emotional, behavioral, familial and cognitive manifestations of addiction.

In fact, adolescents may be more susceptible than adults to dependence on alcohol and drugs, even in the absence of physiological withdrawal. The progression from casual use to dependence can be more rapid in adolescents than in adults. Also, adolescents typically demonstrate a higher degree of co-occurring psychopathology, which may not remit with abstinence. These limitations severely inhibit the ability of adolescents to arrest their addiction and address essential developmental tasks without external assistance and supports.

Adolescents' use of alcohol or other drugs frequently impairs their emotional and intellectual growth. Substance use can prevent a young person from completing the maturational tasks of adolescence, which involve personal relationships, identity formation, individuation, education, employment and family role responsibilities. Because substance use alters the way in which individuals approach and experience interpersonal interactions, the substance-using adolescent's psychological and social development are compromised, as is the formation of a strong positive self-identity.

Younger adolescents have a very narrow view of the world, with little capacity to think of future implications of present actions; nevertheless, they may adopt a pseudomature ("streetwise") posture. The adolescent who lives in a stressed family system, or one with limited intellectual development, may be delayed or impaired in acquiring abstract thinking. Thus, the physician or counselor who attempts to reason with an adolescent about the long-term health effects of substance use often does so futilely because the adolescent is unable to appreciate such long-term consequences.

These and other developmental issues make adolescents particularly vulnerable. As a result, they typically require greater amounts of external assistance and support, both to protect them from the sequelae of substance use and to engage them in the recovery process. Adolescents usually have not yet acquired the skills for independent living and, even without the impairments associated with substance use, they must rely heavily on the guidance of adults. In general, for a given degree of severity or functional impairment, adolescents require more intensive treatment than adults. This difference is reflected in clinical practice—and in the criteria—by a tendency to place adolescents in more intensive levels of care.

Assessment

The adolescent who is using alcohol or other drugs requires a comprehensive and multidimensional assessment. In the course of such an assessment, certain factors should be recognized and addressed. These include more entrenched early stages of readiness to change and accelerated progression of addiction in this age group, a marked prevalence of dual diagnosis and polydrug involvement, the challenges of habilitation as opposed to rehabilitation, and a need to provide comprehensive, individualized, adaptable and interdisciplinary care that incorporates inpatient as well as outpatient treatment and ongoing continuing care.

The assessment should include collateral informants to augment, clarify (and often correct) the history given by the adolescent. Key informants may be adult friends or surrogate parent figures, school and court officials, court-appointed special advocates, social service workers (especially when the child has been involved with the social service system), previous treatment providers, and past assessors. The greater the severity of the adolescent's condition and impairment, the more comprehensive the assessment should be.

A comprehensive biopsychosocial assessment includes all of the following elements (in less severe cases, the assessment should at least involve screening of these elements, as through use of a multidimensional screening instrument). Each area of inquiry contributes to a comprehensive profile of the adolescent, which should be organized according to the six dimensions of the *ASAM Patient Placement Criteria*.

- History of the present episode, including precipitating factors, current symptoms and pertinent present risks

- Family history:

    Family alcohol and drug use history, including past treatment episodes

    Family social history, including profiles of parents (or guardians or other caretakers), home atmosphere, economic status, religious affiliation, cultural influences, leisure activities, monitoring and supervision, and relocations

    Family medical and psychiatric history

- Developmental history, including pregnancy and delivery, developmental milestones and temperament

- Alcohol and drug use history, including onset and pattern of progression, past sequelae and past treatment episodes

- Personal/social history:

    School history
    Peer relationships and friendships
    Leisure activities
    Sexual activity
    Physical or sexual abuse

- Legal history, including past behaviors and their relation to substance use, arrests, adjudications and details of current status

- Psychiatric history, including symptoms and their relation to substance use, current and past diagnoses, treatments and providers

- Medical history, including pertinent medical problems and treatment, surgeries, head injuries, present medications and allergies

- Review of systems, including present and past medical and psychological symptoms

- Mental status examination

- Focused physical examination

- Formulation and diagnoses

- Survey of assets, vulnerabilities and supports

- Treatment recommendations.

All of these assessment elements then contribute to a profile of the adolescent organized by the 6 specific ASAM PPC assessment dimensions.

Diagnosis

In general, all adolescents accepted for the treatment of addiction should meet the diagnostic criteria for a substance-related disorder of the current edition of the *Diagnostic and Statistical Manual of Mental Disorders (DSM)* of the American Psychiatric Association or other standardized and widely accepted criteria. Exceptions would be made for individuals who do not meet the diagnostic criteria but whose symptoms are severe enough to warrant additional assessment.

Treatment

At every level of care, program services for adolescents should be designed to meet their developmental and other special needs. Adaptations of adult treatment models often fall short. Ideally, the treatment environment should be physically separate from that for adult patients. Strategies to engage adolescents, channel their energy, and hold their attention are especially critical. Treatment must address the nuances of adolescent experience, including cognitive, emotional, physical, social and moral development, in addition to involvement with alcohol and other drugs.

Given the current understanding of substance use disorders as having a chronic, long-term, remitting and relapsing course, it should be expected that effective treatment should match this chronic course. In fact, treatment should be regarded as a dynamic, longitudinal process, rather than as a discrete episode of care. While it may encompass one or several acute episodes, it also must endure over the long term. A now outdated approach viewed discrete time-limited episodes of program enrollment as adequate "doses" of treatment. In that view, any further care, also typically time-limited, was regarded as "aftercare" rather than ongoing care—as though the active part of treatment had ended.

The current view of addiction as a chronic disorder supports a stance of therapeutic optimism and an attitude of persistence toward the treatment-refractory patient. It also reinforces the need for chronic attention and vigilance in response to a chronic vulnerability, even in the improved patient. This view is not incompatible with the common experience that a subset of adolescents may respond to more time-limited interventions and seem to "grow out of" their difficulties with developmental maturation.

Ongoing treatment at less intensive levels of care to cement the gains achieved at more intensive levels is a critical feature of successful treatment across a continuum of care. Ongoing active treatment often is required simply to maintain therapeutic gains. This leads to a crucial point regarding the application of the continued service criteria, especially at Level I. The much-needed, frequently long-term (sometimes even indefinite) maintenance phase of treatment, usually in Level I settings, too often is overlooked. Treatment successes such as a period of abstinence or improvement in function should not be interpreted as indicating that treatment is complete. In fact, maintenance strategies such as relapse prevention and strengthening of protective factors are critical components of treatment. Even simple ongoing monitoring (such as checking on parental supervision, scrutinizing school performance or peer relationships, or reviewing warning signs of recurrence of affective disorder etc) is a desirable feature of active outpatient treatment. The *PPC-2R* emphasizes the need for such maintenance and/or monitoring in the new continued service criteria.

Another critical feature of successful treatment across a continuum of care is the ease of transfer back and forth across levels of care. One generally accepted principle is that of gradual step-down through less intensive level of care to consolidate treatment gains achieved at more intensive levels of care. Certainly one reason for longer than appropriate lengths of stay at more intensive levels of care has been the various barriers to step-down at less intensive levels. Reciprocally, acute bursts of intensive treatment may be needed to overcome hurdles at lower levels. It is likely that if providers saw such step-ups as readily available, they would not cling to longer than appropriate lengths of stay. Repeated acute episodes of high intensity care should be an expected (though not necessarily desired) component of care, as they would be in the treatment of any chronic relapsing disorder.

When a treatment plan is unsuccessful, reassessment is required. Such reassessment may indicate the need for more time in the present treatment program or it may indicate that a substantial revision of the treatment plan is required, often involving a change in the strategy, modality or scope of the treatment. It often implies the need for more intensive treatment, but it may suggest that less intensive therapy would be helpful. Unresolved problems—even severe treatment-refractory problems (such as continued use, relapse, lack of treatment attendance or participation)—should not be viewed as synonymous with inability or lack of capacity to solve those problems. Discharge from a level of care *always* should be part of a therapeutic strategy and *never* should reflect futility or therapeutic nihilism.

The Concept of "Imminent Danger"

"Imminent danger" often is used to describe problems that can lead to grave consequences for the individual patient (and possibly others), some of which may be the basis for the legal commitment of an individual to treatment. However, this important concept should be defined more carefully. In fact, three components in combination constitute imminent danger: (a) a strong probability that certain behaviors (such as continued alcohol or drug use or relapse) will occur, (b) the potential for such behaviors to present a significant risk of serious adverse consequences to the individual and/or others (as in a consistent pattern of driving while intoxicated) and (c) the likelihood that such adverse events will occur in the very near future. Clearly, imminent danger does not encompass the universe of possible adverse events.

Confidentiality and Informed Consent

Health care requires informed consent so that the adolescent (and usually the family, significant other or guardian) is made aware of the proposed modalities of treatment, the risks and benefits of such treatment, appropriate alternative treatment modalities and the risks of treatment versus no treatment. Attention should be given to the special requirements for informed consent in the treatment of adolescents.

Before a formal interview begins, certain "ground rules" must be explained to the adolescent and family, as they form the basis for the therapeutic alliance. For example, it should be made clear that all information gathered in the interview becomes part of the adolescent's permanent record and will be shared by treating physicians, social workers, therapists and others. "Secrets" regarding substance use should be avoided. On the other hand, sensitivity to an adolescent's concerns about privacy and confidentiality is very important. The adolescent and parents have a right to refuse to answer any question, although openness and honesty are expected and strongly encouraged because they contribute to a more accurate diagnosis and formulation of an appropriate treatment plan.

Certain confidentiality standards are imposed by federal and possibly state law. For example, the provider may be required to inform the parent, guardian and—under certain circumstances—the police or child protective agencies if a child or adolescent is engaged in behavior that is injurious or life-threatening, or that demonstrates suicidal intent, or if a disclosure of physical or sexual abuse is made to the physician or other clinician, or if there is a strong suspicion of such abuse.

Future Directions Matrix

As a first step toward a possible future configuration of the criteria, a "matrix" format is presented in Appendix B. This Future Directions Matrix takes a significantly different approach to assessment, treatment planning and placement than the present criteria. It emphasizes risk ratings, specifies corresponding types of services and modalities, and indicates the intensity of services and levels of care and settings where the patient's needs are most likely to be met. The goal of the matrix is to promote improved assessment and treatment of dual diagnosis patients by taking an approach that matches specific needs to particular services, rather than matching general needs to a broad level of care. The matrix also continues the process of unbundling treatment services, in recognition of the fact that patients may benefit from variations in the intensity of treatment services they receive to address problems in different dimensions.

ASAM recognizes that current systems of financing care do not support such unbundling, which implies a patient-specific array of services and intensities of care. The experimental matrix does not yet have sufficient detail or specificity, nor has it been field reviewed. Thus, it is *not* intended to be used for patient assessment or placement decisions. It *is* intended to provoke further discussion and, with ongoing expansion and refinement, perhaps to form the foundation for future revisions of the criteria.

References

American Academy of Child and Adolescent Psychiatry, AACAP (1997a). Practice parameters: Assessment of children and adolescents. *Journal of the American Academy of Child and Adolescent Psychiatry* 36(10):45-205.

American Academy of Child and Adolescent Psychiatry, AACAP (1997b). Practice parameters: Assessment and treatment of children and adolescents with substance abuse disorders. *Journal of the American Academy of Child and Adolescent Psychiatry* 36(10 Suppl):140S-156S.

American Psychiatric Association (1994). *Diagnostic and Statistical Manual of Mental Disorders, Fourth Edition (DSM-IV)*. Washington, DC: American Psychiatric Press.

Bauman KE & Ennett ST (1994). Peer influence on adolescent drug use. *American Psychologist* 49:820-822.

Baumrind D & Moselle KA (1985). A developmental perspective on adolescent drug use. *Advances in Alcohol and Substance Abuse* 4:41-67.

Brown SA (1998). Recovery patterns in adolescent substance abuse. In JS Baer, GA Marlatt & RJ McMahon (eds.) *Addictive Behaviors Across the Lifespan. Prevention, Treatment and Policy Issues*. Beverly Hills, CA: Sage Publications Inc., 161-183.

Bukstein O (1995). *Adolescent Substance Abuse: Assessment and Prevention Treatment*. New York, NY: John Wiley and Sons.

Chilcoat HD, Anthony JC, et al. (1996). Impact of parent monitoring on initiation of drug use through later childhood. *Journal of the American Academy of Child and Adolescent Psychiatry* 35(1):91-100.

Clark DB, Kirisci L & Tarter RE (1998). Adolescent versus adult onset and the development of substance use disorders. *Drug and Alcohol Dependence* 49(2):115-121.

Crowley TJ & Riggs PD (1995). Adolescent substance use disorder with conduct disorder and comorbid conditions. In E Rahdert & D Czechowicz (eds.) *Adolescent Drug Abuse: Clinical Assessment and Therapeutic Intervention* (NIDA Research Monograph No. 156). Rockville, MD: National Institute on Drug Abuse, 49-111.

DeWitt DJ, Adlaf EM, et al. (2000). Age of first alcohol use: A risk factor for the development of alcohol disorders. *American Journal of Psychiatry* 157:745-750.

Dishion TJ & Andrews DW (1995). Preventing escalation in problem behavior with high risk young adolescents: Immediate and one-year outcomes. *Journal of Consulting and Clinical Psychology* 63:538-548.

Duff A & Milin R (1996). Case study: Withdrawal syndrome in adolescent chronic cannabis users. *Journal of the American Academy of Child and Adolescent Psychiatry* 35(12):1618-1621.

Hoffmann NG, Mee-Lee D & Arrowood AA (1993). Treatment issues in adolescent substance use and addictions: Options, outcome, effectiveness, reimbursement and admissions criteria. *Adolescent Medicine: State of the Art Reviews* 4(2):371-390.

Hovens JG, Cantwell DP & Kiriakos R (1992). Psychiatric comorbidity in hospitalized adolescent substance abusers. *Journal of the American Academy of Child and Adolescent Psychiatry* 33:476-483.

Hsieh S, Hoffmann NG & Hollister CD (1998). The relationship between pre-, during-, and post-treatment factors and adolescent substance abuse behaviors. *The Journal of Addictive Behaviors* 23:1-12.

Jaffe S, ed. (1996). Adolescent substance abuse and dual disorders. *Child and Adolescent Psychiatric Clinics of North America* 5(1) January.

Johnson JL & Leff M (1999). Children of substance abusers: Overview of research findings. *Pediatrics* 103(5 pt 2):1085-1099.

Kaminer Y (1994). *Adolescent Substance Abuse: A Comprehensive Guide to Theory and Practice*. New York, NY: Plenum Medical Book Co.

Kandel D, Johnson J, et al. (1999). Psychiatric co-morbidity among adolescents with substance use disorders: Findings from the MECA study. *Journal of the American Academy of Child and Adolescent Psychiatry* 138(6):693-699.

Mackenzie RG (1993). Influence of drug use on adolescent sexual activity. *Adolescent Medicine: State of the Art Reviews* 4(2):112-115.

Margolis R (1996). Adolescent chemical dependence: Assessment, treatment and management. In AM Washton (ed.) *Psychotherapy and Substance Abuse: A Practitioner's Handbook*. New York, NY: Guilford Press, 394-412.

Mezzich AC, Tarter RE (1998). Disruptive delinquent and aggressive behavior in female adolescent substance use disorder: Relation to executive functioning. *Journal of Studies on Alcohol* 595:560-567.

Miller WR & Rollnick RK (1991). *Motivational Interviewing*. New York, NY: Guilford Press.

Milin R (1996). Comorbidity of substance abuse and psychotic disorders. *Child and Adolescent Clinics of North America* 5(1):111-131.

Molina BS, Chassin L & Curran RJ (1994). A comparison of mechanisms underlying substance use for early adolescent children of alcoholics and controls. *Journal of Studies on Alcohol* 55(3):269-275.

Monti P, Colby SM, et al. (1998). Brief motivational interviewing in a hospital setting for adolescent smoking: A preliminary study. *Journal of Consulting Clinical Psychology* 66(3):574-578.

Morrison MA, Knauf KJ & Hayes HR (1989). A comprehensive treatment model for chemically dependent adolescents. *Adolescents* (Journal).

National Institute on Drug Abuse, NIDA (1994a). *Assessing Drug Abuse Among Adolescents and Adults: Standardized Instruments (Clinical Report Series)*. Rockville, MD: NIDA.

National Institute on Drug Abuse, NIDA (1994b). *Mental Health Assessment and Diagnosis of Substance Abusers* (Clinical Report Series). Rockville, MD: NIDA.

National Institute on Drug Abuse, NIDA (1996). *Monitoring the Future Study (NIDA Capsule: Facts About Teenagers and Substance Abuse)*. Rockville, MD: NIDA, C83-07.

National Institute on Drug Abuse (1999). *Principles of Drug Addiction Treatment: A Research-Based Guide*. Rockville, MD: NIDA (NIH Publication # 99-4180).

Newcomb MD (1997). Psychosocial predictors and consequences of drug use: A developmental perspective within a prospective study. *Journal of Addictive Diseases* 16(l):51-89.

Patterson GR, et al., (1992). *Antisocial Boys*. Eugene, OR: Castalia Press.

Pickeret SG & Heneggler SW (1996). Multisystemic therapy for adolescent substance abuse and dependence. *Child and Adolescent Psychiatric Clinics of North America* 5(1):201-211.

Rahdert ER & Czechowicz D, eds. (1995). *Adolescent Drug Abuse: Clinical Assessment and Therapeutic Interventions* (NIDA Research Monograph No. 156). Rockville, MD: National Institute on Drug Abuse.

Rahdert ER & Grabowski J, eds. (1998). *Adolescent Drug Abuse: Analysis of Treatment Research* (NIDA Research Monograph 77). Rockville, MD: NIDA.

Reinherz HZ, Giaconia RM, Hauf AM, et al. (2000). General and specific childhood factors for depression and drug disorders by early adulthood. *Journal of the American Academy of Child and Adolescent Psychiatry* 39(2):223-231.

Riggs PD, Boher S, Mikulich SK, et al. (1995). Depression in substance dependent delinquents. *Journal of the American Academy of Child and Adolescent Psychiatry* 34(6):764-771.

Speraw S & Rogers PD (1998). Assessment of the identified substance-abusing adolescent. In AW Graham & TK Schultz (eds.) *Principles of Addiction Medicine, Second Edition*. Chevy Chase, MD: American Society of Addiction Medicine.

Szapocznik J, Peres-Vidal A, Brickman AL, et al. (1998). Engaging adolescent substance abusers and their families in treatment: A strategic structural systems approach. *Journal of Consulting and Clinical Psychology* 56(4):552-557.

Weinberg NZ, Rahdert E, Colliver JD et al. (1998). Adolescent substance abuse: A review of the past 10 years. *Journal of the American Academy of Child and Adolescent Psychiatry* 37(3):252-261.

Wilens TE, Biederman J & Spencer TJ (1996). Attention deficit hyperactivity disorder and psychoactive substance use disorders. *Child and Adolescent Psychiatric Clinics of North America* 5(1):73-91.

Winters KC, ed. (1999a). *Screening and Assessing Adolescents for Substance Use Disorders* (Treatment Improvement Protocol No. 31). Rockville, MD: Center for Substance Abuse Treatment.

Winters KC, ed. (1999b). *Treatment of Adolescents with Substance Use Disorders* (Treatment Improvement Protocol No. 32). Rockville, MD: Center for Substance Abuse Treatment.

Crosswalk of the Adolescent Placement Criteria Levels 0.5 through IV

LEVELS OF CARE

CRITERIA DIMENSIONS	LEVEL 0.5 Early Intervention	LEVEL I Outpatient Treatment	LEVEL II.1 Intensive Outpatient Treatment	LEVEL II.5 Partial Hospitalization
DIMENSION 1: Acute Intoxication and/or Withdrawal Potential	The adolescent is not at risk of withdrawal.	The adolescent is not at risk of withdrawal.	The adolescent is experiencing minimal withdrawal or is at risk of withdrawal.	The adolescent is experiencing mild withdrawal or is at risk of withdrawal.
DIMENSION 2: Biomedical Conditions and Complications	None or very stable	None or very stable	None or stable, or distracting from treatment at a less intensive level of care. Such problems are manageable at Level II.1.	None or stable, or distracting from treatment at a less intensive level of care. Such problems are manageable at Level II.5.
DIMENSION 3: Emotional, Behavioral, or Cognitive Conditions and Complications	The adolescent evidences no or very stable problems in Dimension 3. These are being addressed through concurrent mental health services and do not interfere with addiction treatment at this level of care.	The adolescent's status in Dimension 3 is characterized by all of the following:	The adolescent's status in Dimension 3 features one or more of the following:	The adolescent's status in Dimension 3 features one or more of the following:
(a) Dangerousness/ Lethality		(a) The adolescent is not at risk of harm.	(a) The adolescent is at low risk of harm, and he or she is safe between sessions.	(a) The adolescent is at low risk of harm, but he or she is safe overnight.

ASAM Patient Placement Criteria, Second Edition–Revised

Crosswalk of the Adolescent Placement Criteria Levels 0.5 through IV

LEVELS OF CARE

CRITERIA DIMENSIONS	LEVEL 0.5 Early Intervention	LEVEL I Outpatient Treatment	LEVEL II.1 Intensive Outpatient Treatment	LEVEL II.5 Partial Hospitalization
(b) Interference with Addiction Recovery Efforts		(b) There is minimal interference.	(b) Mild interference requires the intensity of this level of care to support treatment engagement.	(b) Moderate interference requires the intensity of this level of care to support treatment engagement.
(c) Social Functioning		(c) The adolescent evidences minimal to mild impairment.	(c) The adolescent evidences mild to moderate impairment, but can sustain responsibilities.	(c) The adolescent evidences moderate impairment, but can sustain responsibilities.
(d) Ability for Self-Care		(d) The adolescent is experiencing minimal current difficulties with activities of daily living, but there is significant risk of deterioration.	(d) The adolescent is experiencing mild to moderate difficulties with activities of daily living and requires frequent monitoring or interventions.	(d) The adolescent is experiencing moderate difficulties with activities of daily living and requires near-daily monitoring or interventions.
(e) Course of Illness		(e) The adolescent is at minimal imminent risk, which predicts a need for some monitoring or interventions.	(e) The adolescent's history (combined with the present situation) predicts the need for frequent monitoring or interventions.	(e) The adolescent's history (combined with the present situation) predicts the need for near-daily monitoring or interventions.

Crosswalk of the Adolescent Placement Criteria Levels 0.5 through IV

CRITERIA DIMENSIONS	LEVELS OF CARE			
	LEVEL 0.5 Early Intervention	LEVEL I Outpatient Treatment	LEVEL II.1 Intensive Outpatient Treatment	LEVEL II.5 Partial Hospitalization
DIMENSION 4: Readiness to Change	The adolescent is willing to explore how current alcohol or drug use may affect achievement of personal goals.	The adolescent is willing to engage in treatment, and is at least contemplating change, but needs motivating and monitoring strategies.	The adolescent requires close monitoring and support several times a week to promote progress through the stages of change because of variable treatment engagement or a lack of recognition of the need for assistance.	The adolescent requires a near-daily structured program to promote progress through the stages of change because of poor treatment engagement, or escalating use and impairment, or lack of recognition of the role of alcohol or drugs in his or her present problems.
DIMENSION 5: Relapse, Continued Use or Continued Problem Potential	The adolescent needs to gain an understanding of, or skills to change, current use patterns.	The adolescent needs limited support to maintain abstinence or control use and to pursue recovery goals.	The adolescent needs close monitoring and support because of a significant risk of relapse or continued use and deterioration in his or her level of functioning. He or she has poor relapse prevention skills.	The adolescent needs near-daily monitoring and support because of a high risk of relapse or continued use and deterioration in his or her level of functioning. He or she has minimal relapse prevention skills.
DIMENSION 6: Recovery Environment	The adolescent's risk of initiation of or progression in substance use is increased by alcohol or drug use (or values relating to such use) by his or her family, peers or members of his or her social support system.	The adolescent's family and environment can support recovery with limited assistance.	The adolescent's environment is impeding his or her recovery, and the adolescent requires close monitoring and support to overcome that barrier.	The adolescent's environment renders recovery unlikely without near-daily monitoring and support or frequent relief from his or her home environment.

ASAM Patient Placement Criteria, Second Edition–Revised

Crosswalk of the Adolescent Placement Criteria: Levels 0.5 through IV

LEVELS OF CARE

CRITERIA DIMENSIONS	LEVEL III.1 Clinically Managed Low-Intensity Residential Treatment	LEVEL III.5 Clinically Managed Medium-Intensity Residential Treatment	LEVEL III.7 Medically Monitored High-Intensity Residential/ Inpatient Treatment	LEVEL IV Medically Managed Intensive Inpatient Treatment
DIMENSION 1: Acute Intoxication and/or Withdrawal Potential	The adolescent's state of withdrawal (or risk of withdrawal) is being managed concurrently at another level of care.	The adolescent is experiencing mild to moderate withdrawal (or is at risk of withdrawal), but does not need pharmacological management or frequent medical or nursing monitoring.	The adolescent is experiencing moderate to severe withdrawal (or is at risk of withdrawal), but this is manageable at Level III.7-D.	The adolescent is experiencing severe withdrawal (or is at risk of withdrawal) and requires intensive active medical management.
DIMENSION 2: Biomedical Conditions and Complications	None or stable	None or stable; the adolescent is receiving concurrent medical monitoring as needed.	The adolescent requires medical monitoring, but not intensive treatment.	The adolescent requires 24-hour medical and nursing care.
DIMENSION 3: Emotional, Behavioral or Cognitive Conditions and Complications	The adolescent's status in Dimension 3 features one or more of the following:	The adolescent's status in Dimension 3 features one or more of the following:	The adolescent's status in Dimension 3 features one or more of the following:	The adolescent's status in Dimension 3 features one or more of the following:
(a) Dangerousness/ Lethality	(a) The adolescent needs a stable living environment for safety.	(a) The adolescent is at moderate but stable risk of harm and thus needs medium-intensity 24-hour monitoring or treatment for safety.	(a) The adolescent is at moderate risk of harm and needs high-intensity 24-hour monitoring or treatment, or secure containment, for safety.	(a) The adolescent is at severe risk of harm.

Crosswalk of the Adolescent Placement Criteria: Levels 0.5 through IV

CRITERIA DIMENSIONS	LEVELS OF CARE			
	LEVEL III.1 Clinically Managed Low-Intensity Residential Treatment	LEVEL III.5 Clinically Managed Medium-Intensity Residential Treatment	LEVEL III.7 Medically Monitored High-Intensity Residential/ Inpatient Treatment	LEVEL IV Medically Managed Intensive Inpatient Treatment
(b) Interference with Addiction Recovery Efforts	(b) Moderate interference requires limited 24-hour supervision to support treatment engagement.	(b) Moderate to severe interference requires medium-intensity residential treatment to support engagement.	(b) Severe interference requires high-intensity residential treatment to support engagement.	(b) Very severe, almost overwhelming interference renders the adolescent incapable of participating in treatment at a less intensive level of care.
(c) Social Functioning	(c) The adolescent evidences moderate impairment and needs limited 24-hour supervision to sustain responsibilities.	(c) The adolescent evidences moderate to severe impairment and cannot be managed at a less intensive level of care.	(c) The adolescent evidences severe impairment and cannot be managed at a less intensive level of care.	(c) The adolescent evidences very severe, dangerous impairment and requires frequent medical and nursing interventions.
(d) Ability for Self-Care	(d) The adolescent evidences moderate difficulties with activities of daily living and requires limited 24-hour supervision and frequent prompting.	(d) The adolescent evidences moderate to severe difficulties with activities of daily living and requires 24-hour supervision and medium-intensity staff assistance.	(d) The adolescent evidences severe difficulties with activities of daily living and requires 24-hour supervision and high-intensity staff assistance.	(d) The adolescent evidences very severe difficulties with activities of daily living and requires frequent medical and nursing interventions.
(e) Course of Illness	(e) The adolescent's history (combined with the present situation) predicts instability without limited 24-hour supervision.	(e) The adolescent's history (combined with the present situation) predicts destabilization without medium-intensity residential treatment.	(e) The adolescent's history (combined with the present situation) predicts destabilization without high-intensity residential treatment.	(e) The adolescent's history (combined with the present situation) predicts destabilization without inpatient medical management.

ASAM Patient Placement Criteria, Second Edition–Revised

Crosswalk of the Adolescent Placement Criteria: Levels 0.5 through IV

CRITERIA DIMENSIONS	LEVELS OF CARE				
	LEVEL III.1 Clinically Managed Low-Intensity Residential Treatment	LEVEL III.5 Clinically Managed Medium-Intensity Residential Treatment	LEVEL III.7 Medically Monitored High-Intensity Residential/ Inpatient Treatment	LEVEL IV Medically Managed Intensive Inpatient Treatment
DIMENSION 4: Readiness to Change	The adolescent is open to recovery, but needs limited 24-hour supervision to promote or sustain progress.	The adolescent needs intensive motivating strategies in a 24-hour structured program to address minimal treatment engagement or opposition to treatment, or his or her lack of recognition of current severe impairment.	The adolescent needs high-intensity motivating strategies in a 24-hour medically monitored program to address his or her lack of treatment engagement associated with a biomedical, emotional or behavioral condition; or because he or she is actively opposed to treatment, requiring confinement; or because he or she needs high-intensity case management to create linkages that would support outpatient treatment.	The adolescent's problems in Dimension 4 do not qualify him or her for Level IV services.
DIMENSION 5: Relapse, Continued Use or Continued Problem Potential	The adolescent understands the potential for continued use and/or has emerging recovery skills, but needs supervision to reinforce recovery and relapse	The adolescent is unable to control use and avoid serious impairment without a 24-hour structured program because he or she is unable to overcome environmental	The adolescent is unable to interrupt a high severity or high frequency pattern of use and avoid dangerous consequences without high-intensity 24-hour interventions	The adolescent's problems in Dimension 5 do not qualify him or her for Level IV services.

ASAM Patient Placement Criteria, Second Edition–Revised

Crosswalk of the Adolescent Placement Criteria: Levels 0.5 through IV

LEVELS OF CARE

CRITERIA DIMENSIONS	LEVEL III.1 Clinically Managed Low-Intensity Residential Treatment	LEVEL III.5 Clinically Managed Medium-Intensity Residential Treatment	LEVEL III.7 Medically Monitored High-Intensity Residential/ Inpatient Treatment	LEVEL IV Medically Managed Intensive Inpatient Treatment
DIMENSION 5: Relapse, Continued Use or Continued Problem Potential (continued)	prevention skills, or to limit exposure to substances and/or environmental triggers, or to maintain therapeutic gains.	triggers or cravings; or has insufficient supervision between encounters at a less intensive level of care; or has high chronicity and/or poor response to treatment.	(because of an emotional, behavioral or cognitive condition, severe impulse control problems, withdrawal symptoms, and the like).	
DIMENSION 6: Recovery Environment	The adolescent's environment poses a risk to his or her recovery, so that he or she requires alternative residential containment or support.	The adolescent's environment is dangerous to his or her recovery, so that he or she requires residential treatment to promote recovery goals or for protection.	The adolescent's environment is dangerous to his or her recovery, and he or she requires residential treatment to promote recovery goals or for protection, and to help him or her establish a successful transition to a less intensive level of care.	The adolescent's problems in this Dimension 6 do not qualify him or her for Level IV services.

Note: This overview of the Adolescent Criteria is an approximate summary to illustrate the principal concepts and structure of the criteria.

ASAM Patient Placement Criteria, Second Edition–Revised

Continued Service and Discharge Criteria
Adolescent Patient Placement Criteria

In the process of assessing the adolescent patient, certain problems and priorities are identified as justifying admission to a particular level of care. The resolution of those problems and priorities determines when an adolescent can be treated at a different level or discharged from treatment. The appearance of new problems may require services that can be provided effectively at the same level of care, or they may require a more or less intensive level of care.

After the admission criteria for a given level of care have been met, the criteria for continued service, discharge or transfer from that level of care are as follows:

Continued Service Criteria

It is appropriate to retain the adolescent at the present level of care if:

1. The adolescent is making progress, but has not yet achieved the goals articulated in the individualized treatment plan. Continued treatment at the present level of care is assessed as necessary to permit the adolescent to continue to work toward his or her treatment goals;

   or

2. The adolescent is not yet making progress, but has the capacity to resolve his or her problems. He or she is actively working toward the goals articulated in the individualized treatment plan. Continued treatment at the present level of care is assessed as necessary to permit the adolescent to continue to work toward his or her treatment goals;

   and/or

3. New problems have been identified that are appropriately treated at the present level of care. This level is the least intensive at which the adolescent's new problems can be addressed effectively.

To document and communicate the adolescent's readiness for discharge or need for transfer to another level of care, each of the six dimensions of the ASAM criteria should be reviewed. If the criteria apply to the adolescent's existing or new problem(s), he or she should continue in treatment at the present level of care. If not, refer to the Discharge/Transfer Criteria, below.

> **Examples:** Typical findings in each of the six dimensions follow:

Dimension 1, Acute Intoxication/Withdrawal Potential: Signs and symptoms indicate the continued presence of the intoxication or withdrawal problem that required admission to the present level of care. The problem requires monitoring or detoxification services that can be provided effectively only at the present level of care.

> **Example (Continued Service Criterion #1):** An adolescent patient in a Level III.7 program is experiencing improving anxiety, tremors, pulse rate and blood pressure related to withdrawal. However, further detoxification medications and nurse monitoring are needed every 8 hours. Therefore, continued treatment can be provided effectively only at Level III.7.

Dimension 2, Biomedical Condition and Complications: The physical health problem that required admission to the present level of care, or a new problem, requires biomedical services that can be provided effectively only at the present level of care.

> **Example (Continued Service Criterion #2)**: An adolescent patient in a Level III.7 program who has experienced significant weight loss from a co-occurring disorder (anorexia nervosa) has not yet regained sufficient weight to allow safe transfer to a less intensive level of care. However, the adolescent is following through with the treatment plan. He or she needs further medical monitoring and 24-hour nurse management to monitor for insomnia, excessive exercise or purging behavior and to provide dietary structure. These services can be provided effectively only in a Level III.7 program.

Dimension 3, Emotional, Behavioral or Cognitive Conditions and Complications: The emotional, behavioral and/or cognitive problem that required admission to the present level of care continues, or a new problem has appeared. This problem requires interventions than can be provided effectively only at the present level of care.

> **Example (Continued Service Criterion #3)**: Following a methamphetamine binge, an adolescent patient in a Level II.5 program evidences problems with cognition and impulse control. These have persisted beyond what might be expected with a self-limited or substance-induced syndrome. They require consistent behavioral interventions several times a day, several days a week. This can be provided effectively only in a Level II.5 program.

Dimension 4, Readiness to Change: The adolescent continues to demonstrate a need for engagement and motivational enhancement that can be provided effectively only at the present level of care.

> **Example (Continued Service Criterion #1)**: An adolescent patient in a Level II.1 program is attending group sessions, where he has verbalized increasing awareness that marijuana and alcohol use have affected his grades in school and family relationships to a greater extent than he had realized in the past. However, he is not yet implementing the recommended changes. Accordingly, further family work, involvement of school personnel and a probation officer, peer confrontation, education about addiction and attempts at abstinence are needed to improve the adolescent's stage of readiness to change. The motivational enhancement strategies are of such intensity that they can be provided effectively only in a Level II.1 program.

Dimension 5, Relapse, Continued Use or Continued Problem Potential: The adolescent continues to demonstrate a problem, or has developed a new problem, that requires coping skills and strategies to prevent relapse, continued use or continued problems. These strategies can be provided effectively only at the present level of care.

> **Example (Continued Service Criterion #2)**: An adolescent patient in a Level I program continues to experience daily craving for alcohol, but is willing to continue addressing her alcohol problem. She is attending group therapy twice a week and AA meetings four days a week. Although she had a brief "slip" and drank two beers, she talked about the experience in her group session and identified relapse triggers and situations, and made plans to avoid the friends and parties that pose a risk of relapse. The patient requires continued care that can be provided effectively at Level I.

Dimension 6, Recovery Environment: The adolescent continues to demonstrate a problem in his or her recovery environment, or has a new problem, that requires coping skills and support system interventions. These interventions can be provided effectively only at the present level of care.

> **Example (Continued Service Criterion #3)**: In a Level III.5 program, family work has uncovered the fact that an adolescent patient is a victim of incest. As the effects of her use of alcohol, cocaine and marijuana have cleared, the patient has become increasingly distressed, and her alcoholic father has become unwilling to attend family sessions. The individual and group strategies to help the adolescent cope with her emotional distress, as well as her relationship with her father, without reverting to substance use can be provided effectively only in a Level III.5 program. In addition, the family work is sufficiently intense that continued treatment at Level III.5 is necessary until staff can clarify whether the adolescent will require placement outside the family home to permit full recovery.

Discharge/Transfer Criteria

It is appropriate to transfer or discharge the adolescent from the present level of care if he or she meets the following criteria:

1. The adolescent has achieved the goals articulated in his or her individualized treatment plan, thus resolving the problem(s) that justified admission to the present level of care;

    or

2. The adolescent has been unable to resolve the problem(s) that justified admission to the present level of care, despite amendments to the treatment plan. Treatment at another level of care or type of service therefore is indicated;

    or

3. The adolescent has demonstrated a lack of capacity to resolve his or her problem(s). Treatment at another level of care or type of service therefore is indicated;

    or

4. The adolescent has experienced an intensification of his or her problem(s), or has developed a new problem(s), and can be treated effectively only at a more intensive level of care.

To document and communicate the adolescent's readiness for discharge or need for transfer to another level of care, each of the six dimensions of the ASAM criteria should be reviewed. If the criteria apply to the existing or new problem(s), the adolescent should be discharged or transferred, as appropriate. If not, refer to the Continued Service criteria.

> **Examples**: Examples of findings in each of the six dimensions follow:

Dimension 1, Acute Intoxication/Withdrawal Potential: The adolescent's intoxication or withdrawal problem has improved sufficiently to allow monitoring or detoxification services to be provided at a less intensive level of care. Or the adolescent's condition has worsened to a point at which more intensive monitoring or detoxification services are required.

Example (Discharge/Transfer Criterion #1): An adolescent patient in a Level III.7 program is experiencing improving anxiety, tremors, pulse rate and blood pressure related to withdrawal. Nurse monitoring no longer is needed. Therefore, treatment can continue in a Level II.1 program.

Dimension 2, Biomedical Conditions and Complications: The adolescent's physical health has improved sufficiently to allow biomedical services to be provided effectively at a less intensive level of care. Or the adolescent's condition has worsened to a point at which more intensive biomedical services are necessary.

Example (Discharge/Transfer Criterion #2): An adolescent patient in a Level III.7 program has experienced significant weight loss from a co-occurring disorder (anorexia nervosa), which continues to worsen despite behavioral, psychotherapeutic and behavioral interventions and family therapy. As a result, she requires the daily medical management, 24-hour nurse monitoring and dietary structure found in a Level IV program.

Dimension 3, Emotional, Behavioral or Cognitive Conditions and Complications: The adolescent's functioning has improved sufficiently to allow interventions or services to be provided effectively at a less intensive level of care. Or the adolescent's condition has worsened to a point at which more intensive services are necessary.

Example (Discharge/Transfer Criterion #2): An adolescent patient in a Level II.5 program has not been able to resolve his problems with cognition and impulse control, despite behavioral, individual and group therapy and family therapy. Therefore, more specific and structured mental health interventions are required in addition to the addiction treatment. The patient's needs for medical monitoring, 24-hour nurse monitoring, mental health therapy and a structured environment can be provided effectively only in a mental health-oriented "dual diagnosis" Level III.7 program.

Example (Discharge/Transfer Criteria #2 and #3): An adolescent patient in a Level III.7 program is persistently disruptive and overstimulated, and has not developed coping skills to resist the negative peer influences that provoked similar behavior and drug use prior to admission. The adolescent also is unable to integrate or make use of therapeutic activities, materials and behavior management techniques utilized in the program. Further evaluation shows that the adolescent has baseline cognitive impairment in the moderate range of mental retardation. If the Level III.7 program cannot provide the specialty services and programming needed to treat this degree of cognitive impairment, the adolescent should be transferred to a program that offers such specialty treatment (for example, a Level III.7 program, or a Level III.5 program with high-intensity special education services, or a Level II.5 specialty program with adequate home environment supports).

If, after such specialty treatment is provided, the adolescent is assessed as incapable of developing the necessary coping skills because of the cognitive impairment, then an appropriate placement would involve transfer to a program that can provide indefinite monitoring and supervision (such as a Level III.1 group home).

Alternatively, the adolescent could be transferred to a program in which long-term vocational training and/or other habilitative services are provided as substitutes for the internalization of coping skills.

Dimension 4, Readiness to Change: The adolescent's stage of readiness to change has improved sufficiently to allow interventions or strategies to be provided effectively at a less intensive level of care. Or the adolescent has demonstrated regression or lack of progress to such a degree that further interventions at the present level of care will be ineffective and/or decrease the adolescent's willingness to engage in treatment. Transfer to another level of care will permit the use of different strategies to engage the adolescent in treatment and enhance his or her readiness to change.

> **Example (Discharge/Transfer Criterion #2):** An adolescent patient in a Level II.1 program, in response to ongoing early abstinence and distance from drug-using friends, insists that he does not have a problem with substance use and refuses to participate in program activities because they "don't apply to me." The adolescent maintains that he has no thoughts of drug use or urges to use and that he has a good understanding of the effects of drugs on his life. However, he insists that he used only because he was dealing with the pressures involved in moving to a new neighborhood and trying to make friends with what (he now acknowledges) was the "wrong crowd." Despite his parents' and the treatment team's concern that he has a more severe problem that he admits, and despite family therapy, group confrontation and education, the adolescent remains convinced that his drug use was temporary and is now under control. While he is not ready to embrace recovery, he will agree to attend a weekly group session and to participate in random drug screening to demonstrate that he does not have a problem. His family is willing to continue family therapy on a weekly basis. These services can be provided effectively in a Level I program, so the adolescent can be discharged from Level II.1.

> **Example (Discharge/Transfer Criterion #2):** If a marijuana-using adolescent's attendance at a Level 0.5 early intervention session with a school-based substance abuse outreach counselor is sporadic, and if he lacks the support of his (drug-using) parents and his teachers, with the result that he does not accept the fact that he has a problem or listen attentively enough to commit to change, then he should be transferred to a Level I outpatient program for further evaluation.

Dimension 5, Relapse, Continued Use or Continued Problem Potential: The adolescent's coping skills have improved sufficiently that strategies to prevent relapse or continued use can be provided effectively at a less intensive level of care. Or the adolescent has demonstrated regression or lack of progress so significant that further interventions at the present level of care will not enhance his or her ability to prevent relapse or continued use and/or will decrease the adolescent's willingness to engage in treatment. Transfer to another level of service will allow different strategies to be employed to engage the adolescent in treatment and enhance his or her ability to prevent relapse or continued use.

> **Example (Discharge/Transfer Criterion #4):** An adolescent patient who has been in a Level I program for two weeks is unable to cope with thoughts of alcohol and other drug use, craving and impulses to use, and inability to refuse peers' invitations to parties. Her status is deteriorating despite more focused role-playing to enhance peer refusal skills, other behavioral techniques, attendance at AA meetings, and increased individual sessions. Because she easily becomes suicidal when drinking and has been drinking daily and in increasing amounts over the preceding two days, she is transferred to a Level III.5 program.

Dimension 6, Recovery Environment: The adolescent's environment and/or ability to cope with it have improved sufficiently to allow interventions or services to be provided effectively at a less intensive level of care. Or the adolescent's recovery environment and/or ability to cope with it have worsened to such a degree that he or she requires transfer to another level of care, where different interventions or strategies can be provided.

> **Example (Discharge/Transfer Criterion #3):** The physically and sexually abusive father of an adolescent patient in a Level III.5 program continues to use alcohol and refuses attendance at family meetings. There is no foreseeable way of making the patient's home environment safe. She continues to have difficulty in coping with anxiety and stress reactions, but has accommodated to the need for an out-of-home placement. Transfer to a Level III.1 safe living environment, with concurrent Level II.5 services, is needed to strengthen her ability to cope with both her substance use problem and her safety issues with her father.

Level 0.5
Early Intervention

Early intervention is an organized service that may be delivered in a wide variety of settings. Early intervention services are designed to explore and address the adolescent's problems or risk factors that appear to be related to substance use and to assist the adolescent in recognizing the harmful consequences of substance use.

It is important to note that Level 0.5 early intervention services are intended to be a combination of prevention and treatment services for *at-risk* youth. For example, a particularly vulnerable population that warrants special attention at Level 0.5 is the children of substance-abusing parents (COSAP).

Level 0.5 is *not* appropriate for those adolescents who qualify for a diagnosis of substance use disorder. If an adolescent's pattern of substance use has progressed to a point at which it is causing a pattern of impairment, however mild, then the applicable treatment services are best provided at a more intensive level of care.

Length of Service

Length of service varies according to: (a) the adolescent's ability to comprehend the information provided and use that information to make behavior changes and to avoid problems related to substance use and/or (b) the appearance of new problems that require treatment at another level of care.

Adolescent Criteria
Level 0.5: Early Intervention

CHARACTERISTIC	ESSENTIAL FEATURES
EXAMPLES	Level 0.5 services encompass student assistance and school programs, brief intervention counseling with at-risk adolescents, primary care monitoring and interventions, group and/or family therapy with high-risk adolescents, and educational programs for first-time DUI (Driving Under the Influence) offenders.
SETTING	Level 0.5 services may be offered in any age-appropriate setting, including clinical offices or permanent facilities, schools, work sites, community centers, or an adolescent's home.
SUPPORT SYSTEMS	At Level 0.5, necessary support systems include: (a) Referral for ongoing treatment of substance abuse or dependence. (b) Referral for medical, psychological or psychiatric services, including further assessment. (c) Referral for community social services. The adolescent's family may be referred for any of the services listed above.
STAFF	Level 0.5 services may be provided by any professional who is knowledgeable about the biopsychosocial dimensions of substance use and dependence, knowledgeable about adolescent development, experienced in working with and engaging adolescents, able to recognize mental health concerns and substance-related disorders; skilled in alcohol and other drug education, motivational counseling, and brief intervention techniques; and aware of the legal and personal consequences of inappropriate substance use.
INTERVENTIONS	Interventions offered at Level 0.5 may involve individual, group or family counseling, as well as planned educational experiences focused on helping the adolescent recognize and avoid substance use.
ASSESSMENT	At Level 0.5, sufficient assessment is performed to screen for, and rule in or out, substance-related and co-occurring psychiatric disorders. Screening instruments may be used.
DOCUMENTATION	Documentation standards of Level 0.5 programs include progress notes in the adolescent's record that clearly indicate assessment findings, attendance and significant clinical events, particularly those that require further assessment and referral.

ASAM Patient Placement Criteria, Second Edition–Revised

Adolescent Admission Criteria
Diagnostic and Dimensional Criteria

CRITERIA	LEVEL 0.5 Early Intervention
DIAGNOSTIC ADMISSION CRITERIA	The adolescent who is an appropriate candidate for Level 0.5 services evidences problems and risk factors that appear to be related to substance use but do not meet the diagnostic criteria for Substance-Related Disorder as defined in the current *Diagnostic and Statistical Manual of Mental Disorders (DSM)* of the American Psychiatric Association or other standardized and widely accepted criteria.
DIMENSIONAL ADMISSION CRITERIA	The adolescent who is an appropriate candidate for Level 0.5 services meets *one* of the specifications in Dimensions 4, 5 or 6. Any identifiable problems in Dimensions 1, 2 or 3 are stable or are being addressed through appropriate outpatient medical or mental health services.
DIMENSION 1: Acute Intoxication and/or Withdrawal	The adolescent who is an appropriate candidate for Level 0.5 services shows no signs of acute or subacute withdrawal, or risk of acute withdrawal.
DIMENSION 2: Biomedical Conditions and Complications	In Dimension 2, the adolescent's biomedical conditions or problems, if any, are stable or are being actively addressed through appropriate medical services and will not interfere with therapeutic interventions at this level of care.
DIMENSION 3: Emotional, Behavioral or Cognitive Conditions and Complications	In Dimension 3, the adolescent's emotional, behavioral or cognitive conditions or complications, if any, are stable or are being addressed through appropriate mental health services and will not interfere with therapeutic interventions at this level of care.
DIMENSION 4: Readiness to Change	In Dimension 4, the adolescent expresses willingness to gain an understanding of how his or her current use of alcohol or other drugs may be harmful or impair his or her ability to meet responsibilities and achieve personal goals.

Adolescent Admission Criteria
Diagnostic and Dimensional Criteria

CRITERIA	LEVEL 0.5 Early Intervention
DIMENSION 5: **Continued Problem Potential**	The adolescent's status in Dimension 5 is characterized by (a) *or* (b): (a) The adolescent does not understand or accept the need to alter his or her current pattern of use of alcohol or other drugs in order to prevent harm that may be related to such use; *or* (b) The adolescent needs to acquire the specific skills needed to change his or her current pattern of use.
DIMENSION 6: **Living Environment**	The adolescent's status in Dimension 6 is characterized by (a) *or* (b) *or* (c) *or* (d): (a) A significant member of the adolescent's social support system has a pattern of substance use that prevents him or her from meeting social, work, school or family obligations; *or* (b) One or more family members are abusing alcohol or other drugs (or have done so in the past), thereby heightening the adolescent's risk for a substance-related disorder; *or* (c) A significant member of the adolescent's social support system expresses values concerning alcohol or other drug use that pose a risk to the adolescent of initiation of such use or progression of an established pattern of substance use; *or* (d) A significant member of the adolescent's social support system condones or encourages use of alcohol or other drugs.

Level I
Outpatient Treatment

Adolescent Level I encompasses organized outpatient treatment services, which may be delivered in a wide variety of settings. In Level I programs, addiction treatment staff, including addiction-credentialed physicians, provide professionally directed evaluation, treatment and recovery services to adolescents who have substance-related disorders. Such services are provided in regularly scheduled sessions of (usually) fewer than 6 contact hours a week. The services follow a defined set of policies and procedures or clinical protocols.

Level I services are tailored to each patient's level of clinical severity and are designed to help the patient achieve permanent change in his or her alcohol- or other drug-using behaviors. Treatment thus must address major familial, attitudinal, behavioral and cognitive issues that have the potential to undermine the goals of treatment or to impair the adolescent's ability to cope with major life tasks without the use of alcohol or other drugs. Treatment interventions and modalities are tailored to engage adolescents who are at varying levels of developmental maturity.

Treatment at this level of care often requires linkages with other service providers, usually by referral. Examples include psychiatric assessment and treatment, primary care medical assessment and treatment, psychological and/or educational testing for learning disorders, special or alternative education services, family therapies, juvenile justice probation and supervision, foster care support services, and public benefit coordination or other social service agency interventions.

The use of Adolescent Level I services can be appropriate in several different situations:

- Level I may be the initial level of care for an adolescent whose severity of illness warrants this intensity of treatment. Such an adolescent should be able to benefit from professionally directed addiction treatment at this level, using only one level of care, unless (a) an unanticipated event causes a change in his or her level of functioning, leading to a reassessment of the appropriateness of this level of care, or (b) there is recurring evidence that the adolescent is unable to use this level of care (such as repeated episodes of drinking or drug use, even after the treatment plan has been reviewed and revised).

- Level I may represent a "step down" from a more intensive level of care for the adolescent whose progress warrants such a transfer, assuming that he or she meets the criteria for placement in Level I.

- Level I services may be useful for the adolescent patient who is in the early stages of readiness to change and who has not yet committed to recovery. While an adolescent at this stage may require a more intensive level of care (occasionally including coerced treatment) to address high levels of resistance and denial, such an increase in intensity can be counterproductive in certain situations.

  An alternative approach is to use a less intensive level of care to engage the resistant adolescent in treatment by enhancing his or her motivation and/or by modifying the response(s) of the various systems that affect the adolescent. Such an approach may prepare the adolescent for a more intensive level of care, or even forestall the need for more intensive treatment services.

Length of Service

The duration of treatment varies with the severity of the adolescent's illness and his or her response to treatment.

Especially at Level I, ongoing active treatment often is required simply to sustain an adolescent's therapeutic gains. The much-needed maintenance phase of treatment often is long-term (sometimes even indefinite) and too often is overlooked. Treatment successes such as a period of abstinence or improvement in function sometimes are misinterpreted as indicating that treatment is completed. In fact, maintenance strategies such as relapse prevention and strengthening protective factors are critical components of treatment. Even simple ongoing monitoring (such as checking on parental supervision, scrutinizing school performance or peer relationships, reviewing warning signs of recurrence of affective disorder, and the like) is a desirable goal of active outpatient treatment. *It is the clear intention of this revision of the criteria that such maintenance and/or monitoring goals should be expressible in the language of the new continued service criteria.*

Detoxification

Dimension 1 (Acute Intoxication and/or Withdrawal Potential) is the first of the six primary assessment areas to be evaluated in making treatment and placement decisions. The range of clinical severity in this dimension has given rise to a range of detoxification levels. Patients who are experiencing or at risk of an acute withdrawal syndrome should not be treated at Level I. For this reason, the designation "Level I-D" has not been used.

As used here, detoxification refers not only to the attenuation of the physiological and psychological features of withdrawal syndromes, but also to the process of interrupting the momentum of habitual compulsive use in adolescents who are diagnosed with substance *dependence*. Because of the force of this momentum, and the inherent difficulties in overcoming it even when there is no clear withdrawal syndrome *per se*, this phase of treatment frequently requires a greater intensity of services initially in order to establish treatment engagement and patient role induction. This is, of course, critical to the course of treatment because it is impossible to engage an adolescent in treatment while he or she is caught up in a cycle of frequent intoxication and recovery from intoxication. Although the process of interrupting a pattern of high-frequency use may reasonably be attempted at Level I, such efforts often are unsuccessful. In such circumstances, it is safer to place the adolescent at a more intensive level of care.

Adolescent Criteria
Level I: Outpatient Treatment

CHARACTERISTIC	ESSENTIAL FEATURES
EXAMPLES	Level I adolescent program services may be delivered in office practice, school-based health clinics, primary care clinics and child/adolescent behavioral health clinics.
SETTING	Level I adolescent program services may be offered in any age-appropriate setting that meets state licensing or certification criteria.
SUPPORT SYSTEMS	In Level I adolescent programs, necessary support services include: (a) Medical, psychological, psychiatric, laboratory and toxicology, and other necessary services, which are available through consultation or referral. Medical and psychiatric consultation are available within a time appropriate to the severity and urgency of the consultation requested. (b) Direct affiliation with more and less intensive levels of care. In particular, the program is able to facilitate placements at more intensive levels of care as needed, including placements for treatment of intoxication and withdrawal. (c) Emergency services available by telephone 24 hours a day, 7 days a week.
STAFF	Level I adolescent programs are staffed by appropriately credentialed treatment professionals (including physicians, counselors, psychologists, social workers and others), who assess and treat substance-related and co-occurring psychiatric disorders. Staff are able to obtain and interpret information regarding the adolescent's biopsychosocial needs and are knowledgeable about the biopsychosocial dimensions of alcohol and other drug disorders and co-occurring psychiatric disorders. They also are knowledgeable about adolescent development and experienced in working with and engaging adolescents. Clinical staff who assess and treat adolescents are able to recognize the need for specialty evaluation and treatment for intoxication or withdrawal and are able to arrange for such evaluation or treatment in a timely manner.

Adolescent Criteria
Level I: Outpatient Treatment

CHARACTERISTIC	ESSENTIAL FEATURES
THERAPIES	Therapies offered by Level I adolescent programs include individual and group counseling, family therapy, cognitive/behavioral modification, individual and group therapy, educational groups, occupational and recreational therapy, psychotherapy, and other therapies (such as access to a speech therapist or learning disorders specialist). Such services are provided in an amount, frequency and intensity appropriate to the objectives of the individualized treatment plan.
ASSESSMENT/ TREATMENT PLAN REVIEW	In Level I adolescent programs, the assessment and treatment plan review includes: (a) An individual biopsychosocial assessment of every patient. (b) An individualized treatment plan, which involves problem formulation and articulation of treatment goals and measurable treatment objectives. Treatment plan reviews are conducted at specified times, as noted in the plan.
DOCUMENTATION	Documentation standards of Level I adolescent programs include progress notes in the patient record that clearly reflect implementation of the treatment plan and the adolescent's response to treatment, as well as subsequent amendments to the plan.

Adolescent Level I Admission Criteria
Diagnostic and Dimensional Criteria

CRITERIA	LEVEL I Outpatient Services
DIAGNOSTIC ADMISSION CRITERIA	The adolescent who is appropriately placed in a Level I program is assessed as meeting the diagnostic criteria for Substance-Related Disorder, as defined by the current *Diagnostic and Statistical Manual of Mental Disorders (DSM)* of the American Psychiatric Association or other standardized and widely accepted criteria, as well as the dimensional criteria for admission. If the adolescent's presenting alcohol or other drug use history is inadequate to substantiate such a diagnosis, the probability of such a diagnosis may be determined from information submitted by collateral parties (such as family members, legal guardian(s) and significant others).
DIMENSIONAL ADMISSION CRITERIA	The adolescent who is appropriately placed in a Level I program is assessed as meeting specifications in *all* of the following six dimensions.
DIMENSION 1: Acute Intoxication and/or Withdrawal	The adolescent who is appropriately placed in a Level I program is not experiencing acute or subacute withdrawal from alcohol or other drugs, and is not at risk of acute withdrawal; *or* If the adolescent is experiencing very mild withdrawal, the symptoms consist of no more than lingering but improving sleep disturbance. **Nicotine:** Nicotine withdrawal is the exception to the foregoing statement, as it may be marked by more severe symptoms. However, these can be managed in a Level I setting. Nicotine withdrawal symptoms may require either nicotine replacement therapy or non-nicotine pharmacological agents for symptomatic treatment. NOTE: If the adolescent is presenting for treatment after recently experiencing an episode of acute withdrawal without treatment (as opposed to stepping down from a more intensive level of care following a good response to treatment), it is safer to err on the side of greater intensity of services in making a placement. For example, a Level II.1 setting may be indicated if the adolescent is doing poorly or if there are indicators for that level of care in other dimensions.
DIMENSION 2: Biomedical Conditions and Complications	If the adolescent has biomedical conditions and problems in Dimension 2, they are sufficiently stable to permit participation in outpatient treatment.

ASAM Patient Placement Criteria, Second Edition–Revised

Adolescent Level I Admission Criteria
Diagnostic and Dimensional Criteria

CRITERIA	LEVEL I Outpatient Services
DIMENSION 3: **Emotional, Behavioral or Cognitive Conditions and Complications**	The adolescent's status in Dimension 3 is characterized by *all* of the following: (a) *Dangerousness/Lethality*: The adolescent is assessed as not posing a risk of harm to self or others. He or she has adequate impulse control to deal with any thoughts of harm to self or others. (b) *Interference with Addiction Recovery Efforts*: The adolescent's emotional concerns relate to negative consequences and effects of addiction, and he or she is able to view them as part of addiction and recovery. Emotional, behavioral or cognitive symptoms, if present, appear to be related to substance-related problems rather than to a co-occurring psychiatric, emotional or behavioral condition. If they *are* related to such a condition, appropriate additional psychiatric services are provided concurrent with the Level I treatment. The adolescent's mental status does not preclude his or her ability to: [1] understand the materials presented (that is, his or her cognitive abilities are appropriate to the treatment modality and materials used); and [2] participate in the treatment process. (c) *Social Functioning*: Relationships or spheres of social functioning (as with family, friends, and peers at school and work) are impaired but not endangered by substance use (for example, there is no imminent break-up of family, expulsion from home, or imminent failure at school). The adolescent is able to meet personal responsibilities and to maintain stable, meaningful relationships despite the mild symptoms experienced (such as mood swings without aggression or threats of danger, or in-school suspension for lateness but no suspensions for truancy). (d) *Ability for Self-Care*: The adolescent has adequate resources and skills to cope with emotional, behavioral or cognitive problems, with some assistance. He or she has the support of a stable environment and is able to manage the activities of daily living (feeding, personal hygiene, grooming, and the like). (e) *Course of Illness*: The adolescent has only mild signs and symptoms. Any acute problems (such as severe depression, suicidality, aggression or dangerous delinquent behaviors) have been well stabilized, and chronic problems are not serious enough to pose a high risk of vulnerability (such as chronic and stable low-lethality self-injurious behavior, chronic depression without significant impairment or increase in severity, or chronic stable threats without risk of aggression).
DIMENSION 4: **Readiness to Change**	The adolescent's status in Dimension 4 is characterized by (a) *and one of* (b) *or* (c) *or* (d). (a) The adolescent expresses willingness to cooperate with the treatment plan and to attend all scheduled activities. A structured milieu program is not required; *and*

ASAM Patient Placement Criteria, Second Edition–Revised

Adolescent Level I Admission Criteria
Diagnostic and Dimensional Criteria

CRITERIA	LEVEL I Outpatient Services
DIMENSION 4: **Readiness to Change** **(continued)**	(b) The adolescent acknowledges that he or she has an alcohol or other drug problem and wants help to change, but is ambivalent about recovery efforts and requires monitoring and motivating strategies; *or* (c) The adolescent who has co-occurring mental and substance-related disorders is able to acknowledge the psychiatric diagnosis but is resistant to the substance use diagnosis, or vice versa; *or* (d) The adolescent admits that he or she has an alcohol or other drug problem, but is more invested in avoiding a negative consequence than in recovery efforts. He or she requires monitoring and motivating strategies to help with engagement in treatment, to facilitate his or her progress through the stages of change, and to prevent deterioration.
DIMENSION 5: **Relapse, Continued Use or Continued Problem Potential**	In Dimension 5, the adolescent is assessed as being able to significantly reduce his or her substance use or to achieve or maintain abstinence and recovery goals with only minimal support. The adolescent needs regular therapeutic contact to help him or her deal with issues that include, but are not limited to, preoccupation with alcohol or other drug use, craving, peer pressure, impulse control, and lifestyle and attitude changes.
DIMENSION 6: **Recovery Environment**	The adolescent's status in Dimension 6 is characterized by (a) *or* (b) *or* (c): (a) The adolescent's psychosocial environment is sufficiently supportive that outpatient treatment is feasible (for example, significant others are in agreement with the recovery effort; there is a supportive school or work environment or legal coercion; adequate transportation to the program is available; support meeting locations and a non-alcohol/drug-centered work or school environment are located near the home environment and are accessible); *or* (b) The adolescent does not have an ideal primary or social support system to assist with immediate sobriety, but he or she has demonstrated motivation and willingness to obtain such a support system and such efforts are judged to be feasible; *or* (c) The adolescent's family, guardian and/or significant other(s) are supportive but require professional interventions to improve the adolescent's chances of treatment success and recovery. Such interventions may involve assistance in monitoring and supervision techniques, limit-setting, communication skills, a reduction in rescuing behaviors, and the like.

Level II
Intensive Outpatient Treatment/Partial Hospitalization

Adolescent Level II encompasses a structured day or evening treatment program, which may be offered during the day, before or after work or school, in the evening or on a weekend. For appropriately selected patients, Level II programs provide essential education and treatment services while allowing patients to apply their newly acquired skills in "real world" environments.

Level II treatment programs have the capacity to arrange for medical and psychiatric consultation and 24-hour crisis services. They provide comprehensive biopsychosocial assessments and individualized treatment plans that are developed in consultation with the patient. Such plans include problem formulation, treatment goals and measurable treatment objectives. Treatment interventions and modalities also are tailored to engage adolescents who are at varying levels of developmental maturity. Such treatment often requires linkages with other service providers, usually by referral. Examples include psychiatric assessment and treatment, primary care medical assessment and treatment, psychological and/or educational testing for learning disorders, special or alternative education services, family therapies, juvenile justice probation and supervision, foster care support services, public benefit coordination or other social service agency interventions. In addition, the programs have active affiliations with other levels of care and can help the patient access support services such as child care, vocational training and transportation.

Beyond the basic services, many Level II programs provide psychiatric (including psycho-pharmacological) assessment and treatment and have the capacity to effectively treat patients who have complex co-occurring mental and substance-related disorders.

Some programs also can provide overnight housing for adolescents who have problems related to family environment or transportation but who do not need the supervision or 24-hour access to services afforded by a Level III program. Such structured day and evening treatment programs "unbundle" actual clinical treatment from "around-the-clock" supervised living environments that include overnight housing. Alternatively, some programs provide both lodging and services in an integrated fashion that approximates the intensity of a Level III.1 or III.5 program.

Increasingly, distinctions are made among various subtypes of Level II programs. Criteria are offered here for two variations: Intensive Outpatient (Level II.1) and Partial Hospitalization (Level II.5).

Treatment Levels Within Level II

Level II.1: Intensive Outpatient Treatment

Intensive outpatient programs (IOPs) generally provide at *least* 6 hours of structured programming per week, consisting primarily of counseling and education about alcohol and other drug problems. The precise number of hours of service delivered should be adjusted to meet each patient's needs. Six hours per week will be too few for many adolescents who meet the specifications for Level II.1—especially those who are early in their treatment or those who are stepping down from a more intensive level of care. Such adolescents may require 9, 12 or even 15 hours of intensive outpatient services. Other adolescents, who are progressing toward their recovery goals, may taper down to 6 hours.

Different models of intensive outpatient programs have been successfully adapted to variations in local logistics, regulatory requirements, program content and reimbursement limitations. Some programs employ a single fixed schedule of 6 or 9 hours of service per week. Others modify their service hours throughout the stages of treatment, tapering the number of hours according to a prescribed schedule.

Yet another approach is to match intensity and hours of service flexibly with the severity of the patient's problem(s). Using a decimal system to describe these variations, two weekly sessions of three hours each would constitute a Level II.1 program, while three weekly sessions of 3 hours each would be a Level II.2 program, four sessions would be a Level II.3 program, and so on.

The adolescent's needs for psychiatric and medical services are addressed through consultation and referral arrangements if the patient is stable and requires only maintenance monitoring. (Services provided outside the primary program must be tightly coordinated.)

Intensive outpatient treatment differs from partial hospitalization (Level II.5) programs in the intensity of clinical services that are directly available. Specifically, most intensive outpatient programs have less capacity to effectively treat adolescents who have substantial unstable medical and psychiatric problems than do partial hospitalization programs. Adolescent IOPs generally meet before, during or after school or work hours or on weekends.

Level II.5: Partial Hospitalization Programs

Partial hospitalization programs generally feature 20 or more hours of clinically intensive programming per week, as well as daily or near-daily contact, as specified in the patient's treatment plan. Level II.5 partial hospitalization programs often have direct access to or close referral relationships with psychiatric, medical and laboratory services, and thus are better able than Level II.1 programs to meet needs identified in Dimensions 1, 2 and 3, which warrant daily monitoring or management, but which can be appropriately addressed in a structured outpatient setting.

Partial hospitalization often occurs during school hours; such programs typically have access to educational services for their adolescent patients. Programs that do not provide educational services should coordinate with a school system in order to assess and meet their adolescent patients' educational needs.

Adolescents who meet Level III criteria in Dimensions 4, 5 or 6 and who otherwise might be placed in a Level III.1 or III.5 program may be considered for placement in a Level II.5 program if the patient resides in a facility that provides 24-hour support and structure and that limits access to alcohol and other drugs, such as a correctional facility or other licensed health care facility or a supervised living situation.

Length of Service

The duration of treatment varies with the severity of the adolescent's illness and his or her response to treatment.

Detoxification

Dimension 1 (Acute Intoxication and/or Withdrawal Potential) is the first of the six primary assessment areas to be evaluated in making treatment and placement decisions. The range of clinical severity in this dimension has given rise to a range of detoxification levels of service. A patient who is experiencing or at risk of an acute withdrawal syndrome should not be treated at Level II.1. For this reason, the designation of Level II.1-D has not been used. However, it is important to recognize lingering subacute withdrawal symptoms (such as vivid, disturbing dreams associated with marijuana withdrawal), which can be quite disturbing and which are appropriately addressed in a Level II.1 setting.

A patient who is experiencing mild and diminishing acute withdrawal (typically without overt physiological disturbances) can be treated appropriately in a Level II.5-D setting. Level II.5-D services can be offered by certain Level II.5 programs and integrated into the overall treatment program.

As used here, detoxification refers not only to the attenuation of the physiological and psychological features of withdrawal syndromes, but also to the process of interrupting the momentum of habitual compulsive use in adolescents diagnosed with substance *dependence*. Because of the force of this momentum, and the inherent difficulties in overcoming it even when there is no clear withdrawal syndrome *per se*, this phase of treatment frequently requires a greater intensity of services initially in order to establish treatment engagement and patient role induction. This is, of course, critical to the course of treatment because of the impossibility of engaging the adolescent in treatment while he/she is caught up in the cycle of frequent intoxication and recovery from intoxication. In this sense, detoxification is appropriately integrated into treatment at either Level II.1 or II.5; however, it often requires the increased intensity and daily or near-daily contact found in a Level II.5 program.

Essential to this level of care is the availability of appropriately credentialed nurses (registered nurses and/or licensed practical nurses) to monitor adolescent patients.

Adolescent Criteria
Level II: Intensive Outpatient Treatment/Partial Hospitalization

CHARACTERISTIC	LEVEL II.1 Intensive Outpatient Treatment	LEVEL II.5 Partial Hospitalization
EXAMPLES	Examples of Level II.1 adolescent programs are after-school, evening and/or weekend outpatient programs.	Examples of Level II.5 adolescent programs are day treatment programs.
SETTING	Level II.1 adolescent program services may be offered in any age-appropriate setting that meets state licensing or certification criteria.	Level II.5 adolescent programs may be offered in any age-appropriate setting that meets state licensing or certification criteria.
SUPPORT SYSTEMS	In Level II.1 adolescent programs, necessary support services include: (a) Medical, psychological, psychiatric, laboratory and toxicology, educational and occupational services, and other services needed by adolescents are available through consultation or referral. Medical and psychiatric consultation are available within 24 hours by telephone and within 72 hours face-to-face (depending on the urgency of the situation) through on-site services, referral to off-site services, or transfer to another level of care. (b) Emergency services, which are available by telephone 24 hours a day, 7 days a week when the program is not in session. (c) Direct affiliation with more and less intensive levels of care.	In Level II.5 adolescent programs, necessary support services include: (a) Medical, psychological, psychiatric, laboratory and toxicology, educational and occupational services, and other services needed by adolescents are available through consultation or referral. Medical and psychiatric consultation are available within 8 hours by telephone and within 48 hours face-to-face (depending on the urgency of the situation) through on-site services, referral to off-site services, or transfer to another level of care. (b) Emergency services, which are available by telephone 24 hours a day, 7 days a week when the program is not in session. (c) Direct affiliation with more and less intensive levels of care. **Level II.5-D Detoxification** In addition to the foregoing support systems, Level II.5-D support systems feature: (a) Availability of specialized clinical consultation and supervision for biomedical, emotional, cognitive or behavioral problems related to intoxication or detoxification.

Adolescent Criteria
Level II: Intensive Outpatient Treatment/Partial Hospitalization

CHARACTERISTIC	LEVEL II.1 Intensive Outpatient Treatment	LEVEL II.5 Partial Hospitalization
SUPPORT SYSTEMS (continued)		(b) Protocols used to determine the nature of the medical monitoring and/or interventions required (including the need for nursing or physician care and/or transfer to a more intensive level of care) are developed and supported by a physician who is knowledgeable in addiction medicine.
STAFF	Level II.1 adolescent programs are staffed by an interdisciplinary team of appropriately trained clinicians who assess and treat the adolescent's substance-related and co-occurring psychiatric disorders. One or more professional addiction clinicians is on-site during program hours. Staff are knowledgeable about adolescent development and experienced in working with and engaging adolescents.	Level II.5 adolescent programs are staffed by an interdisciplinary team of appropriately trained clinicians who assess and treat the adolescent's substance-related and co-occurring psychiatric disorders. One or more professional addiction clinicians is on-site during program hours. Staff are knowledgeable about adolescent development and experienced in working with and engaging adolescents. **Enhanced Programs (including Level II.5 Detoxification)** Appropriately licensed and credentialed staff are available to administer and/or monitor medications and to provide individual or group education about the medications and their use. The intensity of nursing care is appropriate to the services provided. **Level II.5-D Detoxification** When a Level II.1-D program provides detoxification services to adolescents, it must offer: (a) Appropriately trained personnel who are competent to implement physician-approved protocols for patient observation, supervision, treatment (including the use of over-the-counter medications for symptomatic relief), and determination of the appropriate level of care.

Adolescent Criteria
Level II: Intensive Outpatient Treatment/Partial Hospitalization

CHARACTERISTIC	LEVEL II.1 Intensive Outpatient Treatment	LEVEL II.5 Partial Hospitalization
STAFF (continued)		(b) Nursing and/or medical evaluation and consultation, which are available 24 hours a day to monitor the safety and outcome of detoxification efforts, in accordance with practice guidelines for patient treatment or transfer. (c) Clinicians who assess and treat adolescents are able to obtain and interpret information regarding the signs and symptoms of intoxication and withdrawal, as well as the appropriate treatment and monitoring of those conditions and the best way to facilitate the adolescent's transition to ongoing care.
THERAPIES	Therapies offered by Level II.1 adolescent programs include: (a) A planned format of therapies, delivered on an individual or group basis. Such therapies are designed and adapted to address the adolescent's developmental stage and comprehension level, according to his or her condition. (b) Intensive outpatient programs, which typically provide 6 or more hours of structured programming each week. Skilled treatment services may include individual and group counseling, family therapy, cognitive therapy, behavior modification or educational groups, occupational and recreational therapy, psychotherapy, or other therapies. These are provided in amounts, frequencies and intensities appropriate to achieve the objectives of the treatment plan. (c) Family therapy involving the adolescent's family member(s) or guardian in his or her assessment, treatment and continuing care.	Therapies offered by Level II.5 adolescent programs include: (a) A planned format of therapies, delivered on an individual or group basis. Such therapies are designed and adapted to address the adolescent's developmental stage and comprehension level, according to his or her condition. (b) Partial hospitalization programs, which typically provide a minimum of 20 hours of skilled treatment services each week. Skilled treatment services may include individual and group counseling, family therapy, cognitive therapy, behavior modification or educational groups, occupational and recreational therapy, psychotherapy, or other therapies. These are provided in amounts, frequencies and intensities appropriate to achieve the objectives of the treatment plan. (c) Family therapy involving the adolescent's family member(s) or guardian in his or her assessment, treatment and continuing care.

Adolescent Criteria
Level II: Intensive Outpatient Treatment/Partial Hospitalization

CHARACTERISTIC	LEVEL II.1 Intensive Outpatient Treatment	LEVEL II.5 Partial Hospitalization
THERAPIES (continued)		(d) Educational services (when not available through other resources), which are designed to maintain the educational and intellectual development of the patient and, when indicated, to provide opportunities to remedy deficits in the adolescent's education. **Level II.5-D Detoxification** Clinical services are provided to assess and address the adolescent's withdrawal status and treatment needs. Such clinical services may include nursing and medical monitoring or treatment, use of over-the-counter medications for symptomatic relief, individual or group therapies specific to withdrawal, and withdrawal support.
ASSESSMENT/ TREATMENT PLAN REVIEW	In Level II.1 adolescent programs, elements of the assessment and treatment plan review include: (a) A comprehensive substance use history, obtained as part of the initial assessment, and reviewed by a physician, if necessary. Such determinations are made according to established protocols that include reliance on the adolescent's personal physician when possible, based on the staff's capabilities and the patient's severity, and are approved by a physician. (In states where physician assistants or nurse practitioners are licensed as physician extenders, they may perform the duties designated here for a physician.) (b) An individual biopsychosocial assessment. (c) Information obtained from a parent, guardian or other important resource (such as a teacher or probation officer).	In Level II.5 adolescent programs, elements of the assessment and treatment plan review include: (a) A comprehensive substance use history, obtained as part of the initial assessment, and reviewed by a physician, if necessary. Such determinations are made according to established protocols that include reliance on the adolescent's personal physician when possible, based on the staff's capabilities and the patient's severity, and are approved by a physician. (In states where physician assistants or nurse practitioners are licensed as physician extenders, they may perform the duties designated here for a physician.) (b) An individual biopsychosocial assessment. (c) Information obtained from a parent, guardian or other important resource (such as a teacher or probation officer).

Adolescent Criteria
Level II: Intensive Outpatient Treatment/Partial Hospitalization

CHARACTERISTIC	LEVEL II.1 Intensive Outpatient Treatment	LEVEL II.5 Partial Hospitalization
ASSESSMENT/ TREATMENT PLAN REVIEW (continued)	(d) An individualized treatment plan, including problem formulation and articulation of treatment goals and measurable treatment objectives, as well as activities designed to meet those goals. Treatment plan reviews are conducted at specified times, as noted in the treatment plan.	(d) An individualized treatment plan, including problem formulation and articulation of treatment goals and measurable treatment objectives, as well as activities designed to meet those goals. Treatment plan reviews are conducted at specified times, as noted in the treatment plan. **Level II.5-D Detoxification** In addition to those listed above, elements of the assessment and treatment plan review include: (a) An initial withdrawal assessment, including a medical evaluation at admission (or medical review of an evaluation performed within the 48 hours preceding admission, or within 7 days preceding admission for a patient who is stepping down from a residential setting). (b) Ongoing withdrawal monitoring assessments, performed several times a week. (c) Ongoing screening for medical and nursing needs, with medical and nursing evaluation available through consultation or referral.
DOCUMENTATION	Documentation standards of Level II.1 adolescent programs include progress notes in the patient record that clearly reflect implementation of the treatment plan and the adolescent's response to treatment, as well as subsequent amendments to the plan.	Documentation standards of Level II.5 adolescent programs include progress notes in the patient record that clearly reflect implementation of the treatment plan and the adolescent's response to treatment, as well as subsequent amendments to the plan. **Level II.5-D Detoxification** Detoxification rating scale tables and flow sheets (which may include tabulation of vital signs) are used as needed.

Adolescent Level II Admission Criteria
Diagnostic and Dimensional Criteria

CRITERIA	LEVEL II.1 Intensive Outpatient Treatment	LEVEL II.5 Partial Hospitalization
DIAGNOSTIC ADMISSION CRITERIA	The adolescent who is appropriately placed in a Level II.1 program meets the diagnostic criteria for Substance-Related Disorder or a co-occurring psychiatric disorder, as defined in the current *Diagnostic and Statistical Manual of Mental Disorders (DSM)* of the American Psychiatric Association or other standardized and widely accepted criteria, as well as the dimensional criteria for admission. If the adolescent's presenting alcohol or other drug history is inadequate to substantiate such a diagnosis, the probability of such a diagnosis may be determined from information submitted by collateral parties (such as family members, legal guardian and significant others).	The adolescent who is appropriately placed in a Level II.5 program meets the diagnostic criteria for Substance-Related Disorder or a co-occurring psychiatric disorder, as defined in the current *Diagnostic and Statistical Manual of Mental Disorders (DSM)* of the American Psychiatric Association or other standardized and widely accepted criteria, as well as the dimensional criteria for admission. If the adolescent's presenting alcohol or other drug history is inadequate to substantiate such a diagnosis, the probability of such a diagnosis may be determined from information submitted by collateral parties (such as family members, legal guardian and significant others).
DIMENSIONAL ADMISSION CRITERIA	*Direct admission* to a Level II.1 program is advisable for the adolescent who meets the stability specifications in Dimension 1 (if any withdrawal problems exist) and Dimension 2 (if any biomedical conditions or problems exist) and the severity specifications in *one* of Dimension 3, 4, 5 or 6. *Transfer* to a Level II.1 program is appropriate for the adolescent who has met the objectives of treatment in a more intensive level of care and who requires the intensity of service provided at Level II.1 in at least one dimension. An adolescent also may be transferred to Level II.1 from a Level I program when the services provided at Level I have proved insufficient to address his or her needs or when Level I services have consisted of motivational interventions to prepare the adolescent for participation in a more intensive level of care for which he or she now meets the admission	*Direct admission* to a Level II.5 program is advisable for the adolescent who meets the stability specifications in Dimension 1 (if any withdrawal problems exist) and Dimension 2 (if any biomedical conditions or problems exist) and the severity specifications in *one* of Dimension 1, 3, 4, 5 or 6. *Transfer* to a Level II.5 program is appropriate for the adolescent who has met the objectives of treatment in a more intensive level of care and who requires the intensity of service provided at Level II.5 in at least one dimension. An adolescent also may be transferred to Level II.5 from a Level I or II.1 program when the services provided at those levels have proved insufficient to address his or her needs or when Level I or II.1 services have consisted of motivational interventions to prepare the adolescent for participation in a more intensive level of care for which he or she now meets

Adolescent Level II Admission Criteria
Diagnostic and Dimensional Criteria

CRITERIA	LEVEL II.1 Intensive Outpatient Treatment	LEVEL II.5 Partial Hospitalization
DIMENSIONAL ADMISSION CRITERIA (continued)	criteria. (The adolescent may be transferred to the next higher level of care if the indicated level is not available in the immediate geographic area.)	the admission criteria. (The adolescent may be transferred to the next higher level of care if the indicated level is not available in the immediate geographic area.)
DIMENSION 1: Acute Intoxication and/or Withdrawal	The adolescent who is appropriately placed in a Level II.1 program is not experiencing or at risk of acute withdrawal. At most, the adolescent's symptoms consist of subacute withdrawal marked by minimal symptoms that are diminishing (as during the first several weeks of abstinence following a period of more severe acute withdrawal). The adolescent is likely to attend, engage and participate in treatment, as evidenced by his or her meeting the following criteria: (a) The adolescent is able to tolerate mild subacute withdrawal symptoms. (b) He or she has made a commitment to sustain treatment and to follow treatment recommendations. (c) The adolescent has external supports (family and/or court) that promote engagement in treatment.	The adolescent who is appropriately placed in a Level II.5 program is experiencing acute or subacute withdrawal, marked by mild symptoms that are diminishing (as during the first several weeks of abstinence following a period of more severe acute withdrawal). The adolescent is likely to attend, engage and participate in treatment, as evidenced by meeting the following criteria: (a) The adolescent is able to tolerate mild withdrawal symptoms. (b) He or she has made a commitment to sustain treatment and to follow treatment recommendations. (c) The adolescent has external supports (as from family and/or court) that promote treatment engagement. Drug-specific examples follow: (a) *Alcohol*: Mild withdrawal; no need for sedative-hypnotic substitution therapy; no hyperdynamic state; CIWA-Ar score of ≤ 6; no significant history of regular morning drinking; the adolescent's symptoms are stabilized and he or she is comfortable by the end of each day's active treatment or monitoring.

Adolescent Level II Admission Criteria
Diagnostic and Dimensional Criteria

CRITERIA	LEVEL II.1 Intensive Outpatient Treatment	LEVEL II.5 Partial Hospitalization
DIMENSION 1: **Acute Intoxication and/or Withdrawal** **(continued)**	NOTE: If the adolescent presents for treatment after recently experiencing an episode of acute withdrawal without treatment (as opposed to stepping down from a higher level of care following a good response), it is safer to err on the side of greater intensity of services when making a placement decision. For example, a Level II.5 setting may be indicated if the adolescent is doing poorly or if there are indications in other dimensions that he or she would benefit from that level of care.	(b) *Sedative-hypnotics*: Mild withdrawal; the adolescent may have a history of near-daily sedative-hypnotic use, but no cross-dependence on other substances; no disturbance of vital signs; no unstable complicating exacerbation of affective disturbance; no need for sedative-hypnotic substitution therapy; the adolescent's symptoms are stabilized, and he or she is comfortable by the end of each day's active treatment or monitoring. (c) *Opiates*: Mild withdrawal; the adolescent may need over-the-counter medications for symptomatic relief, but does not need prescription medications or opiate agonist substitution therapy; he or she is comfortable by the end of each day's active treatment or monitoring. The adolescent has sufficient impulse control, coping skills and/or supports to prevent immediate continued use beyond the active treatment day. (d) *Stimulants*: Mild to moderate withdrawal (for example, involving depression, lethargy or agitation), so that the adolescent is likely to need frequent contact and/or higher intensity services to tolerate symptoms, engage in treatment and bolster external supports. The adolescent has sufficient impulse control, coping skills and/or supports to prevent immediate continued use beyond the active treatment day. (e) *Inhalants*: Mild subacute intoxication (involving cognitive impairment, lethargy, agitation and depression), such that the adolescent is likely to need frequent contact and/or higher intensity services to tolerate symptoms, engage in treatment and bolster external supports. The adolescent has

Adolescent Level II Admission Criteria
Diagnostic and Dimensional Criteria

CRITERIA	LEVEL II.1 Intensive Outpatient Treatment	LEVEL II.5 Partial Hospitalization
DIMENSION 1: **Acute Intoxication and/or Withdrawal (continued)**		sufficient impulse control, coping skills and/or supports to prevent immediate continued use beyond the active treatment day. (f) *Marijuana*: Moderate withdrawal (involving irritability, general malaise, inner agitation and sleep disturbance) or sustained subacute intoxication (involving cognitive disorganization, memory impairment and executive dysfunction), such that the adolescent is likely to need frequent contact and/or higher intensity services to tolerate symptoms, engage in treatment and bolster external supports. (g) *Hallucinogens*: Mild persistent intoxication (involving mild perceptual distortion, mild suspiciousness or mild affective instability). The adolescent has sufficient compensatory coping skills to support engagement in treatment.
DIMENSION 2: **Biomedical Conditions and Complications**	In Dimension 2, the adolescent's biomedical conditions and problems, if any, are stable or are being concurrently addressed and will not interfere with treatment at this level of care; *or* The adolescent's biomedical conditions and problems are severe enough to distract from recovery and treatment at a less intensive level of care, but will not interfere with recovery at Level II.1. The biomedical conditions and problems are being addressed concurrently by a medical treatment provider.	In Dimension 2, the adolescent's biomedical conditions and problems, if any, are stable or are being concurrently addressed and will not interfere with treatment at this level of care; *or* The adolescent's biomedical conditions and problems are severe enough to distract from recovery and treatment at a lower level of care, but will not interfere with recovery at Level II.5. The biomedical conditions and problems are being addressed concurrently by a medical treatment provider.

Adolescent Level II Admission Criteria
Diagnostic and Dimensional Criteria

CRITERIA	LEVEL II.1 Intensive Outpatient Treatment	LEVEL II.5 Partial Hospitalization
DIMENSION 3: **Emotional,** **Behavioral or** **Cognitive** **Conditions and** **Complications**	The adolescent's status in Dimension 3 is characterized by at least *one* of the following: (a) *Dangerousness/Lethality*: The adolescent is at mild risk of behaviors endangering self, others or property (for example, he or she has suicidal or homicidal thoughts, but no active plan), and requires frequent monitoring to assure that there is a reasonable likelihood of safety between IOP sessions. However, his or her condition is not so severe as to require daily supervision. (b) *Interference with Addiction Recovery Efforts*: The adolescent's recovery efforts are negatively affected by an emotional, behavioral or cognitive problem, which causes mild interference with and requires increased intensity to support treatment participation and/or compliance. For example, the adolescent requires frequent repetition of treatment materials because of memory impairment associated with marijuana use. (c) *Social Functioning*: The adolescent's symptoms are causing mild to moderate difficulty in social functioning (involving family, friends, school or work), but not to such a degree that he or she is unable to manage the activities of daily living or to fulfill responsibilities at home, school, work or community. For example, the adolescent's problems may involve significantly worsening school performance or in-school detentions, a circle of friends that has narrowed to predominantly drug users, or loss of interest in most activities other than drug use.	The adolescent's status in Dimension 3 is characterized by at least *one* of the following: (a) *Dangerousness/Lethality*: The adolescent is at mild risk of behaviors endangering self, others or property (for example, he or she has suicidal or homicidal thoughts, but no active plan), and requires frequent monitoring to assure that there is a reasonable likelihood of safety between PHP sessions. However, his or her condition is not so severe as to require 24-hour supervision. (b) *Interference with Addiction Recovery Efforts*: The adolescent's recovery efforts are negatively affected by an emotional, behavioral or cognitive problem, which causes moderate interference with and requires increased intensity to support treatment participation and/or compliance. For example, cognitive impairment or significant attention deficit hyperactivity disorder prevents achievement of recovery tasks or goals. (c) *Social Functioning*: The adolescent's symptoms are causing mild to moderate difficulty in social functioning (involving family, friends, school or work), but not to such a degree that the adolescent is unable to manage the activities of daily living or to fulfill responsibilities at home, school, work or community. For example, the adolescent's problems may involve recent arrests or legal charges, or non-compliance with probation, progressive school suspensions or truancy, risk of failing the school year, regular intoxication at school or work, involvement in drug trafficking, or a pattern of intentional property damage.

Adolescent Level II Admission Criteria
Diagnostic and Dimensional Criteria

CRITERIA	LEVEL II.1 Intensive Outpatient Treatment	LEVEL II.5 Partial Hospitalization
DIMENSION 3: **Emotional,** **Behavioral or** **Cognitive** **Conditions and** **Complications** **(continued)**	(d) *Ability for Self-Care*: The adolescent is experiencing mild to moderate impairment in ability to manage the activities of daily living, and thus requires frequent monitoring and treatment interventions. Problems may involve poor hygiene secondary to exacerbation of a chronic mental illness, poor self-care or lack of independent living skills in an older adolescent who is transitioning to adulthood, or in a younger adolescent who lacks adequate family supports. (e) *Course of Illness*: The adolescent's history and present situation suggest that an emotional, behavioral or cognitive condition would become unstable without frequent monitoring and maintenance. For example, he or she may require frequent prompting and monitoring of medication compliance (in an adolescent with a history of medication non-compliance) or frequent prompting and monitoring of behavioral compliance (in an adolescent with a conduct disorder or other serious pattern of delinquent behavior).	Alternatively, the adolescent may be transitioning back to the community as a step-down from an institutionalized setting. (d) *Ability for Self-Care*: The adolescent is experiencing moderate impairment in ability to manage the activities of daily living, and thus requires near-daily monitoring and treatment interventions. Problems may involve disorganization and inability to manage the demands of daily self-scheduling, a progressive pattern of promiscuous or unprotected sexual contacts, or poor vocational or prevocational skills that require habilitation and training provided in the program. (e) *Course of Illness*: The adolescent's history and present situation suggest that an emotional, behavioral or cognitive condition would become unstable without daily or near-daily monitoring and maintenance. For example, signs of imminent relapse may indicate a need for near-daily monitoring of an adolescent with attention deficit hyperactivity disorder and a history of disorganization that becomes unmanageable in school with substance use; or an initial lapse indicates a need for near-daily monitoring in an adolescent whose conduct disorder worsens dangerously within the context of progressive use.
DIMENSION 4: **Readiness to** **Change**	The adolescent's status in Dimension 4 is characterized by (a) *or* (b): (a) The adolescent requires structured therapy and a programmatic milieu to promote progress through the stages of change, as evidenced by behaviors such as the following: [1] the adolescent is verbally compliant, but does not demonstrate	The adolescent's status in Dimension 4 is characterized by (a) *or* (b): (a) The adolescent requires structured therapy and a programmatic milieu to promote progress through the stages of change, as evidenced by behaviors such as the following: [1] the adolescent demonstrates verbal or behavioral opposition to treatment;

Adolescent Level II Admission Criteria
Diagnostic and Dimensional Criteria

CRITERIA	LEVEL II.1 Intensive Outpatient Treatment	LEVEL II.5 Partial Hospitalization
DIMENSION 4: **Readiness to** **Change (continued)**	consistent behaviors; [2] the adolescent is only passively involved in treatment; or [3] the adolescent demonstrates variable compliance with attendance at outpatient sessions or self- or mutual-help meetings or support groups. Such interventions are not feasible or are not likely to succeed in a Level I service; *or* (b) The adolescent's perspective inhibits his or her ability to make progress through the stages of change. For example, he or she has unrealistic expectations that the alcohol or drug problem will resolve quickly and with little or no effort, or does not recognize the need for continued assistance. The adolescent thus requires structured therapy and a programmatic milieu. Such interventions are not feasible or are not likely to succeed in a Level I service.	[2] the adolescent is only minimally involved in treatment; [3] the adolescent demonstrates poor compliance with attendance at outpatient sessions; or [4] the adolescent's alcohol or drug use is escalating, contributing to (for example) school failure, truancy or behaviors leading to suspension from school; *or* (b) The adolescent's perspective and lack of impulse control inhibit his or her ability to make progress through the stages of change. For example, the adolescent attributes his or her alcohol or other drug problem to other persons or external events rather than to an addictive disorder. The adolescent thus requires structured therapy and a programmatic milieu. Such interventions are not feasible or are not likely to succeed in a Level II.1 service. However, the adolescent's resistance is not so high as to render treatment ineffective.
DIMENSION 5: **Relapse, Continued** **Use or Continued** **Problem Potential**	The adolescent's status in Dimension 5 is characterized by (a) *or* (b): (a) The adolescent is at significant risk of relapse or continued use, as well as deterioration in level of functioning, without frequent outpatient monitoring and therapeutic services (as indicated, for example, by difficulty in deferring immediate gratification and related drug-seeking behavior, increasing responsiveness to negative peer influences, or ongoing infrequent lapses); *or*	The adolescent's status in Dimension 5 is characterized by (a) *or* (b): (a) The adolescent is at high risk of relapse or continued use without almost daily outpatient monitoring and structured therapeutic services (as indicated, for example, by susceptibility to relapse triggers, a pattern of frequent or progressive lapses, inability to overcome the momentum of a pattern of habitual use, difficulty in overcoming a pattern of impulsive behaviors, or ambivalence toward or resistance to treatment). Also, treatment at a less intensive level of care has been attempted or given serious consideration and been judged insufficient to stabilize the adolescent's condition; *or*

Adolescent Level II Admission Criteria
Diagnostic and Dimensional Criteria

CRITERIA	LEVEL II.1 Intensive Outpatient Treatment	LEVEL II.5 Partial Hospitalization
DIMENSION 5: **Relapse, Continued Use or Continued Problem Potential** **(continued)**	(b) The adolescent demonstrates impaired recognition and understanding of relapse issues. He or she is able to avoid continued use or relapse only with the moderate treatment support available in a Level II.1 program.	(b) The adolescent demonstrates impaired recognition and understanding of relapse issues. He or she has such poor skills in coping with and interrupting substance use problems, and avoiding or limiting relapse, that the near-daily structure afforded by a Level II.5 program is needed to prevent or arrest significant deterioration in function.
DIMENSION 6: **Recovery Environment**	The adolescent's status in Dimension 6 is characterized by (a) *or* (b) *or* (c): (a) Continued exposure to the adolescent's current school, work or living environment will impede recovery. He or she has insufficient (or severely limited) resources and skills necessary to maintain an adequate level of functioning without the services of a Level II.1 program, but is capable of maintaining an adequate level of functioning between sessions; *or* (b) The adolescent lacks social contacts, or has inappropriate social contacts that jeopardize recovery, or has few friends or peers who do not use alcohol or other drugs. He or she also has insufficient (or severely limited) resources or skills necessary to maintain an adequate level of functioning without the services of a Level II.1 program, but is capable of maintaining an adequate level of functioning between sessions; *or*	The adolescent's status in Dimension 6 is characterized by (a) *or* (b) *or* (c): (a) Continued exposure to the adolescent's current school, work or living environment will render recovery unlikely. He or she lacks the resources and skills necessary to maintain an adequate level of functioning without the services of a Level II.5 program, but is capable of maintaining an adequate level of functioning between sessions; *or* (b) The adolescent lacks social contacts, or has inappropriate social contacts that jeopardize recovery, or has few friends or peers who do not use alcohol or other drugs. He or she also has insufficient (or severely limited) resources or skills necessary to maintain an adequate level of functioning without the services of a Level II.5 program, but is capable of maintaining an adequate level of functioning between sessions; *or*

Adolescent Level II Admission Criteria
Diagnostic and Dimensional Criteria

CRITERIA	LEVEL II.1 Intensive Outpatient Treatment	LEVEL II.5 Partial Hospitalization
DIMENSION 6: **Recovery** **Environment** **(continued)**	(c) The adolescent's family or caretakers are supportive of recovery, but family conflicts and related family dysfunction impede the adolescent's ability to learn the skills necessary to achieve and maintain abstinence. NOTE: The adolescent may require Level II.1 services in addition to an out-of-home placement (for example, at Level III.1 or the equivalent, such as a group home or a non-treatment residential setting such as a detention program). If his or her present environment is supportive of recovery but does not provide sufficient addiction-specific services to foster and sustain recovery goals, the adolescent's needs in Dimension 6 may be met through an out-of-home placement, while other dimensional criteria would indicate the need for care in a Level II.1 program.	(c) Family members and/or significant other(s) living with the adolescent are not supportive of his or her recovery goals and/or are passively opposed to treatment. The adolescent requires structured treatment services and relief from the home environment in order to remain focused on recovery, but he or she may live at home because there is no active opposition to, or sabotaging of, the recovery effort. NOTE: The adolescent may require Level II.5 services in addition to an out-of-home placement (for example, at Level III.1 or the equivalent, such as a group home or a non-treatment residential setting such as a detention program). If his or her present environment is supportive of recovery but does not provide sufficient addiction-specific services to foster and sustain recovery goals, the adolescent's needs in Dimension 6 may be met through an out-of-home placement, while other dimensional criteria would indicate the need for care in a Level II.5 program.

ASAM Patient Placement Criteria, Second Edition–Revised

Level III
Residential/Inpatient Treatment

Adolescent Level III programs offer organized treatment services that feature a planned regimen of care in a 24-hour residential setting. Treatment is delivered in accordance with defined policies, procedures and clinical protocols. Such program are housed in, or affiliated with, permanent facilities where adolescents can reside safely. They are staffed 24 hours a day. Mutual/self-help group meetings are available on-site, or transportation is provided to attend meetings off-site.

While earlier editions of the criteria treated all adolescent residential treatment as one broad undifferentiated level of care, the *PPC-2R* divides Level III into three sublevels:

Level III.1: Clinically Managed Low-Intensity Residential Treatment
Level III.5: Clinically Managed Medium-Intensity Residential Treatment
Level III.7: Medically Monitored High-Intensity Residential/Inpatient Treatment

A characteristic of all Level III programs is that they serve individuals who, because of specific functional deficits, need safe and stable living environments in order to develop their recovery skills. One of the purposes of these programs is to demonstrate aspects of a positive recovery environment. Such a living environment may be housed in the same facility as the treatment services, or they may be in separate facilities that are affiliated with the treatment provider. In the latter situation, the relationship between the living environment and the treatment provider must be sufficiently close to allow specific aspects of the individual treatment plan to be addressed in both facilities.

The sublevels within Level III exist on a continuum ranging from the least intensive residential services to the most intensive medically monitored intensive residential/inpatient services. The intent is not to create just three discrete sublevels of care within Level III, but rather to reflect a range of intensities, with each designated sublevel (such as Level III.5) typifying an approximate point within that range. When a program provides Level III services that exceed the intensity usually ascribed to that level, or can appropriately treat individuals who have a more severe illness than usually is addressed at that level, it should be considered an *enhanced service*.

The term "clinically managed" is used to describe Level III.1 through III.5 programs. Clinically managed services are directed by non-physician addiction specialists rather than medical or psychiatric personnel.

The adolescent who is appropriately placed in a clinically managed program has minimal problems with intoxication or withdrawal (Dimension 1) and few biomedical complications (Dimension 2). Therefore, on-site medical services are not required. Such an adolescent may have problems with emotional, behavioral or cognitive conditions, but these are of sufficient relative stability so as not to require on-site psychiatric services. The adolescent also may have significant deficits in the areas of readiness to change (Dimension 4), relapse, continued use or continued problem potential (Dimension 5) or recovery environment (Dimension 6) and thus be in need of interventions directed by appropriately trained and credentialed addiction treatment staff. He or she also may need case management services to facilitate reintegration into the larger community.

The term "medically monitored" is used to describe Level III.7 programs. Medically monitored program services are provided under the direction of a physician who is a specialist in addiction medicine. The adolescent who is appropriately placed in a medically monitored program may have problems in Dimensions 1, 2, or 3 that require direct medical or nursing services.

Alternatively, he or she may have problems that require the overall high intensity of a Level III.7 program and a treatment milieu that draws on the staffing patterns and availability of an interdisciplinary professional team typically found in a medically monitored program.

Treatment Levels Within Level III

Level III.1: Clinically Managed Low-Intensity Residential Services

Level III.1 programs often are provided in halfway houses and non-therapeutic group homes. Such a program offers at least five hours a week of low-intensity treatment of substance-related disorders (or the number of hours specified by state licensure requirements). Treatment is directed toward applying recovery skills, preventing relapse, improving social functioning and ability for self-care, promoting personal responsibility, developing a social network supportive of recovery, and reintegrating the individual into the worlds of school, work and family life. The services provided may include individual, group and family therapy, educational and vocational counseling and recreational activities. Mutual/self-help meetings either are available on-site or transportation is provided to meetings held off-site.

The care delivered in a Level III.1 program is best understood in its component parts. The treatment services provided by Level III.1 programs, when considered separately from the residential component and other concurrent services, are low-intensity (Level I) outpatient services that often are focused on improving the individual's functioning and coping skills in Dimensions 5 and 6. The other component of care is a structured recovery environment, staffed 24 hours a day, which provides sufficient stability and supervision to prevent or minimize relapse or continued use and continued problem potential (Dimension 5). Interpersonal and group living skills generally are promoted through the use of community or house meetings of residents and staff. When these components are provided together, a Level III.1 program often is appropriate for an adolescent who needs time, structure and low-intensity coaching to practice and integrate recovery and coping skills.

The residential component of a Level III.1 program may be combined with intensive (Level II.1) outpatient services for the adolescent whose living situation is incompatible with his or her recovery goals, if the adolescent meets the dimensional admission criteria for intensive outpatient care.

Some adolescents require the structure of a Level III.1 program to achieve engagement in treatment (Dimension 4). Those who are in the early stages of readiness to change may need to be removed from an unsupportive living environment in order to minimize their continued alcohol or other drug use. In a setting that provides 24-hour structure, supervision and support, the adolescent has an opportunity to develop and practice interpersonal and group living skills, strengthen his or her recovery skills, organize the activities of daily living, participate in concurrent treatment services, engage in and sustain successful concurrent involvement in regular, productive daily activities (such as school or work), and reintegrate into the community and (possibly) family.

Intoxication and withdrawal require separate consideration. Intoxication or very mild withdrawal in an individual who is placed in a Level III.1 program usually represents an isolated relapse associated with problems in applying recovery skills (Dimension 5). The therapeutic response to episodes of lapse or relapse, as well as the ability to manage such episodes, varies considerably across Level III.1 programs. Such matters remain controversial in the field. At the least, episodes of lapse or relapse in Level III.1, and attendant issues in problem recognition or problem solving, require management through additional concurrent Level I or II treatments. Another view suggests that relapse or continued use is *not* appropriately managed at Level III.1, but rather should be managed through transfer to a higher intensity residential level of care.

Treatment at Level III.1 sometimes is warranted as a substitute for or supplement to deficits in the adolescent's recovery environment, such as a chaotic home situation, drug-using caretakers or siblings, or a lack of daily structured activity (such as school). In other cases, an extended period in Level III.1 treatment is needed to sustain and further therapeutic gains made at more intensive levels of care because of the adolescent's functional deficits (including developmental immaturity, greater than average susceptibility to peer influence, or lack of impulse control). Many adolescents evidence a combination of these deficits.

The duration of treatment always depends on individual progress. Because treatment plans should be individualized, lengths of stay should be flexible and individualized to meet the needs of each patient. On the other hand, there may be "threshold" lengths of stay that are associated with certain therapeutic gains. The length of stay in a clinically managed Level III.1 program tends to be longer than in the more intensive residential levels of care. Longer exposure to monitoring, supervision and low-intensity treatment interventions is necessary for adolescents to practice basic living skills and to master the application of coping and recovery skills. In some situations, there is no effective substitute for extended residential containment as reliable protection from the toxic influences of substance exposure, problematic or substance-infested environments, or the cultures of substance-involved and antisocial behaviors.

Level III.1 is not intended to describe or include sober houses, boarding houses or group homes where treatment services are not provided.

Level III.3: Clinically Managed Medium-Intensity Residential Services (Adult)

Adult Level III.3 programming is not included here because the types of programs described as adolescent Level III.5 encompass the range of settings in which adolescent treatment is provided, and the distinction between Levels III.3 and III.5 does not have sufficient specificity in adolescent treatment to merit the added complexity of an additional level.

Level III.5: Clinically Managed Medium-Intensity Residential Services (Adolescent)

Level III.5 programs include medium-intensity settings such as therapeutic group homes, therapeutic community (TC) programs, psychosocial model residential treatment centers, or extended residential rehabilitation programs. These sometimes are referred to simply as "residential programs" without further specificity.

Level III.5 programs are designed to provide relatively extended, subacute treatments that aim to effect fundamental personal change for the adolescent who has significant social and psychological problems. The goals and modalities of treatment focus not only on the adolescent's substance use, but also on a holistic view of the adolescent that takes into account his or her behavior, emotions, attitudes, values, learning, family, culture, lifestyle and overall health. Often, adolescents in Level III.5 programs are in need of *habilitative* rather than rehabilitative approaches, emphasizing the acquisition of new capacities, rather than the restoration of lost ones.

Such programs are characterized by their reliance on the treatment community or milieu as a therapeutic agent of change. These programs utilize 24-hour active programming and containment to create a structure that makes such a community or milieu effective as a tool for acquiring both recovery skills and basic life skills. Critical treatment interventions that require intensity and persistence over extended periods of time, such as modeling prosocial patterns of behavior and adaptive patterns of emotional responsiveness, have sometimes been likened to surrogate or remedial parenting. Just as important can be the induction into a healthy peer group, with the formation of a group identity that emphasizes recovery and overcoming adversity.

The adolescent who is appropriately placed in a Level III.5 program may have problems related to emotional, behavioral and cognitive conditions (Dimension 3), to early stages of treatment engagement and readiness to change (Dimension 4), or to his or her living environment (Dimension 6). In addition to (and intertwined with) substance use, such an adolescent typically has impaired functioning across a broad range of psychosocial domains. These impairments may be expressed as disruptive behaviors, delinquency and juvenile justice involvement, educational difficulties, family conflicts and chaotic home situations, developmental immaturity, and psychological problems.

Such an adolescent may have a variety of psychological or psychiatric problems. Particularly suitable for Level III.5 treatments are the entrenched patterns of maladaptive behavior, extremes of temperament, and developmental or cognitive abnormalities related to mental health symptoms or disorders. Examples of co-occurring disorders that often require extended treatment at Level III.5 are Conduct Disorder and Oppositional Defiant Disorder, as well as the persistent patterns of disruptive behavior that may be associated with other disorders even after they have responded to acute treatment. Level III.5 programs frequently work with aspects of adolescent temperament—including impulsive, extroverted, dramatic, anti-social, thrill-seeking or other personality traits—that may otherwise have the potential to solidify as components of emerging personality disorders.

Level III.5 settings are not intended to encompass treatment for Dimension 3 problems that requires significant medical, psychiatric or nursing monitoring or interventions.

Even adolescents who are not diagnosed with psychiatric disorders (either because they do not meet full diagnostic criteria, or because they have not yet had a formal psychiatric evaluation) may have problems in Dimension 3 that render treatment ineffective at less intensive levels of care. Examples include hyperactivity or distractibility without a diagnosis of ADHD, explosive temper and anger management problems, resistance to limits and authority, patterns of hostility or aggression, impulse control problems, cognitive limitations and learning difficulties. Difficulties with interpersonal relationships (including poor conflict resolution abilities, fighting, social inhibition or withdrawal, and high-risk or indiscriminate sexual activity) frequently are targets of treatment. When treatment in the context of these problems cannot be implemented successfully on an outpatient basis, placement in a Level III.5 program should be considered.

Level III.5 also is appropriate for the adolescent whose problems include delinquency and juvenile justice involvement. In fact, this level of care often is warranted for adolescents who have the constellation of difficulties associated with severe conduct problems, a progressive history of illegal behaviors, a pattern of emerging criminality, or an incipient antisocial value system. In this context, treatment must proceed in a contained, safe and structured environment to allow teaching and practicing of prosocial behaviors and to facilitate healthy reintegration into the community. One of the key purposes of III.5 treatment for this set of problems is assessment and monitoring of safety, with particular attention to issues of *potential* safety outside of the contained setting. Goals of treatment include: overcoming oppositionality through a combination of confrontation, motivational enhancement and supportive limit setting; anger management and acquisition of conflict resolution skills; values clarification and moral habilitation; character molding and education; development of effective behavioral contingency strategies; establishment of a reliable response to external structure; and the internalization of structure through self-regulation skills.

Some Level III.5 programs specialize in the care of adolescents who are involved in the juvenile justice system. In fact, many programs actually are part of, or closely affiliated with, the juvenile justice system (including drug courts) or are located within juvenile justice facilities. Other programs may have a specific track for juvenile justice involved adolescents within the program; while some make no special distinction and integrate their care into the overall program.

Treatment in a Level III.5 program may be used to address problems in treatment engagement and readiness to change (Dimension 4). Many adolescents fail attempts at outpatient treatment out of a lack of engagement, either because of a lack of personal connection to treatment or because the systems surrounding the adolescent (family, school, juvenile justice system, and the like) have not coordinated sufficiently to motivate the adolescent, or both. The immersion experience of a Level III.5 program may be needed to promote treatment role induction and introduce the adolescent into a peer group that is struggling to form a group identity that emphasizes recovery and the need for treatment. For some adolescents, "discovery" may be an appropriate treatment plan. An additional goal of treatment at Level III.5 should be to promote coordination of the multiple systems surrounding the adolescent and to help devise and implement motivational strategies for ongoing engagement in treatment.

Problems in Dimension 6 that would warrant placement in a Level III.5 program include a chaotic home environment in which substance use, illegal behaviors, abuse, neglect or lack of supervision are prominent, or a broader community in which substance use and crime are endemic. These social influences may represent a sense of hopelessness or an acceptance of deviance as normative. There may not be readily apparent role models for the rewards of abstinence. Many adolescents have a social network composed primarily or even exclusively of family or peers who are involved in substance use or criminal behaviors. Some adolescents may have had *no* experience of a living environment conducive to healthy psychosocial development.

Level III.5 programs are found across a spectrum of intensities and program models or styles. They employ a wide variety of treatment methods and modalities. A partial list of common program components would include therapeutic communities, cognitive/behavioral therapies, motivational enhancement techniques, Twelve Step facilitation, discovery and challenge approaches, educational programming (including special education), vocational and/or pre-vocational programming (including work camps), moral reconation techniques, restorative justice approaches, community service, group identity and cultural identity techniques (including rituals and rites of passage), and specific competency building (such as martial arts, wilderness survival skills or expressive arts).

An adolescent may be admitted directly to a Level III.5 program, or transferred from a less intensive level of care. The adolescent also may be transferred for continuing care from a more intensive level of care, for example, when he or she no longer requires the intensity of services or staffing pattern of a Level III.7 program.

Many Level III.5 programs are freestanding. However, many are part of a broader continuum of care, connected to programs of higher and/or lower intensity. In particular, many Level III.5 programs may be connected to Level III.7 programs as "step down" units or tracks. Some Level III.5 programs are directly integrated into Level III.7 programs. In some programs the patients are blended without explicit distinction, except that patients have different acuities and receive somewhat different intensities of service.

Level III.7: Medically Monitored High-Intensity Residential/Inpatient Treatment

Level III.7 programs provide a planned regimen of 24-hour professionally directed evaluation, observation, medical monitoring and addiction treatment in an inpatient setting. They feature permanent facilities, including inpatient beds, and function under a defined set of policies, procedures and clinical protocols. They are appropriate for adolescents whose subacute biomedical and emotional, behavioral or cognitive problems are so severe that they require inpatient treatment, but who do not need the full resources of an acute care general hospital or a medically managed inpatient treatment program.

The services of a Level III.7 program are designed to meet the needs of the adolescent who, among other problems, has functional deficits related to problems in Dimensions 1, 2, or 3. These medically monitored services are provided under the supervision of physicians who are specialists in addiction medicine, and the programs tend to operate under the so-called "medical model." The adolescent who is appropriately placed in a medically monitored program may have problems in Dimensions 1, 2, or 3 that require direct medical or nursing services. Alternatively, he or she may have problems that do not so much require direct medical or nursing services as the overall high intensity of a program and treatment milieu that draws on the staffing pattern and availability of an interdisciplinary professional team that characterize medically monitored programs.

Problems in Dimension 3 probably are the most common reason for admission to Level III.7 programs. Such problems include co-occurring psychiatric disorders (such as Depressive Disorders, Bipolar Disorders, and ADHD) or symptoms (such as hypomania, severe disorganization or impulsiveness, and aggressive behaviors). Because mental health symptoms exist on a continuum of severity, specific problems may fall short of the criteria for diagnoses of specific disorders but still require treatment in a Level III.7 program. For example, an adolescent's high level of inattention and distractibility may significantly interfere with his or her addiction recovery efforts, but not warrant a diagnosis of ADD. An adolescent's behavioral symptom of disruptive behavior may require the high intensity staffing found in a Level III.7 program, but not warrant a diagnosis of a co-occurring Axis I disorder.

In the *PPC-2R*, the organization of the Dimension 3 severity specifications by subdomains emphasizes that placement decisions emerge out of the assessment of symptomatic functional impairment rather than any specific categorical diagnosis. For many high severity adolescents, it is the emotional, behavioral or cognitive sequelae of their substance-related disorders that necessitate Level III.7 treatment, *with or without* an additional diagnosis of a co-occurring psychiatric disorder. Treatment at Level III.7 often is necessary simply to orient an adolescent to the structure of daily life, according to other organizing principles than "getting high" and "being high." Initial abstinence through confinement in a Level III.7 program provides many adolescents who have substance dependence syndromes with a much-needed reintroduction to their own patterns of emotional and cognitive experience without a nearly constant cloud of intoxication.

Problems in Dimension 1 that require Level III.7 services include moderate to severe withdrawal or risk of withdrawal. Adolescents also may need medically monitored treatment because of acute or (more commonly) subacute intoxication.

Lingering drug-induced impairments of cognitive and/or executive function (for example, by inhalants) may lead to disorganization, poor judgement and/or increased impulsivity. These may require periods of close assessment and high-intensity management.

Problems in Dimension 2 that require Level III.7 services include poorly controlled diabetes or asthma, medical non-compliance in a substance-involved HIV-infected adolescent, initial induction of abstinence in a substance-dependent pregnant adolescent, mild to moderate cellulitis requiring close supervision of oral antibiotics in an injection drug-using adolescent, and the like.

The medically monitored care provided in Level III.7 programs is delivered by an interdisciplinary staff of appropriately credentialed treatment professionals, including physicians who are specialists in addiction medicine. Treatment is specific to substance-related disorders, but the skills of the interdisciplinary team and the availability of support services also can accommodate detoxification and/or intensive inpatient treatment of addiction and/or conjoint treatment of co-occurring subacute biomedical and/or emotional, behavioral or cognitive conditions.

The intensity, frequency and type of services provided to patients varies across Level III.7 programs, as well as within a given program from patient to patient. Adolescents who have a more severe illness require use of more intensive staffing patterns and support services. For example, an adolescent who is undergoing medical detoxification or titration of a psychopharmacological regimen typically requires more intensive medical and nursing care than does an adolescent who does not have these problems. Similarly, an adolescent who is undergoing high-intensity behavior modification typically requires more intensive direct care staffing and interventions, with the availability and supervision of medical and nursing care, than does an adolescent who is not undergoing such high-intensity interventions.

With the *PPC-2R*, the requirements for admission to a Level III.7 program have been clarified to indicate that at least *one* of the two specifications must be in Dimensions 1, 2, or 3. An adolescent whose major problems are exclusively in Dimension 4, 5, or 6 may be better served by placement in a clinically managed residential program, such as one at Level III.5.

An adolescent may be admitted directly to a Level III.7 programs or transferred from a less intensive level of care if he or she has been refractory to treatment or as bursts of more intensive services become necessary. An adolescent may be transferred to a Level III.7 program for continuing care from a Level IV program when he or she no longer requires the intensity of services or staffing pattern of a hospital. A fairly common scenario is that of an adolescent who is admitted to a Level IV hospital program on an emergency basis because of a crisis situation and then is transferred to a Level III.7 program for further assessment in a substance-free state to help sort out difficult diagnostic questions regarding subacute intoxication, withdrawal and co-occurring psychiatric disorders.

Length of Service

The duration of treatment always should be determined by the progress of each individual patient. Just as treatment plans should be individualized, lengths of stay should be flexible and individualized to meet the needs of each patient.

There is little data on the dose-response relationship for adolescent residential treatment, and further research is needed to clarify these matters. Nevertheless, there may be certain threshold lengths of stay that are associated with specific therapeutic gains. In particular, the needs of juvenile justice-involved adolescents in public sector programs that use coercive treatment engagement methods (such as a court order or probationary mandate) may be best served by more predictable, though not rigid, lengths of stay. Clinicians and the courts must collaborate closely to assure that the interests of each adolescent patient are assessed and met.

Lengths of stay in clinically managed Level III.5 programs tend to be significantly longer than in medically monitored and medically managed programs. Longer exposure to treatment interventions is necessary for certain adolescents to acquire basic living skills and to master the application of coping and recovery skills. Such patients require the intensity and duration of treatment found in a Level III.5 program to accomplish some of the tasks of habilitation in a temporary "home" that can imprint the features of a recovery environment.

Detoxification

Dimension 1 (Acute Intoxication and/or Withdrawal Potential) is the first of the six primary assessment areas to be evaluated in making treatment and placement decisions. The range of clinical severity in this dimension has given rise to a range of detoxification levels of service.

As used here, detoxification refers not only to the attenuation of the physiological and psychological features of withdrawal syndromes, but also to the process of interrupting the momentum of habitual compulsive use in adolescents diagnosed with substance *dependence*. Because of the force of this momentum, and the inherent difficulties in overcoming it even when there is no clear withdrawal syndrome *per se*, this phase of treatment frequently requires a greater intensity of services initially in order to establish treatment engagement and patient role induction. This is, of course, critical to the course of treatment because it is impossible to engage the adolescent in treatment while he/she is caught up in the cycle of frequent intoxication and recovery from intoxication.

Criteria are provided for two types of Level III residential/inpatient detoxification programs: Level III.5-D and Level III.7-D. The difference between these two levels of detoxification is the intensity of clinical services, particularly as demonstrated by the degree of involvement of medical and nursing professionals.

Level III.5-D: Detoxification provided within a Level III.5 program is an organized service that is delivered by appropriately trained staff, who provide 24-hour supervision, observation and support for the adolescent who is intoxicated or experiencing mild withdrawal. Clinically managed residential detoxification is characterized by its emphasis on staff, peer and social support.

Level III.5-D programs care for adolescents whose intoxication/withdrawal signs and symptoms are significant enough to warrant 24-hour structure and support. However, the medical and nursing services and other resources of a Level III.7-D medically monitored inpatient detoxification program are not present.

Some clinically managed residential detoxification programs are staffed to supervise self-administered over-the-counter medications for the management of withdrawal. All programs at this level rely on established clinical protocols to identify adolescents who are in need of medical services beyond the capability of the program and to transfer such patients to a more appropriate facility.

Level III.7-D: Medically monitored inpatient detoxification is an organized service delivered by medical and nursing professionals, who provide 24-hour medically supervised evaluation and withdrawal management in a permanent facility with inpatient beds. Services are delivered under a defined set of physician-approved policies and physician-monitored procedures or clinical protocols.

Placement in a Level III.7-D program is appropriate for the adolescent whose withdrawal signs and symptoms are moderate to severe and thus require 24-hour inpatient care. Services may be provided in a specialty unit or track within a Level III.7 program. Alternatively, they may involve overlapping the Level III.7 care with Level IV-D (as a step-down service) in a specialty unit of an acute care general or psychiatric hospital where 24-hour observation, monitoring and treatment are available. In either case, the full resources of an acute care general hospital or a medically managed intensive inpatient treatment program are not required.

Adolescent Criteria
Level III: Clinically Managed Residential/Inpatient Treatment

CHARACTERISTIC	LEVEL III.1 Clinically Managed Low-Intensity Residential Treatment	LEVEL III.5 Clinically Managed Medium-Intensity Residential Treatment	LEVEL III.7 Medically Monitored High-Intensity Inpatient Treatment
EXAMPLES	An example of a Level III.1 adolescent program is a halfway house or group home.	An example of a Level III.5 adolescent program is a therapeutic group home, a therapeutic community, a psychosocial model residential program, or an extended rehabilitation program.	An example of a Level III.7 adolescent program is an inpatient or medical model residential treatment program (Intermediate Care Facility or Residential Treatment Center).
SETTING	Level III.1 adolescent programs may be offered in a (usually) freestanding, appropriately licensed facility located in a community setting or a specialty unit within a licensed health care facility.	Level III.5 adolescent programs may be offered in a (usually) freestanding, appropriately licensed facility located in a community setting, or a specialty unit within a licensed health care facility.	Level III.7 adolescent programs may be offered in a freestanding, appropriately licensed health care facility or specialty unit in a general or psychiatric hospital or other licensed health care facility.
SUPPORT SYSTEMS	In Level III.1 adolescent programs, necessary support systems include: (a) Availability of emergency consultation with a physician (by telephone or in person) and emergency services.	In Level III.5 adolescent programs, necessary support systems include: (a) Availability of emergency consultation with a physician (by telephone or in person) and emergency services.	In Level III.7 adolescent programs, necessary support systems include: (a) Physician monitoring and nursing care and observation, available as needed, based on clinical judgment. A physician is available to assess the adolescent in person within 24 hours of admission and thereafter as medically necessary. (In states where physician assistants or nurse practitioners are licensed as physician extenders, they may perform the duties designated here for a physician.) An appropriately trained and licensed nurse conducts an alcohol or other drug-focused nursing assessment at the time

Adolescent Criteria
Level III: Clinically Managed Residential/Inpatient Treatment

CHARACTERISTIC	LEVEL III.1 Clinically Managed Low-Intensity Residential Treatment	LEVEL III.5 Clinically Managed Medium-Intensity Residential Treatment	LEVEL III.7 Medically Monitored High-Intensity Inpatient Treatment
SUPPORT SYSTEMS (continued)			of admission is responsible for monitoring the patient's progress and for medication administration.
	(b) Ability to arrange for appropriate medical procedures, including indicated laboratory and toxicology testing.	(b) Ability to arrange for appropriate medical procedures, including indicated laboratory and toxicology testing.	(b) Additional medical specialty consultation, psychological, laboratory and toxicology services are available through consultation or referral.
	(c) Ability to support and coordinate the adolescent's access to school, work, concurrent treatment services in Level I and Level II addiction treatment programs, as well as other treatment modalities such as outpatient medical and psychiatric programs.	(c) Ability to arrange for appropriate medical and psychiatric treatment through consultation, referral to off-site concurrent treatment services, or transfer to another level of care.	(c) Direct affiliation with other levels of care.
	(d) Direct affiliation with other levels of care.	(d) Direct affiliation with other levels of care.	
		Level III.5-D Detoxification In Level III.5-D programs, support systems feature:	**Level III.7-D Detoxification** In Level III.7-D programs, support systems feature availability of specialized clinical consultation and supervision for biomedical, emotional or behavioral problems related to intoxication and detoxification.

Adolescent Criteria
Level III: Clinically Managed Residential/Inpatient Treatment

CHARACTERISTIC	LEVEL III.1 Clinically Managed Low-Intensity Residential Treatment	LEVEL III.5 Clinically Managed Medium-Intensity Residential Treatment	LEVEL III.7 Medically Monitored High-Intensity Inpatient Treatment
SUPPORT SYSTEMS (continued)		(a) Availability of specialized clinical consultation and supervision for biomedical and emotional/behavioral problems related to intoxication and detoxification. (b) Protocols used to determine the nature of the medical monitoring and other interventions required (including nursing and physician care and/or transfer to a medically monitored facility or an acute care hospital) are developed and supported by a physician knowledgeable in addiction medicine.	
STAFF	Level III.1 adolescent programs are staffed by: (a) Allied health professional staff, such as counselor aides or group living workers, who are on-site 24 hours a day or as required by licensing regulations.	Level III.5 programs are staffed by: (a) Allied health professional staff, such as counselor aides or group living workers, who are on-site 24 hours a day or as required by licensing regulations. One or more professional addiction clinicians is on-site at least 40 hours a week.	Level III.7 programs are staffed by: (a) An interdisciplinary staff of appropriately trained clinicians (including physicians, nurses, counselors and psychologists), who are able to assess and treat the adolescent and to obtain and interpret information regarding the adolescent's needs.

Adolescent Criteria
Level III: Clinically Managed Residential/Inpatient Treatment

CHARACTERISTIC	LEVEL III.1 Clinically Managed Low-Intensity Residential Treatment	LEVEL III.5 Clinically Managed Medium-Intensity Residential Treatment	LEVEL III.7 Medically Monitored High-Intensity Inpatient Treatment
STAFF (continued)	(b) Clinical staff who are knowledgeable about the biological and psychosocial dimensions of substance use disorders. Staff are knowledgeable about adolescent development and experienced in working with and engaging adolescents.	(b) Clinical staff who are knowledgeable about the biological and psychosocial dimensions of substance use disorders, and who have specialized training in behavioral management techniques. Staff are knowledgeable about adolescent development and experienced in working with and engaging adolescents.	(b) Clinical staff who are knowledgeable about the biological and psychosocial dimensions of substance use and psychiatric disorders, and who have specialized training in behavioral management techniques. Staff are knowledgeable about adolescent development and experienced in working with and engaging adolescents.
	(c) Appropriately trained staff who are available to supervise the self-administration of medications.	(c) Appropriately trained staff who are available to supervise the self-administration of medications.	(c) Appropriately licensed or credentialed staff who are available to administer and monitor medications.
		(d) Nursing care at a level of intensity that is appropriate to the services provided by the program, or as required by local licensing and regulations.	(d) Registered or licensed practical nurses who are available for primary nursing care and observation 24 hours a day. The intensity of nursing care is appropriate to the severity of patients' needs.
		(e) Appropriately trained addiction counselors or licensed, certified or registered addiction clinicians, who provide a planned treatment regimen of 24-hour professionally directed evaluation, care and treatment for adolescent patients and their families.	(e) Appropriately trained addiction counselors or licensed, certified or licensed, certified addiction clinicians, who provide a planned treatment regimen of 24-hour professionally directed evaluation, care and treatment for adolescent patients and their families.

Adolescent Criteria
Level III: Clinically Managed Residential/Inpatient Treatment

CHARACTERISTIC	LEVEL III.1 Clinically Managed Low-Intensity Residential Treatment	LEVEL III.5 Clinically Managed Medium-Intensity Residential Treatment	LEVEL III.7 Medically Monitored High-Intensity Inpatient Treatment
STAFF (continued)	**Enhanced Programs** Appropriately licensed or credentialed staff are available to administer medications in accordance with a physician prescription order. The intensity of nursing services is appropriate to the services provided by the program.	**Enhanced Programs** Appropriately licensed or credentialed staff are available to administer medications in accordance with a physician prescription order. Facility-approved addiction counselors or licensed, certified or registered addiction clinicians provide a planned treatment regimen of 24-hour professionally directed evaluation, care and treatment services for adolescents and their families. **Level III.5-D Detoxification** When a Level III.5-D program provides detoxification services to adolescents (typically without on-site access to medical and nursing personnel), it must provide (in addition to the therapies listed above): (a) Clinicians who are able to obtain and interpret information regarding the signs and symptoms of intoxication and withdrawal, as well as the appropriate monitoring and treatment of those conditions and how to facilitate entry into ongoing care; *and*	**Level III.7-D Detoxification** When a Level III.7 program provides detoxification services to adolescents, it must provide (in addition to the therapies listed above) a physician who is routinely available by telephone 24 hours a day. In states where physician assistants or nurse practitioners are licensed as physician extenders, they may perform the duties designated for a physician.

ASAM Patient Placement Criteria, Second Edition–Revised

Adolescent Criteria
Level III: Clinically Managed Residential/Inpatient Treatment

CHARACTERISTIC	LEVEL III.1 Clinically Managed Low-Intensity Residential Treatment	LEVEL III.5 Clinically Managed Medium-Intensity Residential Treatment	LEVEL III.7 Medically Monitored High-Intensity Inpatient Treatment
STAFF (continued)		(b) Appropriately trained staff who are competent to implement physician-approved protocols for patient observation, supervision and treatment (including over-the-counter medications for symptomatic relief), determination of the appropriate level of care, and facilitation of the patient's transition to continuing care; *and* (c) Access, as needed, medical evaluation and consultation, which are available 24 hours a day to monitor the safety and outcome of detoxification in this setting, in accordance with treatment/transfer practice guidelines.	
THERAPIES	Therapies offered by Level III.1 adolescent programs include: (a) Supervision and sufficient structure to promote abstinence, improve the adolescent's ability to manage and organize the activities of daily living, sustain participation in concurrent treatment services (as needed), and sustain	Therapies offered by Level III.5 adolescent programs include: (a) A structured therapeutic milieu in which behavior modification techniques are used to foster group living skills and an atmosphere of individual participation in a community of recovery.	Therapies offered by Level III.7 programs include: (a) A structured therapeutic milieu in which behavior modification techniques are used to foster group living skills and an atmosphere of individual participation in a community of recovery.

Adolescent Criteria
Level III: Clinically Managed Residential/Inpatient Treatment

CHARACTERISTIC	LEVEL III.1 Clinically Managed Low-Intensity Residential Treatment	LEVEL III.5 Clinically Managed Medium-Intensity Residential Treatment	LEVEL III.7 Medically Monitored High-Intensity Inpatient Treatment
THERAPIES (continued)	successful concurrent involvement in regular, productive daily activity (such as school or work). (b) Planned clinical program activities that are designed to foster group living skills, develop and apply recovery skills (including relapse prevention), and promote development of a social network supportive of recovery and successful reintegration into the community. Program activities may include (but are not limited to) individual and group counseling, family counseling, educational groups, and occupational or recreational activities. (c) Random drug screening, used to shape behaviors and reinforce treatment gains, as appropriate to the adolescent's individualized treatment plan.	(b) Trained clinical staff provide services—adapted to the adolescent's developmental and cognitive level—to assess and address the adolescent's individual needs. Such services encompass individual and group counseling, psychotherapy, family therapy, educational services, low-intensity medical treatment, low-intensity psychiatric treatment, expressive therapies, occupational or recreational activities, vocational rehabilitation services, and the like. (c) Planned clinical program activities that are designed to develop and apply recovery skills (including relapse prevention), promote development of a social network supportive of recovery, reinforce prosocial values, enhance the adolescent's understanding of addiction, promote successful involvement in regular, productive daily activity (such as school or work), enhance personal responsibility and	(b) Trained clinical staff provide services—adapted to the adolescent's developmental and cognitive level—to assess and address the adolescent's individual needs. Such services encompass individual and group counseling, psychotherapy, family therapy, educational services, medical treatment, psychiatric treatment, expressive therapies, occupational or recreational activities, vocational rehabilitation services, and the like. (c) Planned clinical program activities that are designed to develop and apply recovery skills (including relapse prevention), promote development of a social network supportive of recovery, reinforce prosocial values, enhance the adolescent's understanding of addiction, promote successful involvement in regular, productive daily activity (such as school or work), enhance personal responsibility and

Adolescent Criteria
Level III: Clinically Managed Residential/Inpatient Treatment

CHARACTERISTIC	LEVEL III.1 Clinically Managed Low-Intensity Residential Treatment	LEVEL III.5 Clinically Managed Medium-Intensity Residential Treatment	LEVEL III.7 Medically Monitored High-Intensity Inpatient Treatment
THERAPIES (continued)		developmental maturity and, as indicated, promote successful reintegration into community living. (d) Family therapy involves significant family members or guardians in the assessment, treatment and continuing care of the adolescent. (e) Educational services are provided in accordance with local regulations (typically on-site) and are designed to maintain the educational and intellectual development of the adolescent and, when indicated, to provide opportunities to remedy deficits in the educational level of adolescents who have fallen behind because of their involvement with alcohol and other drugs. (f) Random drug screening, used to shape behaviors and reinforce treatment gains, as appropriate to the adolescent's individualized treatment plan. **Level III.5-D Detoxification** Trained clinicians provide daily clinical services to assess and address the adolescent's withdrawal status and service needs. Such clinical services may include nursing or	developmental maturity and, as indicated, promote successful reintegration into community living. (d) Family therapy involves significant family members or guardians in the assessment, treatment and continuing care of the adolescent. (e) Educational services are provided in accordance with local regulations (typically on-site) and are designed to maintain the educational and intellectual development of the adolescent and, when indicated, to provide opportunities to remedy deficits in the educational level of adolescents who have fallen behind because of their involvement with alcohol and other drugs. (f) Relevant health and illness education services are provided. **Level III.7-D Detoxification** An interdisciplinary team provide daily clinical services to assess and address the adolescent's withdrawal status and service needs. Such clinical services may include

Adolescent Criteria
Level III: Clinically Managed Residential/Inpatient Treatment

CHARACTERISTIC	LEVEL III.1 Clinically Managed Low-Intensity Residential Treatment	LEVEL III.5 Clinically Managed Medium-Intensity Residential Treatment	LEVEL III.7 Medically Monitored High-Intensity Inpatient Treatment
THERAPIES (continued)		medical monitoring, use of medications to alleviate symptoms, individual or group therapy specific to withdrawal, and withdrawal support.	nursing or medical monitoring, pharmacologic therapies as needed, individual or group therapy specific to withdrawal, and withdrawal support. Frequent nurse monitoring of the adolescent's progress in detoxification and medication administration are available, if needed.
ASSESSMENT/ TREATMENT PLAN REVIEW	In Level III.1 adolescent programs, the assessment and treatment plan review include: (a) An individualized biopsychosocial assessment, which is conducted or updated to confirm the appropriateness of placement in this level of care and to help guide the individualized treatment planning process. (b) An individualized treatment plan, which is formulated and updated at specified intervals to document the adolescent's clinical problems, measurable goals and objectives, and planned interventions.	In Level III.5 adolescent programs, the assessment and treatment plan review include: (a) An individualized biopsychosocial assessment, which is conducted or updated to confirm the appropriateness of placement in this level of care and to help guide the individualized treatment planning process. (b) An individualized treatment plan, which is formulated and updated at specified intervals to document the adolescent's clinical problems, measurable treatment goals and objectives, and planned therapeutic interventions.	In Level III.7 adolescent programs, the assessment and treatment plan review include: (a) A comprehensive biopsychosocial assessment (including addiction, mental health, family and educational assessments), which is begun at the time of assessment to help guide the individualized treatment planning process. (b) A physical examination, performed by a physician within 24 hours of admission, or evaluation by a physician within 24 hours of admission of the record of a physical examination conducted no more than 7 days prior to admission. A psychiatric assessment is performed in a timely

Adolescent Criteria
Level III: Clinically Managed Residential/Inpatient Treatment

CHARACTERISTIC	LEVEL III.1 Clinically Managed Low-Intensity Residential Treatment	LEVEL III.5 Clinically Managed Medium-Intensity Residential Treatment	LEVEL III.7 Medically Monitored High-Intensity Inpatient Treatment
ASSESSMENT/ TREATMENT PLAN REVIEW (continued)			fashion, as clinically indicated. (In states where physician assistants or nurse practitioners are licensed as physician extenders, they may perform the duties designated for a physician.)
	(c) Planning that reflects case management and coordination of related addiction treatment, health care, mental health, and social, vocational and housing services provided concurrently, as well as the integration of services in this and other levels of care.	(c) Planning that reflects case management conducted by on-site staff and coordination of related addiction treatment, health care, mental health, and social, vocational and housing services provided concurrently, as well as the integration of services in this and other levels of care.	(c) An individualized treatment plan, which is formulated and updated at specified intervals to document the adolescent's clinical problems, measurable treatment goals and objectives, and planned therapeutic interventions. (d) Ongoing assessment and continuing updates of the treatment plan to reflect the adolescent's clinical progress, reviewed by an interdisciplinary treatment team.
		Level III.5-D Detoxification In addition to those listed above, elements of the assessment and treatment plan review should include: (a) An initial withdrawal assessment, including a medical evaluation and referral within the 48 hours preceding admission (or if a step-down from another residential setting, within 7 days preceding admission).	**Level III.7-D Detoxification** In addition to those listed above, elements of the assessment and treatment plan review should include: (a) An initial withdrawal assessment within 24 hours of admission, or earlier if clinically warranted.

Adolescent Criteria
Level III: Clinically Managed Residential/Inpatient Treatment

CHARACTERISTIC	LEVEL III.1 Clinically Managed Low-Intensity Residential Treatment	LEVEL III.5 Clinically Managed Medium-Intensity Residential Treatment	LEVEL III.7 Medically Monitored High-Intensity Inpatient Treatment
ASSESSMENT/ TREATMENT PLAN REVIEW (continued)		(b) Daily withdrawal monitoring assessments. (c) Ongoing screening for medical and nursing needs, with such medical and nursing services available as needed through consultation or referral.	(b) Daily nursing withdrawal monitoring assessments and continuous availability of nursing evaluation. (c) Daily availability of medical evaluation, with continuous on-call coverage.
DOCUMENTATION	Documentation standards of Level III.1 programs include progress notes in the patient record that clearly reflect implementation of the treatment plan, as well as subsequent amendments to the plan.	Documentation standards of Level III.5 programs include progress notes in the patient record that clearly reflect implementation of the treatment plan and the adolescent's response to treatment, as well as subsequent amendments to the plan. **Level III.5-D Detoxification** Detoxification rating scale tables and flow sheets (which may include tabulation of vital signs) are used as needed.	Documentation standards of Level III.7 programs include progress notes in the patient record that clearly reflect implementation of the treatment plan and the adolescent's response to treatment, as well as subsequent amendments to the plan. **Level III.7-D Detoxification** Detoxification rating scale tables and flow sheets (which may include tabulation of vital signs) are used as needed.

Adolescent Level III Admission Criteria
Diagnostic and Dimensional Criteria

CRITERIA	LEVEL III.1 Clinically Managed Low-Intensity Residential Treatment	LEVEL III.5 Clinically Managed Medium-Intensity Residential Treatment	LEVEL III.7 Medically Monitored High-Intensity Inpatient Treatment
DIAGNOSTIC ADMISSION CRITERIA	The adolescent who is appropriately placed in a Level III.1 program meets the diagnostic criteria for Substance-Related Disorder, as defined by the current *Diagnostic and Statistical Manual of Mental Disorders (DSM)* of the American Psychiatric Association or other standardized and widely accepted criteria, as well as the dimensional criteria for admission.	The adolescent who is appropriately placed in a Level III.5 program meets the diagnostic criteria for Substance-Related Disorder, as defined by the current *Diagnostic and Statistical Manual of Mental Disorders (DSM)* of the American Psychiatric Association or other standardized and widely accepted criteria, as well as the dimensional criteria for admission.	The adolescent who is appropriately placed in a Level III.7 program meets the diagnostic criteria for Substance-Related Disorder, as defined by the current *Diagnostic and Statistical Manual of Mental Disorders (DSM)* of the American Psychiatric Association or other standardized and widely accepted criteria, as well as the dimensional criteria for admission.
DIMENSIONAL ADMISSION CRITERIA	The adolescent who is appropriately placed in a Level III.1 program meets specifications in *two* of Dimensions 1 through 6.	The adolescent who is appropriately placed in a Level III.5 program meets specifications in *two* of Dimensions 1 through 6.	The adolescent who is appropriately placed in a Level III.7 program meets specifications in *two* of Dimensions 1 through 6, with at least one in Dimensions 1, 2, or 3.
DIMENSION 1: Acute Intoxication and/or Withdrawal	The adolescent's status in Dimension 1 is characterized by problems with intoxication or withdrawal (if any) that are being managed through concurrent placement at another level of care for detoxification (typically Level I, Level II.1 or Level II.5).	The adolescent's status in Dimension 1 is characterized by the following: (a) The adolescent is at risk of or experiencing acute or subacute intoxication or withdrawal, with mild to moderate symptoms. He or she needs containment and increased treatment intensity (without frequent access to medical or nursing services) to support engagement in treatment, ability to tolerate withdrawal,	The adolescent's status in Dimension 1 is characterized by the following: The adolescent is experiencing or at risk of acute or subacute intoxication or withdrawal, with moderate to severe signs and symptoms. He or she needs 24-hour treatment services, including the availability of active medical and nursing monitoring to manage withdrawal, support engagement in treatment,

ASAM Patient Placement Criteria, Second Edition–Revised

Adolescent Level III Admission Criteria
Diagnostic and Dimensional Criteria

CRITERIA	LEVEL III.1 Clinically Managed Low-Intensity Residential Treatment	LEVEL III.5 Clinically Managed Medium-Intensity Residential Treatment	LEVEL III.7 Medically Monitored High-Intensity Inpatient Treatment
DIMENSION 1: **Acute Intoxication and/or Withdrawal (continued)**	If residential placement in a Level III.1 program is being used to support detoxification at a non-residential level of care, then the adolescent is considered to have met specifications in Dimension 1.	and prevention of immediate continued use. Alternatively, the adolescent has a history of failure in treatment at the same or a less intensive level of care. Problems with intoxication or withdrawal are manageable at this level of care. Drug-specific examples follow: (a) *Alcohol*: Mild acute withdrawal or moderate subacute withdrawal, with symptoms that require 24-hour support and extended monitoring and non-pharmacological management; no abnormal vital signs; no need for sedative-hypnotic substitution detoxification; a CIWA-Ar score of <8; no significant history of regular morning drinking. (b) *Sedative-hypnotics*: Mild to moderate withdrawal, with symptoms that require 24-hour support and extended monitoring; may have a recent history of low-level daily sedative-hypnotic use, but no cross-dependence on other substances; may have a need for extended agonist substitution therapy, but only with a stable taper regimen in the context of a step-down from a higher level	and prevention of immediate continued use. Alternatively, the adolescent has a history of failure in treatment at the same or a less intensive level of care. Problems with intoxication or withdrawal are manageable at this level of care. Drug-specific examples follow: (a) *Alcohol*: Moderate withdrawal, with significant symptoms that require access to nursing and medical monitoring. The patient may have a history of daily drinking or drinking to self-medicate withdrawal, or regular morning drinking. He or she may require sedative-hypnotic substitution therapy, but typically this can be managed with a standing taper without the need for extensive titration. (b) *Sedative-hypnotics*: Moderate withdrawal, with significant symptoms that require access to nursing and medical monitoring. The adolescent may be cross-dependent on other substances and may require detoxification with tapering substitute agonist therapy and/or pharmacological management of symptoms.

Adolescent Level III Admission Criteria
Diagnostic and Dimensional Criteria

CRITERIA	LEVEL III.1 Clinically Managed Low-Intensity Residential Treatment	LEVEL III.5 Clinically Managed Medium-Intensity Residential Treatment	LEVEL III.7 Medically Monitored High-Intensity Inpatient Treatment
DIMENSION 1: Acute Intoxication and/or Withdrawal (continued)		of care, where the regimen has been titrated and established; no abnormal vital signs; no unstable complicating exacerbation of affective disorder. (c) *Opiates*: Mild to moderate withdrawal, with symptoms requiring 24-hour support and extended monitoring and non-pharmacological or over-the-counter medication for symptomatic relief; no need for prescription pharmacological treatments or agonist substitution therapy. (d) *Stimulants*: Mild to moderate to severe withdrawal (involving lethargy, apathy, agitation, depression, suspiciousness, fearfulness, or hypervigilance) of sufficient intensity that the patient needs 24-hour containment and increased intensity of treatment to support the ability to tolerate symptoms, support treatment engagement, and bolster external supports.	(c) *Opiates*: Moderate to severe withdrawal, usually in the context of daily opiate use. The patient requires access to nursing and medical monitoring, may require use of prescription medications or agonist substitution therapy, and may need monitoring for induction of antagonist therapy (as with naltrexone). Severe craving states or affective instability typical of withdrawal may require high-intensity 24-hour treatment to support engagement. (d) *Stimulants*: Severe withdrawal (involving sustained affective or behavioral disturbances or mild psychotic symptoms), which requires access to nursing and medical monitoring. Severe craving states or affective instability typical of withdrawal may require high-intensity 24-hour treatment to support engagement.

Adolescent Level III Admission Criteria
Diagnostic and Dimensional Criteria

CRITERIA	LEVEL III.1 Clinically Managed Low-Intensity Residential Treatment	LEVEL III.5 Clinically Managed Medium-Intensity Residential Treatment	LEVEL III.7 Medically Monitored High-Intensity Inpatient Treatment
DIMENSION 1: **Acute Intoxication and/or Withdrawal (continued)**		With the high craving states typical of withdrawal, the adolescent may require 24-hour containment and increased intensity of treatment because of lack of sufficient impulse control, coping skills, or supports to prevent immediate continued use. (e) *Inhalants*: Moderate subacute intoxication (involving cognitive impairment, lethargy, agitation, and depression) of sufficient intensity that the patient needs 24-hour containment and increased treatment intensity to support the ability to tolerate symptoms, support engagement in treatment, and bolster external supports. (f) *Marijuana*: Moderate to severe withdrawal symptoms (involving irritability, general malaise, inner agitation, severe sleep disturbance, and severe craving) or sustained susceptibility subacute intoxication states (involving cognitive disorganization, memory impairment, executive dysfunction, and the like), such that the patient needs 24-hour containment and increased treatment intensity to support the adolescent's ability to tolerate symptoms, support engagement in treatment, and	(e) *Inhalants*: Severe subacute intoxication (involving mild delirium or other serious cognitive impairment, lethargy, agitation, and depression) of sufficient intensity that the patient requires access to nursing and medical monitoring. (f) *Marijuana*: Severe sustained intoxication (involving mild psychosis, coarse cognitive disorganization, agitation, and the like), which requires access to nursing and medical monitoring.

Adolescent Level III Admission Criteria
Diagnostic and Dimensional Criteria

CRITERIA	LEVEL III.1 Clinically Managed Low-Intensity Residential Treatment	LEVEL III.5 Clinically Managed Medium-Intensity Residential Treatment	LEVEL III.7 Medically Monitored High-Intensity Inpatient Treatment
DIMENSION 1: **Acute Intoxication and/or Withdrawal (continued)**		bolster external supports. The patient may be using or likely to use marijuana in order to relieve withdrawal from other substances, and may need containment to prevent immediate continued use. (g) *Hallucinogens*: Moderate to severe persistent intoxication (involving perceptual distortion, moderate non-delusional suspiciousness, moderate affective instability, and the like), which requires 24-hour containment and increased intensity of treatment to support the adolescent's ability to tolerate symptoms, support engagement in treatment, and bolster external supports.	(g) *Hallucinogens*: Severe persistent intoxication (involving mild delirium, mild psychosis, agitation, moderate to severe affective instability, cognitive disorganization, and the like), which requires access to nursing and medical monitoring.
DIMENSION 2: **Biomedical Conditions and Complications**	The adolescent's status in Dimension 2 is characterized by *one* of the following: (a) Biomedical conditions distract from recovery efforts and require limited residential supervision to ensure their adequate treatment or to provide support to overcome the distraction. Adequate nursing or medical monitoring can be provided through an arrangement with another provider. The adolescent is	The adolescent's status in this Dimension 2 is characterized by *one* of the following: (a) Biomedical conditions distract from recovery efforts and require residential supervision (that is unavailable at a less intensive level of care) to ensure their adequate treatment, or they require medium-intensity residential treatment to provide support to overcome the distraction. Adequate nursing or medical	The adolescent's status in Dimension 2 is characterized by *one* of the following: (a) A biomedical complication of addiction or a co-occurring biomedical condition that requires active nursing or medical monitoring, which can be provided directly by the program or through an arrangement with another provider and which does not require the resources of an acute care hospital; *or*

Adolescent Level III Admission Criteria
Diagnostic and Dimensional Criteria

CRITERIA	LEVEL III.1 Clinically Managed Low-Intensity Residential Treatment	LEVEL III.5 Clinically Managed Medium-Intensity Residential Treatment	LEVEL III.7 Medically Monitored High-Intensity Inpatient Treatment
DIMENSION 2: Biomedical Conditions and Complications (continued)	capable of self-administering any prescribed medications or procedures, with available supervision; *or*	monitoring can be provided through an arrangement with another provider. The adolescent is capable of self-administering any prescribed medications or procedures, with available supervision; *or*	
	(b) Continued substance use would place the adolescent at risk of serious damage to his or her physical health because of a biomedical condition (such as pregnancy or HIV) or an imminently dangerous pattern of high-risk use (such as continued use of shared injection apparatus). Adequate nursing or medical monitoring for biomedical conditions can be provided through an arrangement with another provider. The adolescent is capable of self-administering any prescribed medications or procedures, with available supervision.	(b) Continued substance use would place the adolescent at risk of serious damage to his or her physical health because of a biomedical condition (such as pregnancy or HIV) or an imminently dangerous pattern of high-risk use (such as continued use of shared injection apparatus). Adequate nursing or medical monitoring for biomedical conditions can be provided through an arrangement with another provider. The adolescent is capable of self-administering any prescribed medications or procedures, with available supervision.	(b) Continued alcohol or drug use places the adolescent at imminent risk of serious damage to physical health because of a biomedical condition (such as brittle diabetes, pregnancy, or HIV), which requires active nursing or medical monitoring.
	Enhanced Program The adolescent has a biomedical problem that requires a degree of staff attention (as through monitoring of medications or assistance with mobility) that is provided directly by the program or by a Level I or II service outside of the Level III.1 program.	**Enhanced Program** The adolescent has a biomedical problem that requires a degree of staff attention (as through monitoring of medications or assistance with mobility) that is provided directly by the program or by a Level I or II service outside of the Level III.5 program.	

Adolescent Level III Admission Criteria
Diagnostic and Dimensional Criteria

CRITERIA	LEVEL III.1 Clinically Managed Low-Intensity Residential Treatment	LEVEL III.5 Clinically Managed Medium-Intensity Residential Treatment	LEVEL III.7 Medically Monitored High-Intensity Inpatient Treatment
DIMENSION 3: Emotional, Behavioral or Cognitive Conditions and Complications	The adolescent's status in Dimension 3 is characterized by *one* of the following (requiring 24-hour supervision):	The adolescent's status in Dimension 3 is characterized by *one* of the following (requiring 24-hour supervision and a medium-intensity therapeutic milieu):	The adolescent's status in this Dimension 3 is characterized by *one* of the following (requiring 24-supervision and a high-intensity therapeutic milieu, with access to nursing and medical monitoring and treatment):
	(a) *Dangerousness/Lethality*: The adolescent is at risk for dangerous consequences because of the lack of a stable living environment (for example, exposure to the elements, risk of assault, risk of prostitution, and the like). He or she needs a stable residential setting for protection.	(a) *Dangerousness/Lethality*: The adolescent is at moderate but stable risk of imminent harm to self or others, and needs medium-intensity 24-hour monitoring and/or treatment for protection and safety. However, he or she does not require access to medical or nursing services.	(a) *Dangerousness/Lethality*: The adolescent is at moderate (and possibly unpredictable) risk of imminent harm to self or others and needs 24-hour monitoring and/or treatment in a high-intensity programmatic milieu and/or enforced containment for safety.
	(b) *Interference with Addiction Recovery Efforts*: The adolescent needs a stable living environment to promote a sustained focus on recovery tasks (for example, recovery efforts are hindered by the adolescent's preoccupying worries about shelter).	(b) *Interference with Addiction Recovery Efforts*: The adolescent's recovery efforts are negatively affected by his or her emotional, behavioral or cognitive problems in significant and distracting ways. He or she requires 24-hour structured therapy and/or a programmatic milieu to promote sustained focus on recovery tasks because of active symptoms.	(b) *Interference with Addiction Recovery Efforts*: The adolescent's recovery efforts are negatively affected by his or her emotional, behavioral or cognitive problems in significant and distracting ways. He or she requires 24-hour structured therapy and/or a high-intensity programmatic milieu to stabilize unstable emotional or behavioral problems (as through ongoing medical or nursing evaluation, behavior modification, titration of medications, and the like).

Adolescent Level III Admission Criteria
Diagnostic and Dimensional Criteria

CRITERIA	LEVEL III.1 Clinically Managed Low-Intensity Residential Treatment	LEVEL III.5 Clinically Managed Medium-Intensity Residential Treatment	LEVEL III.7 Medically Monitored High-Intensity Inpatient Treatment
DIMENSION 3: Emotional, Behavioral or Cognitive Conditions and Complications (continued)	(c) *Social Functioning*: The adolescent's emotional, behavioral or cognitive problem results in moderate impairment in social functioning. He or she therefore needs limited 24-hour supervision, which can be provided by program staff or in combination with a Level I or Level II program. This might involve protection from antisocial peer influences in a motivated adolescent, reinforcement of improving behavior self-management techniques, support of increasingly independent functions (such as school or work), and the like.	(c) *Social Functioning*: The adolescent has significant impairments, with moderate to severe symptoms (such as poor impulse control, disorganization, and the like). These seriously impair his or her ability to function in family, social, school or work settings, and cannot be managed at a less intensive level of care. This might involve, for example, a recent history of high-risk runaway behavior, inability to resist antisocial peer influences, a need for consistent boundaries unavailable in the home environment or inability to sustain school attendance, and the like.	(c) *Social Functioning*: The adolescent has significant impairments, with severe symptoms (such as poor impulse control, disorganization, and the like), which seriously impair his or her ability to function in family, social, school or work settings and which cannot be managed at a less intensive level of care. These might involve a recent history of aggressive or severely disruptive behavior, severe inability to manage peer conflict, or a recurrent or persistent pattern of runaway behavior requiring enforced confinement, and the like.
	(d) *Ability for Self-Care*: The adolescent has moderate impairment in his or her ability to manage the activities of daily living and thus needs limited 24-hour supervision, which can be provided by program staff or through coordination with a Level I or Level II program. The adolescent's impairments might require the provision of food and shelter, prompting for self-care, or supervised self-adminstration of medications.	(d) *Ability for Self-Care*: The adolescent has moderate impairment in his or her ability to manage the activities of daily living and thus requires 24-hour supervision and staff assistance, which can be provided by the program. The adolescent's impairments may involve a need for intensive modeling and reinforcement of personal grooming and hygiene, a pattern of continuing indiscriminate or unprotected sexual contacts in an adolescent with a history of sexually transmitted diseases, moderate dilapidation and self-neglect in the context of advanced alcohol	(d) *Ability for Self-Care*: The adolescent has a significant lack of personal resources and moderate to severe impairment in ability to manage the activities of daily living. He or she thus needs 24-hour supervision and significant staff assistance, including access to nursing or medical services. The adolescent's impairments may involve progressive and severe dilapidation and self-neglect in the context of advanced substance dependence, the need for observation after eating to prevent self-induced vomiting, the need for intensive

Adolescent Level III Admission Criteria
Diagnostic and Dimensional Criteria

CRITERIA	LEVEL III.1 Clinically Managed Low-Intensity Residential Treatment	LEVEL III.5 Clinically Managed Medium-Intensity Residential Treatment	LEVEL III.7 Medically Monitored High-Intensity Inpatient Treatment
DIMENSION 3: Emotional, Behavioral or Cognitive Conditions and Complications (continued)		or drug dependence, a need for intensive teaching of personal safety techniques in an adolescent who has suffered physical or sexual assault, and the like.	reinforcement of medication compliance, the need for intensive modeling of adequate self-care during pregnancy, the need for intensive training for self-care in a cognitively impaired patient, and the like.
	(e) *Course of Illness*: The adolescent's history and present situation suggest that an emotional, behavioral or cognitive condition would become unstable without 24-hour supervision (for example, an adolescent who experiences rapid dangerous exacerbation if he or she misses a few doses of medicine or if he or she has even a minor relapse to substance use); *or* The adolescent's emotional, behavioral or cognitive condition suggests the need for low-intensity and/or longer-term reinforcement and practice of recovery skills in a controlled environment.	(e) *Course of Illness*: The adolescent's history and present situation suggest that an emotional, behavioral or cognitive condition would become unstable without 24-hour supervision and a medium-intensity structured programmatic milieu. These may involve, for example, an adolescent whose substance use has been associated with a dangerous pattern of criminal or delinquent behaviors and who needs monitoring to assess safety and the likelihood of successful treatment on an outpatient basis before being returned to the community following release from a juvenile justice setting, or an adolescent with a recent lapse or relapse, whose history suggests that this is likely to result in disruptive behavior that will impede participation in treatment at a less intensive level of care, and the like.	(e) *Course of Illness*: The adolescent's history and present situation suggest that an emotional, behavioral or cognitive condition would become unstable without 24-hour supervision and a high-intensity structured programmatic milieu, with access to nursing or medical monitoring or treatment. These may be required to treat an adolescent who, for example, requires containment or enforced abstinence for reinstatement or titration of a pharmacological treatment regimen; or an adolescent whose substance use has been associated with a dangerous pattern of aggressive/violent behaviors and who needs monitoring to assess safety and likelihood of outpatient treatment success before returning to the community following release from a juvenile justice setting; or an adolescent who requires intensive monitoring or treatment because ongoing substance use prevents

Adolescent Level III Admission Criteria
Diagnostic and Dimensional Criteria

CRITERIA	LEVEL III.1 Clinically Managed Low-Intensity Residential Treatment	LEVEL III.5 Clinically Managed Medium-Intensity Residential Treatment	LEVEL III.7 Medically Monitored High-Intensity Inpatient Treatment
DIMENSION 3: Emotional, Behavioral or Cognitive Conditions and Complications (continued)			adequate or safe treatment or diagnostic clarification for an emotional, behavioral or cognitive condition that may or may not be substance-induced; or an adolescent whose history suggests rapid escalation of dangerousness/lethality when using alcohol or drugs and who is in relapse or at imminent risk of relapse.
DIMENSION 4: Readiness to Change	The adolescent's status in Dimension 4 is characterized by *both* of the following: (a) The adolescent is open to recovery but requires limited 24-hour supervision to promote or sustain progress through the stages of change; *and*	The adolescent's status in Dimension 4 is characterized by *one* of the following: (a) The adolescent requires 24-hour supervision and a structured programmatic milieu to promote progress through the stages of change, as evidenced by a lack of previous treatment engagement and/or extensive functional impairment. For example, the adolescent has not engaged or followed through with motivational enhancement interventions in outpatient treatment, or the adolescent's substance use and/or related functional impairment has contributed to his or her leaving school without an alternate structured daily activity; or the adolescent with juvenile justice involvement has failed in previous attempts to mandate or coerce treatment at a less intensive level of care and	The adolescent's status in Dimension 4 is characterized by *one* of the following: (a) The adolescent has not related his or her problems to substance use or has not accepted the need to change. Therefore, treatment is likely to succeed only at Level III.7. For example, the adolescent does not recognize that substance use causes his or her disorganization and thus cannot adequately manage his or her diabetes or other chronic illness; or the adolescent does not acknowledge that he or she is impaired by overuse of opioid analgesics and therefore cannot adequately manage his or her sickle cell disease; or the adolescent does not recognize the ways in which substance use exacerbates his or her aggressiveness, and therefore cannot avoid dangerous altercations, and the like; *or*

Adolescent Level III Admission Criteria
Diagnostic and Dimensional Criteria

CRITERIA	LEVEL III.1 Clinically Managed Low-Intensity Residential Treatment	LEVEL III.5 Clinically Managed Medium-Intensity Residential Treatment	LEVEL III.7 Medically Monitored High-Intensity Inpatient Treatment
DIMENSION 4: **Readiness to Change (continued)**		requires a Level III.5 program to initiate engagement in treatment and role induction; *or*	
	(b) The adolescent is cooperative and likely to engage in treatment at this level of care.	(b) The adolescent has not related his or her problems to substance use or has not accepted the need to change and thus is in need of intensive motivating strategies, activities and processes available only in a setting with 24-hour supervision and a medium-intensity milieu. For example, the adolescent does not believe that there is a need for further treatment or recovery work following detoxification, even though he or she is at imminent risk of resuming a recent pattern of theft and thus requires intensive motivation to prepare for compliance or follow-through with outpatient treatment; *or*	(b) The adolescent has not demonstrated sufficient readiness to change and thus is in need of intensive motivating strategies, activities and processes available only in a 24-hour high-intensity structured milieu or medically monitored setting to promote or sustain treatment engagement or readiness to change. For example, the adolescent may need the availability of intensive behavior modification, with access to "time out" or a quiet room or therapeutic holds to manage his or her disruptive response to treatment; or intensive motivational enhancement therapies requiring this level of staffing, monitoring and 24-hour structure, or intensive case management to link and prepare relevant participants such as family, probation officer, or school for implementation of a plan to sustain treatment engagement at a less intensive level of care.
		(c) Despite serious consequences to his or her life, the adolescent does not believe that there is any problem in daily substance use.	

Adolescent Level III Admission Criteria
Diagnostic and Dimensional Criteria

CRITERIA	LEVEL III.1 Clinically Managed Low-Intensity Residential Treatment	LEVEL III.5 Clinically Managed Medium-Intensity Residential Treatment	LEVEL III.7 Medically Monitored High-Intensity Inpatient Treatment
DIMENSION 5: Relapse/ Continued Use Potential	The adolescent's status in Dimension 5 is characterized by *one* of the following, requiring low-intensity 24-hour supervision to prevent relapse or attenuate continued use: (a) The lack of monitoring or supervision between treatment encounters at a less intensive level of care has been a major barrier to abstinence; *or*	The adolescent's status in Dimension 5 is characterized by *one* of the following, requiring medium-intensity 24-hour supervision to prevent relapse or attenuate continued use: (a) The lack of monitoring or supervision between treatment encounters at a less intensive level of care has been a major barrier to abstinence and achievement of recovery goals. The adolescent's continued substance use poses a high risk of serious impairment in the absence of 24-hour monitoring and structured support; *or*	The adolescent's status in Dimension 5 is characterized by *one* of the following, requiring high-intensity 24-hour supervision and structured programmatic milieu with access to nursing and medical monitoring and treatment, to prevent relapse or attenuate continued use: (a) The adolescent is unable to interrupt a high frequency/ high severity pattern of use, with imminent severe risk of dangerous consequences. For example, the adolescent has severe and persistent problems with impulse control that require stabilization through high-intensity interventions; or he or she has issues with intoxication or withdrawal that require stabilization in a medically monitored setting; or there is imminent risk of danger to self or others with relapse or continued use; or there is a likelihood of self-medication of recurrent symptoms of a mood disorder, which require stabilization in a medically monitored setting. Treatment at a less intensive level of care has been attempted or given serious consideration; *or*

Adolescent Level III Admission Criteria
Diagnostic and Dimensional Criteria

CRITERIA	LEVEL III.1 Clinically Managed Low-Intensity Residential Treatment	LEVEL III.5 Clinically Managed Medium-Intensity Residential Treatment	LEVEL III.7 Medically Monitored High-Intensity Inpatient Treatment
DIMENSION 5: Relapse/ Continued Use Potential (continued)	(b) The adolescent's recovery skills are not yet sufficient to overcome environmental triggers such as peer substance use or internal triggers such as craving; *or*	(b) The adolescent requires residential containment, treatment and a structured programmatic milieu to further develop recovery skills that are not yet sufficient to overcome environmental triggers (such as peer substance use or family stressors) or internal triggers (such as craving). The adolescent's continued use poses a high risk of serious impairment in the absence of 24-hour monitoring and structured support; *or*	(b) The modality of treatment requires Level III.7 care. For example, Level III.7 care is required to safely and effectively initiate antagonist therapy (such as naltrexone for opioid dependence), or agonist substitution therapy (such as methadone or buprenorphine for opioid dependence), or aversion therapy (such as disulfiram for alcoholism); or Level III.7 care is required for the monitoring, case management and documentation needed to arrange a less intensive level of care or other needed treatment resources (such as a group home, special education placement, and the like).
	(c) The adolescent's history of chronic substance use, repeated relapse and/or resistance to treatment predicts continued use or relapse without residential containment.	(c) The adolescent's history of chronic substance use, repeated relapse and/or resistance to treatment predicts continued use or relapse without residential treatment and a structured programmatic milieu. For such an adolescent, the intensity of a Level III.5 setting is required to promote and prepare for treatment response and relapse prevention at a less intensive level of care.	

Adolescent Level III Admission Criteria
Diagnostic and Dimensional Criteria

CRITERIA	LEVEL III.1 Clinically Managed Low-Intensity Residential Treatment	LEVEL III.5 Clinically Managed Medium-Intensity Residential Treatment	LEVEL III.7 Medically Monitored High-Intensity Inpatient Treatment
DIMENSION 5: Relapse/ Continued Use Potential (continued)		(d) The adolescent's likelihood of relapse and/or continued use poses a high risk of serious impairment in the absence of 24-hour monitoring and structured support. Such an adolescent may be at high risk of relapse/continued use because of ongoing exposure to substances in the context of trafficking, involvement with a gang or other delinquent or drug-involved peers.	
DIMENSION 6: Recovery Environment	The adolescent's status in Dimension 6 is characterized by *one* of the following: (a) The adolescent has been living in an environment in which there is a high risk of neglect, or initiation or repetition of physical, sexual or severe emotional abuse, such that the adolescent is assessed as being unable to achieve or maintain recovery without residential containment; *or*	The adolescent's status in Dimension 6 is characterized by *one* of the following: (a) The adolescent has been living in an environment in which there is a high risk of neglect, or initiation or repetition of physical, sexual or severe emotional abuse, such that the adolescent is assessed as being unable to achieve or maintain recovery without residential treatment; *or*	The adolescent's status in Dimension 6 is characterized by *one* of the following: (a) The adolescent has been living in an environment in which supports that might otherwise have enabled treatment at a less intensive level of care are unavailable. For example, the family undermines the adolescent's treatment, or is unable to sustain treatment attendance at a less intensive level of care, or family members have active substance use disorders and/or facilitate access to alcohol or other drugs, or the home environment is dangerously chaotic or abusive, or the family is unable to adequately supervise medications, or the family is unable to adequately implement a needed behavior management plan. Level III.7

Adolescent Level III Admission Criteria
Diagnostic and Dimensional Criteria

CRITERIA	LEVEL III.1 Clinically Managed Low-Intensity Residential Treatment	LEVEL III.5 Clinically Managed Medium-Intensity Residential Treatment	LEVEL III.7 Medically Monitored High-Intensity Inpatient Treatment
DIMENSION 6: **Recovery Environment (continued)**	(b) The adolescent has a family or other household member who has an active substance use disorder, or substance use is endemic in his or her home environment or broader social network, so that recovery goals are assessed as unachievable without residential containment; *or* (c) The adolescent's home environment or social network is too chaotic or ineffective to support or sustain treatment goals, so that recovery is assessed as unachievable without residential support. For example, the adolescent's family reinforces antisocial norms and values, or the family cannot sustain treatment engagement or school attendance, or the family is experiencing significant social isolation or withdrawal; *or*	(b) The adolescent has a family or other household member who has an active substance use disorder, or substance use is endemic in his or her home environment or broader social network, so that recovery goals are assessed as unachievable without residential treatment; *or* (c) The adolescent's home environment or social network is too chaotic or ineffective to support or sustain treatment goals, so that recovery is assessed as unachievable without residential treatment. For example, the adolescent's family reinforces antisocial norms and values, or the family cannot sustain treatment engagement or school attendance, or the family is experiencing significant social isolation or withdrawal; *or*	care thus is needed to effect a change in the home environment so as to establish a successful transition to a less intensive level of care; *or* (b) Logistical impediments (such as distance from a treatment facility, mobility limitations, lack of transportation, and the like) preclude participation in treatment at a less intensive level of care, and Level III.7 care is necessary to establish a successful transition to a less intensive level of care.

Adolescent Level III Admission Criteria
Diagnostic and Dimensional Criteria

CRITERIA	LEVEL III.1 Clinically Managed Low-Intensity Residential Treatment	LEVEL III.5 Clinically Managed Medium-Intensity Residential Treatment	LEVEL III.7 Medically Monitored High-Intensity Inpatient Treatment
DIMENSION 6: Recovery Environment (continued)	(d) Logistical impediments (such as distance from a treatment facility, mobility limitations, lack of transportation, and the like) preclude participation in treatment at a less intensive level of care.	(d) Logistical impediments (such as distance from a treatment facility, mobility limitations, lack of transportation, and the like) preclude participation in treatment at a less intensive level of care.	

Level IV
Medically Managed Intensive Inpatient Treatment

Adolescent Level IV medically managed intensive inpatient treatment is an organized service, delivered in an acute care inpatient setting. It is appropriate for adolescents whose acute biomedical, emotional, behavioral and cognitive problems are so severe that they require primary medical and nursing care.

Level IV program services are delivered by an interdisciplinary staff of addiction-credentialed physicians and other appropriately credentialed treatment professionals. Such a program encompasses a planned regimen of 24-hour medically directed evaluation and treatment services, provided under a defined set of policies, procedures and clinical protocols.

Treatment is provided 24 hours a day in a permanent facility with inpatient beds. The full resources of a general acute care or psychiatric hospital are available. Although treatment is specific to substance dependence disorders, the skills of the interdisciplinary team and the availability of support services allow the conjoint treatment of any co-occurring biomedical conditions and mental disorders that need to be addressed.

Length of Service

The duration of treatment varies with the severity of the adolescent's illness and his or her response to treatment.

Detoxification

Dimension 1 (Acute Intoxication and/or Withdrawal Potential) is the first of the six primary assessment areas to be evaluated in making treatment and placement decisions. The range of clinical severity in this dimension has given rise to a range of detoxification levels of service.

As used here, detoxification refers not only to the attenuation of the physiological and psychological features of withdrawal syndromes, but also to the process of interrupting the momentum of habitual compulsive use in adolescents diagnosed with substance *dependence*. Because of the force of this momentum, and the inherent difficulties in overcoming it even when there is no clear withdrawal syndrome *per se*, this phase of treatment frequently requires a greater intensity of services initially in order to establish treatment engagement and patient role induction. This is, of course, critical to the course of treatment because it is impossible to engage the adolescent in treatment while he/she is caught up in the cycle of frequent intoxication and recovery from intoxication.

Level IV-D services are delivered under a defined set of physician-approved policies and physician-managed procedures or medical protocols. This level is appropriate for the adolescent whose withdrawal signs and symptoms are so severe that he or she needs primary medical and nursing care services, including 24-four hour observation, monitoring and treatment.

The treatment is specific to acute medical detoxification. However, the call for a multidisciplinary team and the availability of support services emphasize the importance of assessing and developing a care plan for any treatment priorities identified in Dimensions 2 through 6.

Adolescent Criteria
Level IV: Medically Managed Intensive Inpatient Treatment

CHARACTERISTIC	ESSENTIAL FEATURES
EXAMPLES	Level IV adolescent programs typically are housed in the following settings: [1] an acute care general hospital, [2] an acute psychiatric hospital or psychiatric unit within an acute care general hospital, and [3] an appropriately licensed chemical dependency specialty hospitals with acute care medical and nursing staff and life support equipment.
SETTING	Level IV adolescent program services may be offered in any age-appropriate, licensed acute care setting that offers intensive biomedical and/or psychiatric services and a defined program of addiction treatment.
	Such a program must offer medically directed acute detoxification and related treatment aimed at alleviating acute emotional, behavioral, cognitive or biomedical distress resulting from an adolescent's use of alcohol or other drugs. The program may provide life support care and treatment, as needed, either directly or through transfer of the adolescent to another service within the facility or to another medical facility equipped to provide such care.
	Adolescents who meet the criteria for Dimension 1 may be placed in a Level IV program in an acute care general hospital, a psychiatric hospital, or a chemical dependency specialty hospital; those meeting criteria in Dimension 2 would be placed in a Level IV program in an acute care general hospital; and those meeting the criteria in Dimension 3 might be placed in a Level IV program in a psychiatric specialty hospital or a psychiatric specialty unit in a general hospital.
	Level IV-D Detoxification Level IV-D detoxification services may be offered in any appropriately licensed acute care setting that is able to provide medically directed acute detoxification and related treatment aimed at alleviating acute emotional, behavioral or biomedical distress resulting from the adolescent's use of alcohol or other drugs.
	At least three types of settings provide this level of care:
	(a) An acute care general hospital.
	(b) An acute care psychiatric hospital with ready access to the full resources of an acute care general hospital, or a psychiatric unit in an acute care general hospital.
	(c) An appropriately licensed chemical dependency specialty hospital with acute care medical and nursing staff and life support equipment, or an acute care addiction treatment unit in an acute care general hospital.

Adolescent Criteria
Level IV: Medically Managed Intensive Inpatient Treatment

CHARACTERISTIC	ESSENTIAL FEATURES
SUPPORT SYSTEMS	In Level IV adolescent programs, necessary support systems include a full range of acute care services, specialty consultation, indicated laboratory and toxicology testing, and intensive care.
STAFF	Level IV adolescent programs are staffed by: (a) An interdisciplinary team of appropriately credentialed clinical staff (including addiction-credentialed physicians, nurses, counselors, psychologists and social workers) who assess and treat adolescents with substance-related disorders or addicted adolescents with concomitant acute biomedical, emotional or behavioral disorders. Staff are knowledgeable about the biopsychosocial dimensions of adolescent addiction and the biomedical and emotional, behavioral and cognitive disorders. (In states where physician assistants or nurse practitioners are licensed as physician extenders, they may perform the duties designated here for a physician.) (b) A team of appropriately trained and credentialed professionals who provide daily medical management by physicians 24 hours a day, primary nursing care and observation 24 hours a day, and professional counseling services daily. (c) Facility-approved addiction counselors or licensed, certified or registered addiction clinicians who administer planned interventions according to the assessed needs of the adolescent.
THERAPIES	Therapies offered by Level IV adolescent programs include: (a) A highly individualized program of treatment for the substance dependence disorder and any concurrent biomedical, emotional, behavioral or cognitive problems, delivered by an interdisciplinary treatment team. (b) Cognitive, behavioral, medication and other therapies, provided on an individual or group basis, depending on the adolescent's needs. For the adolescent who has a severe biomedical disorder, biomedical interventions are available to supplement addiction treatment. For the adolescent who has a severe psychiatric problem, psychiatric interventions complement addiction treatment. (c) Health education services. (d) Planned clinical interventions that are designed to enhance the adolescent's acceptance of his or her substance dependence problem. (e) Services for the adolescent's family, guardian or significant other(s).

Adolescent Criteria
Level IV: Medically Managed Intensive Inpatient Treatment

CHARACTERISTIC	ESSENTIAL FEATURES
THERAPIES (continued)	**Level IV-D Detoxification** Level IV-D detoxification is provided by an interdisciplinary team provides daily clinical services to assess the adolescent patient's withdrawal status and provide treatment as needed. Clinical services involve medical management (including pharmacological treatments, as appropriate) and individual and/or group therapy specific to withdrawal and withdrawal support. Frequent nurse monitoring of the adolescent's progress in detoxification is available. Medication administration is available as needed.
ASSESSMENT/ TREATMENT PLAN REVIEW	In Level IV adolescent programs, elements of the assessment and treatment plan review include: (a) A comprehensive nursing assessment, conducted at the time of admission. (b) Physician approval of the admission. (c) A comprehensive history and physical examination, performed by a physician, usually at the time of admission. (d) A comprehensive biopsychosocial assessment, begun at the time of admission. (e) An educational assessment, performed to assist in the design of an appropriate educational program. (f) Referral arrangements for continuing treatment at another level of care, as needed. (g) An individualized treatment plan, which includes problem formulation and articulation of treatment goals and measurable treatment objectives. Treatment plan reviews are conducted at specified times, as noted in the treatment plan. **Level IV-D Detoxification** In addition to the assessment and treatment plan activities described above, elements of the Level IV-D assessment and treatment plan review include: (a) An initial withdrawal assessment by a physician or nurse, conducted at the time of admission. (b) Daily assessment of the adolescent's withdrawal symptoms and progress during detoxification, as well as any amendments to the treatment plan.

Adolescent Criteria
Level IV: Medically Managed Intensive Inpatient Treatment

CHARACTERISTIC	ESSENTIAL FEATURES
DOCUMENTATION	Documentation standards of Level IV adolescent programs include progress notes in the patient record that clearly reflect implementation of the treatment plan and the adolescent's response to treatment, as well as subsequent amendments to the plan. **Level IV-D Detoxification** Detoxification rating scale tables and flow sheets (which may include tabulation of vital signs) are used as needed.

Adolescent Level IV Admission Criteria
Diagnostic and Dimensional Criteria

CRITERIA	LEVEL IV Medically Managed Intensive Inpatient Services
DIAGNOSTIC ADMISSION CRITERIA	The adolescent who is appropriately placed in a Level IV program is assessed as meeting the diagnostic criteria for Substance-Related Disorder, as defined by the current *Diagnostic and Statistical Manual of Mental Disorders (DSM)* or other standardized and widely accepted criteria, as well as the dimensional criteria for admission. If the adolescent's presenting alcohol or drug use history is inadequate to substantiate such a diagnosis, the probability of such a diagnosis may be determined from information submitted by collateral parties (such as family members, legal guardian and significant others).
DIMENSIONAL ADMISSION CRITERIA	The adolescent who is appropriately placed in a Level IV program meets specifications in at least *one* of Dimensions 1, 2 or 3.
DIMENSION 1: Acute Intoxication and/or Withdrawal	The adolescent who is appropriately placed in a Level IV program is experiencing acute withdrawal, with severe signs or symptoms, and is at risk for complications that require 24-hour intensive medical services. Such complications may involve delirium, hallucinosis, seizures, high morbidity medical complications, pregnancy, severe agitation, psychosis, unremitting suicide risk, and the like; *or* There is recent (within 24 hours) serious head trauma or loss of consciousness, with persistent mental status or neurological changes, resulting in the need to closely observe the adolescent at least hourly; *or* Drug overdose or intoxication has compromised the adolescent's mental status, cardiac function or other vital signs or functions; *or* The adolescent has a significant acute biomedical disorder that poses substantial risk of serious or life-threatening consequences during withdrawal (such as significant hypertension or esophageal varices).
DIMENSION 2: Biomedical Conditions and Complications	The adolescent's status in Dimension 2 is characterized by *one* of the following: (a) Biomedical complications of the addictive disorder require medical management and skilled nursing care (examples include delirium, seizures, GI bleeding, pancreatitis, stupor/coma, renal failure, rhabdomyolysis, severe cellulitis, endocarditis, and the like); *or* (b) A concurrent biomedical illness or other condition (such as pregnancy) requires stabilization and intensive medical management (as through daily primary nursing interventions, IV therapy, 24-hour observation, intensive medication regimens, or intensive investigations); *or*

Adolescent Level IV Admission Criteria
Diagnostic and Dimensional Criteria

CRITERIA	LEVEL IV Medically Managed Intensive Inpatient Services
DIMENSION 2: **Biomedical Conditions and Complications** **(continued)**	(c) A concurrent biomedical condition is so severe that continued drinking or drug use present an immediate danger to life or severe danger to health (including pregnancy).
DIMENSION 3: **Emotional, Behavioral or Cognitive Conditions and Complications**	The adolescent's status in Dimension 3 is characterized by *one* of the following: (a) *Dangerousness/Lethality*: The adolescent presents an imminent risk of suicidal, homicidal or other violent behavior, or is at risk of a psychosis with unpredictable, disorganized or agitated behavior that endangers self or others. Such a patient may require a locked unit. (b) *Interference with Addiction Recovery Efforts*: The adolescent is unable to focus on recovery tasks because of unstable, overwhelming psychiatric problems (for example, a schizophrenic patient who has gravely regressed to a lower level of functioning, or a bipolar youth who is manic, or a juvenile diabetic whose uncontrolled glucose levels are causing his or her confusion). (c) *Social Functioning*: The adolescent is unable to cope with family, school, work or friends, or has severely impaired ability to function in family, social, work or school settings because of an overwhelming mental health problem (such as a thought disorder or severe mood lability that places the patient at risk). (d) *Ability for Self-Care*: The adolescent has insufficient resources and skills to maintain an adequate level of functioning and requires daily medical and nursing care (for example, an adolescent with head injury, mental retardation, severe depression, eating disorder and severe cachexia). (e) *Course of Illness*: The adolescent's history and present situation suggest that, in the absence of medical management, the patient's emotional, behavioral or cognitive condition will become unstable. The unfolding course of the adolescent's illness, with ensuing changes in symptoms or mental status, is likely to lead to imminently dangerous consequences. (Examples include an adolescent in relapse who has a history of severe psychosis with intoxication, or an adolescent who requires detoxificaiton and has become acutely suicidal during past attempts at withdrawal, or an adolescent who is experiencing a recurrence of severe depression and who has had a dangerous relapse to alcohol or drug use, with attendant high-severity, high-risk behaviors and episodes of depression in the past.)
DIMENSION 4: **Readiness to Change**	Only an adolescent who meets criteria in Dimensions 1, 2 or 3 is appropriately placed in a Level IV program. Problems in Dimensions 4, 5 or 6 alone are not sufficient for placement at Level IV.

Adolescent Level IV Admission Criteria
Diagnostic and Dimensional Criteria

CRITERIA	LEVEL IV Medically Managed Intensive Inpatient Services
DIMENSION 5: **Relapse, Continued Use or Continued Problem Potential**	Only an adolescent who meets criteria in Dimensions 1, 2 or 3 is appropriately placed in a Level IV program. Problems in Dimensions 4, 5 or 6 alone are not sufficient for placement at Level IV.
DIMENSION 6: **Recovery Environment**	Only an adolescent who meets criteria in Dimensions 1, 2 or 3 is appropriately placed in a Level IV program. Problems in Dimensions 4, 5 or 6 alone are not sufficient for placement at Level IV.

Appendices

Appendix A
Matrix for Matching Multidimensional Risk with Type and Intensity of Service Needs—Adult

The Work Group on Co-Occurring Mental and Substance-Related Disorders developed an experimental "Matrix" format and criteria that take a significantly different approach to assessment, treatment planning, and placement of the individual with co-occurring mental and substance-related disorders. The Matrix format accompanies the criteria with "Risk Ratings" that can be matched with the types of services and modalities needed, as well as the intensity of services required and the treatment settings in which such services might appropriately be delivered.

The goal of the Matrix format is to promote improved assessment and treatment of patients with co-occurring disorders by adopting a more holistic, multidimensional approach that matches the patient's needs to specific treatment services, rather than to broader levels of care.

It is presented here as a possible "future directions" format as a potential alternative to, or supplement to the traditional Level of Service format. As the field experiments with this format, the feedback received will assist in determining the usefulness of this approach in working with patients who have co-occurring mental and substance-related disorders. Because there have not been validity or reliability studies with this matrix, users should understand the piloting, field testing nature of this matrix and provide feedback and guidance accordingly.

Concepts Underlying the Matrix

Individuals with mental and substance-related disorders can be viewed as suffering from biopsychosocial illnesses that, to varying degrees, have biological and medical, psychological and psychiatric, and sociocultural origins and clinical features. Treatment of these individuals is most effective and efficient when it addresses the individual's specific biopsychosocial issues in a manner that will stabilize the acute episode, arrest further deterioration of function, and help promote recovery.

To optimize the use of treatment and financial resources, patient care must be individualized rather than driven by the patient's diagnosis or the availability of certain levels of care or types of treatment programs. Diagnosis is a necessary, but not sufficient, determinant of service needs. Just as with patients who are diagnosed with cancer, hypertension or diabetes, it is the severity of the patient's illness and the degree of the patient's impairment—not merely the diagnosis—that determine the patient's specific treatment needs and thus drive the treatment plan.

Professionals working in the addiction and mental health fields have yet to achieve consensus on how to assess clinical risk. As a result, a variety of criteria and decision rules have been developed for matching patients to treatment services and care settings. The ensuing confusion adversely affects communications among professionals, with patients and their families, and with care managers and payers. It also dissipates limited resources.

Multidimensional Risk Profile

As a step toward consensus—or at least toward minimizing confusion about assessment of patients with co-occurring disorders—the Work Group on Co-Occurring Disorders has articulated the following principles:

1. Risk is multidimensional and biopsychosocial. Addressing a particular patient's risk may require more than one treatment component (e.g., stabilizing a psychosis or detoxifying a patient while also addressing an unstable or abusive living environment).

2. Risk relates to the patient's history. For example, the patient whose withdrawal always results in seizures has different treatment needs from the patient whose withdrawal involves only mild symptoms of anxiety. Or the patient who in the past has acted on suicidal impulses by hanging has needs different from the patient who acted on suicidal impulses by superficially scratching a wrist.

3. Risk is expressed in current status. For example, a patient who develops elevated vital signs in response to discontinuation of alcohol use requires different treatment services from a calm patient who is not currently using alcohol or other drugs. Similarly, an actively psychotic patient who is hallucinating needs more intensive services than a patient who is chronically psychotic but currently stable.

4. Risk involves a degree of change from baseline or premorbid functioning. For example, a previously outgoing and fully functioning individual who suddenly withdraws from social contact needs more intensive services than does an individual who is chronically withdrawn and barely able to function outside a supportive living environment.

5. Risk assessment must integrate the patient's history, changing situation and current status.

Developing a multidimensional Risk Profile involves integrating biopsychosocial data from the patient's history and current status into a succinct summary. The Matrix attempts to facilitate this task by presenting descriptions in each of the biopsychosocial dimensions to use in determining the types of services/modalities and intensity of services needed.

For each assessment dimension (which correspond to Dimensions 1 to 6 of the traditional Patient Placement Criteria), the risk description and rating suggest the severity of the patient's problem in that dimension. The treatment priorities represented by the Types of Services/Modalities Needed suggest the specific types of treatment services/modalities the patient requires, as well as the intensity with which those services should be delivered to appropriately address the patient's multidimensional service needs.

The corresponding rating in the Intensity of Service/Level of Service/Setting quadrant suggests the intensity of the level of care and setting that appropriately allows the treatment and service plan to be effectively delivered. Each dimension is considered separately ("unbundled") from the other dimensions to allow independent assessment of all areas of potential concern.

The Matrix allows the intensity of clinical services to be "delinked" from the intensity of social and case management services, so as to promote the most efficient use of clinical care. It is at the point of developing the placement decision that these "unbundled" or "delinked" assessments must be re-integrated into a comprehensive treatment plan. The Work Group anticipates that the widening array of treatment services, modalities and settings will allow more specific matching of patient needs to type and intensity of service and setting.

The Work Group offers the Matrix and Multidimensional Risk Profiles in the hope that they will provide a basis for common understanding among mental health and addiction treatment professionals.

Characteristics of the Matrix

The Matrix is multidimensional. It employs the six assessment dimensions of the ASAM *Patient Placement Criteria* (PPC), first developed in 1991 and since modified to be applicable to dual diagnosis populations. These six assessment dimensions make explicit the components of a biopsychosocial assessment and promote comprehensive assessment of all the areas in which a patient's needs are likely to require services in order to achieve an optimal outcome.

The Matrix provides some benchmarks for rating Risk, for determining priorities in Types of Services/Modalities Needed, and for assessing the Intensity of Services needed.

The Matrix helps to identify potential services, modalities and resources even as the inventory of those services grows through improved treatment matching research and expansion of treatment options and interventions in the provider network.

The Matrix promotes individualized treatment by matching the Risk Rating in each of six dimensions with the most appropriate treatment modalities and services.

Risk Description. Each Risk Description provides both a numerical rating of risk (on a scale of 0 to 4) and a narrative description of risk in terms of signs and symptoms that indicate the individual's severity and level of function in a particular assessment dimension. The risk descriptions and ratings within each assessment dimension help staff determine the immediacy and scope of the service plan by guiding what types and modalities of service are needed. They also indicate the intensity or level of service at which the patient can be treated with safety and efficacy.

Risk Domains. A Risk Domain is an assessment subcategory within Dimension 3, as described below:

- **Dangerousness/Lethality.** This Risk Domain describes how impulsive an individual may be with regard to homicide, suicide, or other forms of harm to self or others and/or to property. The seriousness and immediacy of the individual's ideation, plans and behavior—as well as his or her ability to act on such impulses—determine the patient's risk rating and the type and intensity of services he or she needs.

- **Interference with Addiction Recovery Efforts.** This Risk Domain describes the degree to which a patient is distracted from addiction recovery efforts by emotional, behavioral and/or cognitive problems and, conversely, the degree to which a patient is able to focus on addiction recovery. (Note that high risk and severe impairment in this domain do not, in themselves, require services in a Level IV program.)

- **Social Functioning.** This Risk Domain describes the degree to which an individual's relationships (e.g., coping with friends, significant others or family; vocational or educational demands; and ability to meet personal responsibilities) are affected by his or her substance use and/or other emotional, behavioral and cognitive problems. (Note that high risk and severe impairment in this domain do not, in themselves, require services in a Level IV program.)

- **Ability for Self-Care.** This Risk Domain describes the degree to which an individual's ability to perform activities of daily living (such as grooming, food and shelter) are affected by his or her substance use and/or other emotional, behavioral and cognitive problems. (Note that high risk and severe impairment in this domain do not, in themselves, require services in a Level IV program.)

- **Course of Illness.** This Risk Domain employs the history of the patient's illness and response to treatment to interpret the patient's current signs, symptoms and presentation and predict the patient's likely response to treatment. Thus, the domain assesses the interaction between the chronicity and acuity of the patient's current deficits. A high risk rating is warranted when the individual is assessed as at significant risk and vulnerability for dangerous consequences either because of severe, acute life-threatening symptoms, or because a history of such instability suggests that high intensity services are needed to prevent dangerous consequences.

    For example, a patient may present with medication compliance problems, having discontinued antipsychotic medication two days ago. If a patient is known to rapidly decompensate into acute psychosis when medication is stopped, his or her rating is high. However, if it is known that he or she slowly isolates without any rapid deterioration when medication is stopped, the risk rating would be less. Another example could be the patient who has been depressed, socially withdrawn, staying in bed and not bathing. If this has been a problem for six weeks, the risk rating is much higher than for a patient who has been chronically withdrawn and isolated for six years with a severe and persistent schizophrenic disorder.

How to Use the Matrix to Match Multidimensional Risk with Type and Intensity of Service Needs

Step 1: Assess all six dimensions to determine whether the patient has immediate needs related to imminent danger, as indicated by a Risk Rating of "4" in any of the six dimensions. The Dimension with the highest risk rating determines the immediate service needs and placement decision. For example, if in Dimension 1, the patient has a risk rating of 4 due to severe withdrawal posing imminent risk of seizures and delirium tremens, then placement in a Level IV-D, medically managed intensive inpatient detoxification service is required. Further assessment of all six dimensions proceeds once placement has been achieved.

Step 2: If the patient is not in imminent danger, determine the patient's Risk Rating in each of the six dimensions. (For patients who have "dual diagnosis" problems, assess Dimensions 4, 5 and 6 separately for the mental and substance-related disorders. This assists in identifying differential mental health and addiction treatment service needs and helps determine the kind of dual diagnosis program most likely to meet the patient's needs.)

Step 3: Identify the appropriate Types of Services and Modalities needed for all dimensions with any clinically significant risk ratings. Not all dimensions may have sufficient severity to warrant service needs at the time of the assessment.

    For example, a patient may have risk ratings of zero in Dimensions 1 and 2 and need no detoxification or biomedical services. However Dimensions 3 and 6 may have risk ratings of 2 and 3 respectively. The patient needs mental health and medication management and monitoring for the Dimension 3 depressive symptoms and rapidly deteriorating work functioning. For the Dimension 6 problems with a drinking, unsupportive spouse, the patient may need assertive assistance in coping with the living environment.

Step 4: Use the Multidimensional Risk Profile produced by this assessment in Steps 2 and 3 to develop an initial treatment plan and placement recommendation. This is achieved by identifying in which level of care the variety of service needs in all relevant dimensions can effectively and efficiently be provided. The appropriate Intensity of Service, Level of Care, and Setting may be the highest Risk Rating across all the dimensions. (Consider, however, that the interaction of needs across all dimensions may require more intensive services than the highest Risk Rating alone. For example, in Risk rating 2 for Dimension 5, Relapse/Continued Use/Continued Problem Potential, the Intensity of Service/Level of Service/Setting is listed as Level II.1 or II.5. The patient may require Level II.5 because of the interaction between the addiction treatment needs and the mental health needs of a person with cocaine dependence and a chronically disabling, albeit currently stabilized psychotic disorder.)

Step 5: Make ongoing decisions about the patient's continued service needs and placement by repeating Steps 1 through 4. Keep in mind that movement into and through the continuum of care should be a fluid and flexible process that is driven by continuous monitoring of the patient's changing Multidimensional Risk Profile.

Appendix A
Adult Criteria: Matrix for Matching Multidimensional Risk with Type and Intensity of Services

Risk Rating and Description	Types of Services and Modalities Needed	Intensity of Service/ Level of Care/Setting
(Clinical descriptors of Risk Ratings 0 through 4)	(Indicates which service(s) match the assessed risk rating)	(Indicates where the service can most safely and efficiently be delivered)
Risk Rating: 0 = *Indicates full functioning; no severity; no risk in this Dimension*	*Indicates no need for specific services in this Dimension*	**Intensity: 0** = *Indicates no need for any intensity or level of service in this Dimension*
Risk Rating: 1-4 = *Indicates various levels of functioning and severity and the level of risk in this Dimension.* *(NOTE: A higher number indicates a greater level of severity.)*	*Indicates the range of specific services needed in the treatment plan to match the patient's functioning and severity in this Dimension.*	**Intensity: 1-4** = *Indicates the intensity or level of service that can deliver the service plan safely and efficiently for in Dimension.* *(NOTE: A higher number indicates a greater level of intensity.)*

Dimension 1: Acute Intoxication/Withdrawal Potential
(DSM-IV Dependence Tolerance and Withdrawal Items; Abuse Items)

Risk Rating and Description (NOTE: A higher number indicates a greater level of severity or intensity.)	Types of Services and Modalities Needed	Intensity of Service/ Level of Care/Setting
Risk Rating: 0 = The patient is fully functioning and demonstrates good ability to tolerate and cope with withdrawal discomfort. No signs or symptoms of intoxication or withdrawal are present, or signs or symptoms are resolving. For patients on Opioid Maintenance Therapy (OMT), the dose is well-stabilized, with no opioid intoxication or withdrawal.	No immediate intoxication monitoring or detoxification services are needed. The patient on OMT requires opioid maintenance medications, such as methadone or LAAM.	**Intensity: 0** = Does not affect the placement decision. OMT patients continue in Level I Outpatient OMT.
Risk Rating: 1 = The patient demonstrates adequate ability to tolerate and cope with withdrawal discomfort. Mild to moderate intoxication or signs and symptoms interfere with daily functioning, but do not pose an imminent danger to self or others. There is minimal risk of severe withdrawal (e.g., as a continuation of detoxification at other levels of service, or in the presence of heavy alcohol or sedative-hypnotic use with minimal seizure risk). For patients on Opioid Maintenance Therapy (OMT), the dose is inadequately stabilized and the patient has mild symptoms of withdrawal, or occasional compensatory use of opiates or other drugs.	Low-intensity intoxication monitoring or detoxification services are needed. For patients who require intensive mental health services (a Dimension 3 Risk Rating of 2 or higher), low-intensity detoxification can be provided in a mental health setting with ongoing case management to coordinate care. The patient on OMT requires dose adjustment, counseling services to assess and address readiness to change and relapse issues, and random urine testing.	**Intensity: 1** = Level I-D ambulatory detoxification without extended on-site monitoring. OMT patients continue in Level I Outpatient OMT. **LOC/Setting:** Outpatient primary care, or an addiction or mental health service.

ASAM Patient Placement Criteria, Second Edition–Revised

Dimension 1: Acute Intoxication/Withdrawal Potential
(DSM-IV Dependence Tolerance and Withdrawal Items; Abuse Items)

Risk Rating and Description (NOTE: A higher number indicates a greater level of severity or intensity.)	Types of Services and Modalities Needed	Intensity of Service/ Level of Care/Setting
Risk Rating: 2 = The patient has some difficulty tolerating and coping with withdrawal discomfort. Intoxication may be severe, but responds to support and treatment sufficiently that the patient does not pose an imminent danger to self or others. Moderate signs and symptoms, with moderate risk of severe withdrawal (e.g., as a continuation of detoxification at other levels of service, or in the presence of heavy alcohol or sedative-hypnotic use with minimal seizure risk, or many signs and symptoms of opiate or stimulant withdrawal). For patients on Opioid Maintenance Therapy (OMT), the dose is inadequately stabilized and the patient has moderate symptoms of withdrawal, or frequent compensatory use of opiates or other drugs.	Moderate-intensity intoxication monitoring or detoxification services are needed. For patients who require partial hospital or more intensive mental health services (a Dimension 3 Risk Rating of 2 or 3 or higher), moderate-intensity detoxification can be provided in a mental health setting with ongoing case management to coordinate care. The patient on OMT requires dose adjustment, counseling services to assess and address readiness to change and relapse issues, and random urine testing.	**Intensity: 2** = Level II-D ambulatory detoxification with extended on-site monitoring. OMT patients continue in Level I Outpatient OMT. **LOC/Setting:** Outpatient primary care, or an addiction or mental health service.
Risk Rating: 3 = The patient demonstrates poor ability to tolerate and cope with withdrawal discomfort. Severe signs and symptoms of intoxication indicate that the patient may pose an imminent danger to self or others, and intoxication has not abated at less intensive levels of service. There are severe signs and symptoms, or risk of severe but manageable withdrawal; or withdrawal is worsening despite detoxification at a less intensive level of care (e.g., as a continuation of detoxification at other levels of service, or in the presence of opiate withdrawal with cravings and impulsive behaviors).	Moderately high-intensity intoxication monitoring or detoxification services are needed. Nursing and medical monitoring may be needed for more severe withdrawal. For patients who require medically monitored and nurse-managed mental health services (a Dimension 3 Risk Rating of 3 or higher), moderately high-intensity detoxification can be provided in a mental health setting with ongoing case management to coordinate care.	**Intensity: 3** = Level III.2-D clinically managed residential detoxi-fication or Level III.7-D medically monitored inpatient detoxification. OMT patients continue in Level I Outpatient OMT. **LOC/Setting:** A general, addiction or mental health facility.

Dimension 1: Acute Intoxication/Withdrawal Potential
(DSM-IV Dependence Tolerance and Withdrawal Items; Abuse Items)

Risk Rating and Description (NOTE: A higher number indicates a greater level of severity or intensity.)	Types of Services and Modalities Needed	Intensity of Service/ Level of Care/Setting
For patients on Opioid Maintenance Therapy (OMT), the dose is inadequately stabilized and the patient has severe symptoms of withdrawal, or frequent, significant and ongoing compensatory use of opiates or other drugs.	The patient on OMT requires dose adjustment, counseling services to assess and address readiness to change and relapse issues, and random urine testing.	
Risk Rating: 4 = The patient is incapacitated, with severe signs and symptoms. Severe withdrawal presents danger, as of seizures. Continued use poses an imminent threat to life (e.g., liver failure, GI bleed, or fetal death). For patients on Opioid Maintenance Therapy (OMT), the dose is inadequately stabilized, and the patient has repeated, significant concurrent use of opiates or other drugs. Such use is unresponsive to treatment interventions, dose adjustments and increasing sanctions.	High-intensity intoxication monitoring or detoxification services are needed, with monitoring and management more often than hourly. The patient on OMT requires dose adjustment, counseling services to assess readiness to change and explore long-term outpatient detoxification from the OMT medication.	**Intensity: 4** = Level IV-D medically managed intensive inpatient detoxification. OMT patients continue in Level I Outpatient OMT. **LOC/Setting:** A general, addiction or mental health acute inpatient unit.

Dimension 2: Biomedical Conditions and Complications
(DSM-IV Axis III)

Risk Rating and Description (NOTE: A higher number indicates a greater level of severity or intensity.)	Types of Services and Modalities Needed	Intensity of Service/ Level of Care/Setting
Risk Rating: 0 = The patient is fully functioning and demonstrates good ability to cope with physical discomfort. No biomedical signs or symptoms are present, or biomedical problems (such as hypertension or chronic pain) are stable.	No immediate biomedical services (except for long-term monitoring) are needed.	**Intensity: 0** = Does not affect the placement decision.
Risk Rating: 1 = The patient demonstrates adequate ability to tolerate and cope with physical discomfort. Mild to moderate signs or symptoms (such as mild to moderate pain) interfere with daily functioning.	Low-intensity biomedical services are needed, including case management to coordinate addiction and mental health care.	**Intensity: 1** = Level I outpatient services. **LOC/Setting:** Outpatient primary care, or an addiction or mental health service that incorporates specific services for "dual diagnosis" patients and access to or coordination with primary care.
Risk Rating: 2 = The patient has some difficulty tolerating and coping with physical problems and/or has other biomedical problems. These problems may interfere with recovery and mental health treatment. The patient neglects to care for serious biomedical problems. Acute, non-life threatening medical signs and symptoms (such as acute episodes of chronic, distracting pain, or signs of malnutrition or electrolyte imbalance) are present.	Moderate-intensity biomedical services are needed, including case management to ensure further biomedical evaluation and treatment as part of the overall treatment plan. For patients with significant mental health impairments (a Dimension 3 Risk Rating of 1 or 2 or higher), case management may be needed to coordinate the patient's addiction, mental health and biomedical care.	**Intensity: 2** = Level I or II outpatient or intensive outpatient/partial hospitalization services. **LOC/Setting:** Outpatient primary care, or an addiction or mental health service that incorporates specific services for "dual diagnosis" patients and access to or coordination with primary care.

Dimension 2: Biomedical Conditions and Complications
(DSM-IV Axis III)

Risk Rating and Description (NOTE: A higher number indicates a greater level of severity or intensity.)	Types of Services and Modalities Needed	Intensity of Service/ Level of Care/Setting
Risk Rating: 3 = The patient demonstrates poor ability to tolerate and cope with physical problems, and/or his or her general health condition is poor. The patient has serious medical problems, which he or she neglects during outpatient or intensive outpatient treatment. Severe medical problems (such as severe pain requiring medication or brittle diabetes) are present but stable.	Moderately high-intensity biomedical services are needed, including medical and nursing monitoring to ensure stabilization. For patients with significant mental health impairments (a Dimension 3 Risk Rating of 1 or 2 or higher), case management may be needed to coordinate the patient's addiction, mental health and biomedical care.	**Intensity: 3** = Level III.7 medically monitored inpatient services. **LOC/Setting:** A general, addiction or mental health facility that incorporates specific services for "dual diagnosis" patients and access to or coordination with primary care.
Risk Rating: 4 = The patient is incapacitated, with severe medical problems (such as extreme pain, uncontrolled diabetes, GI bleeding, or infection requiring IV antibiotics).	High-intensity biomedical services are needed for stabilization and medication management, including medical and nursing close observation and 24-hour management.	**Intensity: 4** = Level IV medically managed intensive inpatient services. **LOC/Setting:** A general, addiction or mental health acute inpatient unit that incorporates specific services for "dual diagnosis" patients. For patients with severe mental health impairments (a Dimension 3 Risk Rating of 3 or higher), this may require inpatient psychiatric care or a medical/psychiatric setting.

Dimension 3: Emotional, Behavioral or Cognitive Conditions and Complications
(DSM-IV Dependence Impairment Items; Abuse Items; Axes IV and V)

Risk Rating and Description, by Risk Domains (a) (NOTE: Individuals need not match descriptions in all of the subdomains within any one risk rating category.)	Types of Services and Modalities Needed (b)	Intensity of Service/ Level of Care/Setting (c)
Risk Rating: 0 = The patient either has no mental health problems or has a diagnosed but stable mental disorder. *Dangerousness/Lethality*: Good impulse control and coping skills. *Interference with Addiction Recovery Efforts*: Ability to focus on recovery, identify appropriate supports and reach out for help. *Social Functioning*: Full functioning in relationships with significant others, work and friends, et al. *Ability for Self-Care*: Full functioning, with good resources and skills to cope with emotional problems. *Course of Illness*: No emotional or behavioral problems, or problems identified are stable (e.g., depression that is stable and managed with antidepressants). No recent serious or high-risk vulnerability.	No immediate mental health services are needed.	**Intensity: 0** = Does not affect the placement decision.

ASAM Patient Placement Criteria, Second Edition–Revised

Dimension 3: Emotional, Behavioral or Cognitive Conditions and Complications
(DSM-IV Dependence Impairment Items; Abuse Items; Axes IV and V)

Risk Rating and Description, by Risk Domains (a) (NOTE: Individuals need not match descriptions in all of the subdomains within any one risk rating category.)	Types of Services and Modalities Needed (b)	Intensity of Service/ Level of Care/Setting (c)
Risk Rating: 1 = The patient has a diagnosed mental disorder that requires intervention, but does not significantly interfere with addiction treatment. *Dangerousness/Lethality*: Adequate impulse control and coping skills to deal with any thoughts of harm to self or others. *Interference with Addiction Recovery Efforts*: Emotional concerns relate to negative consequences and effects of addiction. The patient is able to view these as part of addiction and recovery. *Social Functioning*: Relationships or spheres of social functioning (as with significant others, friends, work) are being impaired but not endangered by patient's substance use (e.g., no imminent divorce, job loss, or coping in homeless situations). The patient is able to meet personal responsibilities and maintain stable meaningful relationships despite the mild symptoms experienced (e.g., mood or anxiety symptoms subthreshold for DSM-IV diagnosis or, if meeting diagnostic criteria, patient is able to continue in essential roles). *Ability for Self-Care*: Adequate resources and skills to cope with emotional or behavioral problems. *Course of Illness*: Mild to moderate signs and symptoms (e.g., dysphoria, relationship problems, work or school problems, or problems coping in the	Low-intensity mental health services are needed, including case management to coordinate addiction and mental health care, medication monitoring, psychoeducation about mental disorders and psychotropic medications, and self/mutual help and dual diagnosis support and recovery groups to deal with emotional aspects of recovery.	**Intensity: 1** = Level I outpatient services. **LOC/Setting**: Outpatient primary care, or an addiction or mental health service that incorporates specific services for "dual diagnosis" patients, or addiction treatment services with psychiatric integration, consultation/liaison and/or collaboration; or mental health care with addiction integration, consultation/liaison or collaboration.

Dimension 3: Emotional, Behavioral or Cognitive Conditions and Complications
(DSM-IV Dependence Impairment Items; Abuse Items; Axes IV and V)

Risk Rating and Description, by Risk Domains (a) (NOTE: Individuals need not match descriptions in all of the subdomains within any one risk rating category.)	Types of Services and Modalities Needed (b)	Intensity of Service/ Level of Care/Setting (c)
community, with good response to treatment in the past. Any past serious problems have a long period of stability (e.g., serious depression and suicidal behavior 15 years ago) or past problems are chronic but not severe enough to pose any high risk vulnerability (e.g., superficial wrist scratching, but no previous hospitalization or life-threatening behavior).		
Risk Rating: 2 = Patients are of two types. The first exhibits this level of impairment only during acute impairment. The second demonstrates this level of decompensation at baseline. This Risk Rating implies persistent mental illness, with symptoms and disability that cause significant interference with addiction treatment, but do not constitute an immediate threat to safety and do not prevent independent functioning. *Dangerousness/Lethality:* Suicidal ideation; violent impulses; significant history of suicidal or violent behavior requires more than routine monitoring.	Moderate-intensity mental health services are needed, including case management to ensure monitoring and evaluation of emotional, behavioral, and cognitive status as part of the treatment plan, medication management and monitoring, and medical and nursing monitoring and management as needed. For acute decompensation patients, activities to address the substance use disorder may need to be postponed until the patient's mental health symptoms are more stable.	**Intensity: 2** = Level II.1 intensive outpatient or Level II.5 partial hospitalization services. **LOC/Setting:** Intensive mental health treatment with integrated addiction services, or "dual diagnosis" intensive outpatient services. Partial hospitalization mental health treatment with integrated addiction services, or "dual diagnosis" partial hospitalization services. For baseline patients, the range of settings may include outpatient case management to intensive outpatient, partial hospitalization and Level III.1 for supportive living.

Dimension 3: Emotional, Behavioral or Cognitive Conditions and Complications
(DSM-IV Dependence Impairment Items; Abuse Items; Axes IV and V)

Risk Rating and Description, by Risk Domains (a) (NOTE: Individuals need not match descriptions in all of the subdomains within any one risk rating category.)	Types of Services and Modalities Needed (b)	Intensity of Service/ Level of Care/Setting (c)
Interference with Addiction Recovery Efforts: Emotional, behavioral or cognitive problems distract the patient from recovery efforts. *Social Functioning*: Relationships or spheres of social functioning (as with significant others, friends, work) are being impaired by substance use, but also are linked to a psychiatric disorder (e.g., a patient with depression or anxiety disorder is unable to sleep or socialize). Symptoms are causing moderate difficulty in managing relationships with significant others, social, work or school functioning, or coping in the community, but not to a degree that they pose a significant danger to self or others, or that the patient is unable to manage activities of daily living or basic responsibilities in the home, work, school, or community. *Ability for Self-Care*: Poor resources, with moderate or minimal skills to cope with emotional or behavioral problems. *Course of Illness*: Frequent and/or intensive symptoms (e.g., frequent suicidal or homicidal ideation; vegetative signs; agitation or retardation; inconsistent impulse control), with a history that indicates significant problems that are not well-stabilized (e.g., psychotic episodes with frequent periods of decompensation). Acute or acute-on-chronic problems pose some risk of harm to self or others, but the patient is not imminently	For baseline patients, the patient's substance use disorder may be addressed in psychiatrically enhanced addiction services, staffed by mental health professionals with smaller caseloads. For patients with high Risk Ratings in Dimension 4, motivational enhancement therapies may be integrated into ongoing mental health services.	

ASAM Patient Placement Criteria, Second Edition–Revised

Dimension 3: Emotional, Behavioral or Cognitive Conditions and Complications
(DSM-IV Dependence Impairment Items; Abuse Items; Axes IV and V)

Risk Rating and Description, by Risk Domains (a) (NOTE: Individuals need not match descriptions in all of the subdomains within any one risk rating category.)	Types of Services and Modalities Needed (b)	Intensity of Service/ Level of Care/Setting (c)
dangerous (e.g., hallucinations and delusions invoke homicidal ideation, but the patient has no plan or means to harm others).		
Risk Rating: 3 = Patients are of two types. The first exhibits this level of impairment only during acute impairment. The second demonstrates this level of decompensation at baseline. This Risk Rating is characterized by severe psychiatric symptomatology, disability and impulsivity, but the patient has sufficient control that he or she does not require involuntary confinement. *Dangerousness/Lethality*: Frequent impulses to harm self or others which are potentially destabilizing, but the patient is not imminently dangerous in a 24-hour setting. *Interference with Addiction Recovery Efforts*: Recovery efforts are negatively affected by the patient's emotional, behavioral or cognitive problems in significant and distracting ways, up to and including inability to focus on recovery efforts. *Ability for Self-Care*: Insufficient or severe lack of capacity to cope with emotional or behavioral problems. Uncontrolled behavior, confusion or	Moderately high-intensity mental health services are needed, including daily monitoring and ready access to medical management, and medication management if symptoms become acute but not dangerous. Assertive case management and community outreach are needed for the severely and persistently mentally ill patient. Supportive living arrangements, with 24-hour supervision, are needed. For acute decompensation patients, activities to address the substance use disorder (other than detoxification and discharge planning) may need to be postponed until the patient's mental health symptoms are stabilized. For baseline patients, the patient's substance use disorder may be addressed in addiction-treatment enhanced mental health services.	**Intensity: 3** = Level III.5 clinically managed residential services or Level III.7 medically monitored inpatient services. **LOC/Setting:** A free-standing residential "dual diagnosis" service, or subacute residential psychiatric unit with medical monitoring and integrated addiction services.

Dimension 3: Emotional, Behavioral or Cognitive Conditions and Complications
(DSM-IV Dependence Impairment Items; Abuse Items; Axes IV and V)

Risk Rating and Description, by Risk Domains (a) (NOTE: Individuals need not match descriptions in all of the subdomains within any one risk rating category.)	Types of Services and Modalities Needed (b)	Intensity of Service/ Level of Care/Setting (c)
disorientation, which limit the patient's capacity for self-care. Inadequate activities of daily living. *Course of Illness*: Acute course of illness dominates the clinical presentation so that symptoms may involve impaired reality testing, communication, thought processes, judgment, or attention to personal hygiene, which significantly compromise the patient's ability to adjust his or her life in the community, or previous treatment has not achieved stabilization or complete remission of symptoms. The patient has limited ability to follow through with treatment recommendations, thus demonstrating risk of and vulnerability to dangerous consequences.	For patients with high Risk Ratings in Dimension 4, motivational enhancement therapies may be integrated into ongoing mental health services.	
Risk Rating: 4 = Patients have severe psychiatric symptomatology, disability and impulsivity, and requires involuntary confinement. *Dangerousness/Lethality*: Severe psychotic, mood or personality disorder, which presents acute risk to the patient, such as immediate risk of suicide, psychosis with unpredictable, disorganized or violent behavior, or gross neglect of self-care.	High-intensity mental health services are needed, including 24-hour medical and nursing monitoring and management, medication management, ECT or secure services, and close observation more often than hourly. Appropriate addiction services (such as detoxification and motivational enhancement therapies) can be integrated into mental health services.	**Intensity: 4** = Level IV medically managed intensive inpatient services. **LOC/Setting:** A psychiatric acute inpatient unit. For addicted patients who are somewhat ready to engage in recovery, a dual diagnosis specialty unit is ideal.

Dimension 3: Emotional, Behavioral or Cognitive Conditions and Complications
(DSM-IV Dependence Impairment Items; Abuse Items; Axes IV and V)

Risk Rating and Description, by Risk Domains (a) (NOTE: Individuals need not match descriptions in all of the subdomains within any one risk rating category.)	Types of Services and Modalities Needed (b)	Intensity of Service/ Level of Care/Setting (c)
Interference with Addiction Recovery Efforts: Risk in this domain does not influence type and intensity of services needed. *Social Functioning*: Risk in this domain does not influence type and intensity of services needed. *Ability for Self-Care*: Risk in this domain does not influence type and intensity of services needed. *Course of Illness*: High risk and significant vulnerability for dangerous consequences. The patient exhibits severe and acute life-threatening symptoms (e.g., dangerous or impulsive behavior or cognitive functioning) that pose imminent danger to self or others. Symptoms of psychosis include command hallucinations or paranoid delusions. History of instability is such that high-intensity services are needed to prevent dangerous consequences (e.g., the patient is not responding to daily changes in medication at less intensive levels of service, with escalating psychosis).		

NOTES:

(a) Consider dangerousness and/or lethality, interference with addiction recovery efforts, social functioning, capacity for self-care, and course of illness (history of present illness—the pattern of symptoms and response to treatment up to, and including, the present illness—and pattern of treatment response).

(b) Consider acute stabilization, medical management and monitoring, mental health consultation and integration of mental health and addiction services, skills training, case management, medication management and monitoring, and systems intervention and coordination.

(c) Consider traditional addiction and mental health services, availability of addiction services coordinated with mental health services or mental health services coordinated with addiction treatment, integrated inpatient or outpatient "dual diagnosis" services, assertive case management and community outreach services.

Dimension 4: Readiness to Change

Risk Rating and Description (NOTE: A higher number indicates a greater level of severity or intensity.)	Types of Services and Modalities Needed	Intensity of Service/ Level of Care/Setting
Risk Rating: 0 = *Substance Use Disorders*: The patient is willingly engaged in treatment as a proactive, responsible participant, and is committed to change his or her alcohol and/or other drug use. *Mental Disorders*: The patient is willingly engaged in treatment as a proactive, responsible participant, and is committed to change his or her mental functioning and behavior.	No immediate engagement or motivational enhancement strategies or services are needed.	**Intensity: 0 =** Self/mutual help groups support referral into an appropriate addiction treatment service, depending on Risk Ratings in the other dimensions. For dual diagnosis patients with a Dimension 3 Risk Rating of 2 or higher at baseline, active addiction treatment may be integrated into a mental health setting, according to the intensity of service required by the patient's Risk Ratings in Dimensions 5 and 6.
Risk Rating: 1 = *Substance Use Disorders*: The patient is willing to enter treatment and to explore strategies for changing his or her substance use, but is ambivalent about the need for change. He or she is willing to explore the need for treatment and strategies to reduce or stop substance use (e.g., the patient views his or her substance use problem as caused by depression or another psychiatric diagnosis). Or the patient is willing to change his or her substance use, but believes it will not be difficult to do so, or will not accept a full recovery treatment plans. *Mental Disorders*: The patient is willing to enter treatment and to explore strategies for changing his or her mental functioning, but is ambivalent about the need for change. He or she is willing to explore the need for treatment and strategies to deal with mental disorders. The patient's participation in mental health treatment	In any addiction/dual diagnosis setting, low-intensity engagement or motivational strategies are needed. These include education about the illness(es), education of family and significant others, and legal, work or school system reinforcement of the need for treatment. For patients with impairment in Dimension 3, motivational enhancement is integrated into continuing care management at any degree of intensity, as well as into specific treatment episodes.	**Intensity: 1 =** Level I outpatient services for motivational enhancement strategies. **LOC/Setting:** An outpatient addiction or mental health service.

Dimension 4: Readiness to Change

Risk Rating and Description (NOTE: A higher number indicates a greater level of severity or intensity.)	Types of Services and Modalities Needed	Intensity of Service/ Level of Care/Setting
is sufficient to avert mental decompensation (e.g., a bipolar patient who is ambivalent about taking mood-stabilizing medications, but who generally follows through with treatment recommendations).		
Risk Rating: 2 = *Substance Use Disorders*: The patient is reluctant to agree to treatment for substance use problems. He or she is able to articulate the negative consequences of substance use, but has low commitment to change his or her use of alcohol or other drugs. The patient is assessed as having low readiness to change and is only passively involved in treatment, is variably compliant with attendance at outpatient sessions or meetings of self/mutual help or other support groups. *Mental Disorders*: The patient is reluctant to agree to treatment for mental disorders. He or she is able to articulate the negative consequences of his or her mental health problems, but has low commitment to therapy. The patient is assessed as having low readiness to change and is only passively involved in treatment (e.g., is variable in follow through with use of psychotropic medications or attendance at therapy sessions).	Moderate-intensity engagement or motivational strategies are needed, with active support from family, significant others, legal, work or school systems to set and follow through with clear, consistent limits and consequences. Assertive case management or assertive community treatment (ACT) may be needed.

For patients who face legal consequences, court-mandated treatment (as through drug court) may be indicated. For patients with Dimension 3 baseline Risk Ratings of 2 or higher, intensive case management may be required to integrate motivational enhancement therapies and continuing mental health care. | **Intensity: 1** = Level I outpatient services for motivational enhancement strategies, coupled with Level II services for assertive case management if the case management involves more than 9 hours per week.

LOC/Setting: An outpatient addiction or mental health service, with assertive case management or an assertive community treatment (ACT) team.

High-intensity residential addiction services are not recommended, unless appropriate legal consequences promote patient motivation. The patient may require outpatient motivational enhancement therapies in an addiction or mental health treatment setting, with coordinated mental health care (Dimension 3, Risk Rating 1), or outpatient motivational enhancement therapies and active treatment integrated into a mental health setting (Dimension 3, Risk Ratings 2 to 4). |

Dimension 4: Readiness to Change

Risk Rating and Description (NOTE: A higher number indicates a greater level of severity or intensity.)	Types of Services and Modalities Needed	Intensity of Service/ Level of Care/Setting
Risk Rating: 3 = *Substance Use Disorders*: The patient exhibits inconsistent follow-through and shows minimal awareness of his or her substance use disorder and need for treatment. He or she appears unaware of the need to change, and thus is unwilling or only partially able to follow through with treatment recommendations. *Mental Disorders*: The patient exhibits inconsistent follow-through and shows minimal awareness of his or her mental disorder and need for treatment. He or she appears unaware of the need to change, and thus is unwilling or only partially able to follow through with treatment recommendations.	Moderately high-intensity engagement or motivational enhancement strategies are needed to engage the patient in treatment. Effort should be focused on any available systems leverage (family, school, work, or legal system) to align incentives that promote treatment engagement and investment by the patient. If treatment resistance is caused by psychosis, IM injections of a depot antipsychotic may be needed. Assertive case management or assertive community treatment (ACT) may be needed. For patients with a Dimension 3 Risk Rating of 2 to 4, intensive case management or assertive community treatment (ACT) may be required.	**Intensity: 1** = Level I outpatient services for motivational strategies with families and significant others, and/or Level II services for education and engagement strategies and for assertive case management with the patient (if the case management involves more than 9 hours per week). **LOC/Setting:** An outpatient addiction or mental health service, or an outpatient "dual diagnosis" service, with assertive case management or an assertive community treatment (ACT) team. High-intensity residential addiction services are not recommended. Instead, the patient may require outpatient motivational enhancement therapies integrated into ongoing treatment.
Risk Rating: 4a = (No immediate action required.) *Substance Use Disorders:* The patient is unable to follow through, has little or no awareness of substance use problems and any associated negative consequences, knows very little about addiction, and sees no connection between his/her suffering and substance use. He or she is not imminently dangerous or unable to care for self, is not willing to explore change, and is in denial regarding his or her illness and its implications (for example, he or she blames others for legal or family problems, and rejects treatment).	The patient needs high-intensity engagement or motivational strategies to try to engage him or her in treatment. Any available systems leverage (as through family, school, work or the judicial system) should be used to align incentives to promote the patient's engagement and investment in treatment. Preferred strategies involve assertive community treatment rather than intensive therapy aimed at breaking through denial.	**Intensity: 1** = Level I outpatient treatment for motivational strategies with family and significant others and/or Level II.1 services for education and engagement strategies with the patient, if necessary, and for assertive case management (if the case management involves more than 9 hours per week). **LOC/Setting:** An outpatient addiction or mental health service or an outpatient dual diagnosis service with assertive case management or assertive community treatment teams.

Dimension 4: Readiness to Change

Risk Rating and Description (NOTE: A higher number indicates a greater level of severity or intensity.)	Types of Services and Modalities Needed	Intensity of Service/ Level of Care/Setting
Mental Disorders: The patient is unable to follow through, has little or no awareness of a mental disorder and any associated negative consequences, knows very little about mental illness, and sees no connection between his or her suffering and mental health problems. He or she is not imminently dangerous or unable to care for self, is not willing to explore change, and is in denial regarding his or her illness and its implications.		
Risk Rating: 4b = (Immediate action required.) *Substance Use Disorders:* The patient is unable to follow through with treatment recommendations. As a result, his or her behavior represents an imminent danger of harm to self or others, or he or she is unable to function independently and to engage in self-care. For example, the patient repeatedly demonstrates inability to follow through with treatment and continues to use alcohol and/or other drugs and to become violent or suicidal or to drive dangerously. *Mental Disorders:* The patient is unable to follow through with treatment recommendations. As a result, his or her behavior represents an imminent danger of harm to self or others, or he or she is unable to function independently and to engage in self-care. For example, the patient refuses all medications and is overtly psychotic, so that his or her judgment and impulse control is severely impaired.	The patient needs containment for stabilization while imminently dangerous. If treatment resistance is caused by psychosis, involuntary commitment and placement in a secure unit may be necessary. If treatment resistance is caused by severe, acute intoxication, close observation may be needed until the patient is less toxic.	**Intensity: 4** = Level IV medically managed intensive inpatient services, or Level III.3 clinically managed medium-intensity residential services, or Level III.7 medically monitored intensive inpatient services may be required. **LOC/Setting:** A hospital-based acute care unit may be required if a secure unit is needed. The patient also may be placed in a freestanding residential dual diagnosis service or a subacute inpatient psychiatric unit with medical monitoring and integrated addiction services.

Dimension 5: Relapse/Continued Use/ Continued Problem Potential

Risk Rating and Description (NOTE: A higher number indicates a greater level of severity or intensity.)	Types of Services and Modalities Needed	Intensity of Service/ Level of Care/Setting
Risk Rating: 0 = *Substance Use Disorders*: The patient has no potential for further substance use problems, or has low relapse potential and good coping skills. *Mental Disorders*: The patient has no potential for further mental health problems, or has low potential and good coping skills.	No immediate relapse prevention services are needed. The patient may need self/mutual help or a non-professional support group.	**Intensity: 0** = Self/mutual help groups.
Risk Rating: 1 = *Substance Use Disorders*: The patient has minimal relapse potential, with some vulnerability, and has fair self-management and relapse prevention skills. *Mental Disorders*: The patient has minimal relapse potential, with some vulnerability, and has fair self-management and relapse prevention skills.	Low-intensity relapse prevention services are needed to reinforce coping skills until the patient is integrated into continuing care or a self/mutual help or non-professional group. Medication management may be needed (as with anti-craving, opioid maintenance or antipsychotic medications).	**Intensity: 1** = Level I outpatient services. **LOC/Setting:** An outpatient addiction or mental health service. For patients with a Dimension 3 Risk Rating of 2 to 4, these services may be provided in a mental health setting, or addiction treatment may be integrated into continuing care mental health services.
Risk Rating: 2 = *Substance Use Disorders*: The patient has impaired recognition and understanding of substance use relapse issues, but is able to self-manage with prompting. *Mental Disorders*: The patient has impaired recognition and understanding of mental illness relapse issues, but is able to self-manage with prompting.	Moderate-intensity relapse prevention services are needed to monitor and strengthen the patient's coping skills. The patient also needs relapse prevention education and help with integration into self/mutual help and community support groups, assertive case management and assertive community treatment (ACT). Medication management may be needed (as with anti-craving, opioid maintenance or antipsychotic medications).	**Intensity: 2** = Level II.1 intensive outpatient services or Level II.5 partial hospitalization services for clinical care, coupled with Level II assertive case management or assertive community treatment. **LOC/Setting:** An outpatient addiction or mental health service or a partial hospital "dual diagnosis" service, coupled with intensive case management or assertive community treatment.

Dimension 5: Relapse/Continued Use/ Continued Problem Potential

Risk Rating and Description (NOTE: A higher number indicates a greater level of severity or intensity.)	Types of Services and Modalities Needed	Intensity of Service/ Level of Care/Setting
	The patient may need addiction treatment coupled with continuing outpatient mental health and/or addiction care (routine or intensive). For patients with a Dimension 3 Risk Rating of 1 to 2, continuing coordinated and integrated mental health care is required while intensive addiction treatment is provided. For patients with a Dimension 3 Risk Rating of 2 or (especially) 3, intensive case management services may be required to coordinate and integrate addiction treatment into continuing mental health care.	For patients with a Dimension 3 Risk Rating of 2 to 3, higher intensity addiction treatment services may be required (such as Level III residential services), or the patient may need psychiatrically enhanced services or to be integrated into a higher intensity mental health setting. Patients with a combination of addiction and mental impairments may require more intensive services than would either disorder alone.
Risk Rating: 3 = *Substance Use Disorders*: The patient has little recognition and understanding of substance use relapse issues, and has poor skills to cope with and interrupt addiction problems, or to avoid or limit relapse. *Mental Disorders*: The patient has little recognition and understanding of mental illness relapse issues, and has poor skills to cope with and interrupt mental health problems, or to avoid or limit relapse.	Moderately high-intensity relapse prevention services are needed, including structured coping skills training, motivational strategies, and exploration of family and/or significant others' ability to align incentives to consolidate engagement in treatment and possible assistance in finding a supportive living environment. The patient also needs assertive case management and assertive community treatment (ACT). Medication management may be needed (as with anti-craving, opioid maintenance or antipsychotic medications).	**Intensity: 2 or 3** = Level II.5 partial hospitalization services with Level III.1 clinically managed low-intensity residential services, combined with coordinated outpatient mental health or addiction care. **LOC/Setting:** An outpatient addiction or mental health service or a partial hospital "dual diagnosis" service, coupled with a supportive living arrangement. For patients with a Dimension 3 Risk Rating of 2 to 3, these services need to be psychiatrically enhanced or integrated into an intensive mental health setting (such as Level II.5 or Level III.1 residential).

Dimension 5: Relapse/Continued Use/ Continued Problem Potential

Risk Rating and Description (NOTE: A higher number indicates a greater level of severity or intensity.)	Types of Services and Modalities Needed	Intensity of Service/ Level of Care/Setting
	The patient may need addiction treatment coupled with continuing outpatient mental health and/or addiction care (routine or intensive). For patients with a Dimension 3 Risk Rating of 1 to 2, continuing coordinated and integrated addiction treatment and mental health care is required. For patients with a Dimension 3 Risk Rating of 2 to 3 at baseline, assertive community treatment or other intensive case management services may be required.	Patients with a combination of addiction and mental impairments may require more intensive services than would either disorder alone.
Risk Rating: 4a = (No immediate action required.) ***Substance Use Disorders:*** Repeated treatment episodes have had little positive effect on the patient's functioning. He or she has no skills to cope with and interrupt addiction problems, or to prevent or limit relapse. However, the patient is not in imminent danger and is able to care for self (e.g., the patient has undergone repeated detoxifications but is unable to cope with continued cravings to use). ***Mental Disorders:*** Repeated treatment episodes have had little positive effect on the patient's functioning. He or she has no skills to cope with and interrupt mental health problems, or to prevent or limit relapse. However, the patient	Exploration of systems incentives to consolidate the patient's engagement in treatment is required. The patient needs motivational strategies, structured coping skills, assertive case management and community outreach, assistance in finding supportive living arrangements, and assertive community treatment (ACT). Medication management may be needed (as with anti-craving, opioid maintenance or antipsychotic medications). The patient may need addiction treatment coupled with continuing outpatient mental health and/or addiction care (routine or intensive).	**Intensity: 1 to 3** = A range of levels, depending on the degree of danger the patient poses to self or others and his or her stage of readiness to change. These could involve Level I outpatient services for appropriate individual therapy, Level II services for clinical therapies and/or assertive case management and ACT, Level III.1 clinically managed low-intensity residential services, Level III.3 or Level III.5. **LOC/Setting:** An outpatient addiction or mental health service, or an outpatient "dual diagnosis" service, with assertive case management or assertive community treatment (ACT) team, supportive living arrangements, and residential services.

Dimension 5: Relapse/Continued Use/ Continued Problem Potential

Risk Rating and Description (NOTE: A higher number indicates a greater level of severity or intensity.)	Types of Services and Modalities Needed	Intensity of Service/ Level of Care/Setting
is not in imminent danger and is able to care for self (e.g., the patient is severely and persistently mentally ill, with chronic dysfunction and inability to arrest psychotic episodes).	For patients with a Dimension 3 Risk Rating of 2 or higher, coordinated and integrated addiction treatment and mental health case management and/or assertive community treatment may be indicated.	For patients who are ready to change, Level III.1, III.3 or III.5 services may be indicated, with a degree of mental health enhancement that reflects the patient's Dimension 3 Risk Rating. For patients who are at an early stage of readiness to change, continuing outpatient case management (at an intensity that reflects the patient's Dimension 3 Risk Rating) with motivational enhancement therapy is indicated, in a mental health/dual diagnosis outpatient setting or a more intensive mental health setting.
Risk Rating: 4b = (Immediate action required.) *Substance Use Disorders*: The patient has no skills to arrest the addictive disorder, or to prevent relapse to substance use. His or her continued addictive behavior places the patient and/or others in imminent danger (e.g., a patient whose continued drug use leads to impulsive, psychotic and aggressive behaviors).	The patient needs containment for stabilization while imminently dangerous. If the relapse and/or dangerousness is due to psychosis, placement in a secure unit and/or involuntary commitment may be necessary. If continued use is due to severe, acute intoxication, close observation may be needed until the patient is less toxic.	**Intensity: 4** = Level IV medically managed intensive inpatient services (for the patient who needs psychiatric close observation because of dangerous, impulsive behavior), or Level III.3 or III.5 clinically managed residential services (if the patient's degree of impulsivity requires 24-hour structure but not medical or psychiatric close observation).

Dimension 5: Relapse/Continued Use/ Continued Problem Potential

Risk Rating and Description (NOTE: A higher number indicates a greater level of severity or intensity.)	Types of Services and Modalities Needed	Intensity of Service/ Level of Care/Setting
Mental Disorders: The patient has no skills to arrest the mental illness, or to prevent relapse to mental health problems. His or her continued psychiatric disorder places the patient and/or others in imminent danger (e.g., a patient whose depression and feelings of hopelessness cause strong impulses to slash his or her wrists, or who has paranoid delusions with command hallucinations to harm others).	Medication management may be needed (as with anti-craving, opioid maintenance or antipsychotic medications). When the patient is stabilized, a supportive living arrangement will be needed. For patients with a Dimension 3 Risk Rating of 2 or higher at baseline, continuing mental health and addiction treatment with intensive case management also is required.	**LOC/Setting:** A hospital-based acute care unit if a secure setting is needed. If not, a free-standing residential "dual diagnosis" service for stabilization. Once the patient is stabilized, a supervised supportive living arrangement is appropriate.

Dimension 6: Recovery Environment

Risk Rating and Description (NOTE: A higher number indicates a greater level of severity or intensity.)	Types of Services and Modalities Needed	Intensity of Service/ Level of Care/Setting
Risk Rating: 0 = *Substance Use Disorders*: The patient has a supportive environment or is able to cope with poor supports. *Mental Disorders*: The patient has a supportive environment or is able to cope with poor supports.	No immediate supportive living or skills training services are needed.	**Intensity: 0** = Self/mutual help groups allow the patient to access needed addiction or mental health treatment from his or her current living environment. For patients with severe mental impairment, Level III.1 residential support may assist with such access.
Risk Rating: 1 = *Substance Use Disorders*: The patient has passive support or significant others are not interested in his or her addiction recovery, but he or she is not too distracted by this situation and is able to cope. *Mental Disorders*: The patient has passive support or significant others are not interested in an improved mental health environment, but he or she is not too distracted by this situation and is able to cope.	The patient needs assistance in finding a supportive living environment or skills training, vocational training, child care and transportation. For patients with a Dimension 3 Risk Rating of 1 or higher, coordination of mental health and addiction care may support functioning in the current recovery environment.	**Intensity: 1** = Level I outpatient services may allow the patient to live independently while obtaining needed treatment. **LOC/Setting:** An outpatient addiction or mental health service. For patients with severe mental impairment, mental health and case management support may be needed to structure access to and participation in treatment.
Risk Rating: 2 = *Substance Use Disorders*: The patient's environment is not supportive of addiction recovery but, with clinical structure, the patient is able to cope most of the time. *Mental Disorders*: The patient's environment is not supportive of good mental health but, with clinical structure, the patient is able to cope most of the time.	The patient needs assistance in finding a supportive living environment or skills training, vocational training, child care and transportation, assertive case management and assertive community treatment (ACT). The range of services needed depends on the interaction among Dimensions 3, 4 and 5. For example, a stabilized, depressed, alcoholic patient who is ready for recovery and active in self/mutual help groups may need only individual or group counseling once a week, whereas a psychotic patient who is addicted to intravenous cocaine and who is not	**Intensity: 1 to 3** = Level I outpatient services, Level II.1 intensive outpatient services, or Level II.5 partial hospitalization services, coupled with Level III.1 clinically managed low-intensity residential services. **LOC/Setting:** An outpatient addiction or mental health service or a partial hospital "dual diagnosis" service, coupled with a supportive living environment, assertive case management or assertive community treatment (ACT) team visiting the patient in his or her home as needed.

Dimension 6: Recovery Environment

Risk Rating and Description (NOTE: A higher number indicates a greater level of severity or intensity.)	Types of Services and Modalities Needed	Intensity of Service/ Level of Care/Setting
	motivated for recovery and has few skills to cope with craving may need more intensive services.	For patients with a Dimension 3 Risk Rating of 2 to 3, psychiatric enhancement of addiction treatment services may be required. Such a patient also needs continuing mental health support in the living environment. Depending on the patient's Dimension 4 Risk Rating, the mental health supported living environment may be "wet" (continued active substance use is tolerated); "damp" (intoxication or recent use is tolerated); or "dry" (detoxification and abstinence are required). Appropriate case management and motivational enhancement therapies are provided.
Risk Rating: 3 = *Substance Use Disorders*: The patient's environment is not supportive of addiction recovery and he or she finds coping difficult, even with clinical structure. *Mental Disorders*: The patient's environment is not supportive of good mental health and he or she finds coping difficult, even with clinical structure.	The patient needs assertive assistance in finding a supportive living environment or skills training (depending on the patient's coping skills and impulse control), structured vocational rehabilitation, assertive case management and community outreach, and assertive community treatment (ACT). The range of services needed depends on the interaction among Dimensions 3, 4 and 5, as described above.	**Intensity: 2 to 3 =** Level II intensive outpatient services or Level II.5 partial hospitalization services, coupled with Level III.1 clinically managed low-intensity residential services, or equivalent support through case management and community outreach teams. **LOC/Setting:** A halfway house or "dual diagnosis" supportive living group home with assertive case management, or an ACT team visiting the patient in his or her home as needed. For patients with a Dimension 3 Risk Rating of 2 to 3, psychiatric enhancement of addiction treatment services may be required. Such a patient also needs continuing mental health support in the living environment. Depending on the

Dimension 6: Recovery Environment

Risk Rating and Description (NOTE: A higher number indicates a greater level of severity or intensity.)	Types of Services and Modalities Needed	Intensity of Service/ Level of Care/Setting
		patient's Dimension 4 Risk Rating, the mental health supported living environment may be "wet" (continued active substance use is tolerated); "damp" (intoxication or recent use is tolerated); or "dry" (detoxification and abstinence are required). Appropriate case management and motivational enhancement therapies are provided.
Risk Rating: 4a = (No immediate action required.) *Substance Use Disorders*: The patient's environment is not supportive and is chronically hostile and toxic to addiction recovery or treatment progress (e.g., the patient has many drug-using friends, or drugs are readily available in the home environment, or there are chronic lifestyle problems but not acute conditions). The patient is unable to cope with the negative effects of this environment on his or her recovery. *Mental Disorders*: The patient's environment is not supportive and is chronically hostile and toxic to good mental health (e.g., the patient is homeless and unemployed and has chronic lifestyle problems but not acute conditions). The patient is unable to cope with the negative effects of this environment on his or her recovery.	The patient needs highly assertive assistance in finding a supportive living environment or skills training and impulse control services, or need for protection, assertive case management and community outreach, and assertive community treatment (ACT). The range of services needed depends on the interaction among Dimensions 3, 4 and 5, as described above. For example, an alcoholic patient with panic disorder who is motivated for recovery may need Level III.1 services, while a severely and persistently psychotic schizophrenic patient who drinks daily and lives on the street may need more ACT team contact than is available at Level III.1.	**Intensity: 3** = Level III.1 clinically managed low-intensity residential services, or equivalent support through case management and community outreach teams. **LOC/Setting:** A halfway house or "dual diagnosis" supportive living group home with assertive case management, or an ACT team monitoring the patient in his or her home or other living environment through frequent visits. For patients with a Dimension 3 Risk Rating of 2 to 3, psychiatric enhancement of addiction treatment services may be required. Such a patient also needs continuing mental health support in the living environment. Depending on the patient's Dimension 4 Risk Rating, the mental health supported living environment may be "wet" (continued active substance use is tolerated); "damp" (intoxication or recent use is tolerated); or "dry" (detoxification and abstinence are required). Appropriate case management and motivational enhancement therapies are provided.

Dimension 6: Recovery Environment

Risk Rating and Description (NOTE: A higher number indicates a greater level of severity or intensity.)	Types of Services and Modalities Needed	Intensity of Service/ Level of Care/Setting
Risk Rating: 4b = (Immediate action required.) *Substance Use Disorders*: The patient's environment is not supportive and is actively hostile to addiction recovery, posing an immediate threat to the patient's safety and well-being (e.g., the patient lives with a drug dealer who offers drugs daily). *Mental Disorders*: The patient's environment is not supportive or is actively hostile to a safe mental health environment, posing an immediate threat to the patient's safety and well-being (e.g., the patient lives with a physically abuse alcohol partner).	The patient needs immediate separation from a toxic environment and placement in a temporary supportive living environment. The range of services needed depends on the interaction among Dimensions 3, 4 and 5, as described above. For example, a psychotic patient who is not motivated for recovery or an impulsive heroin addict may need a more intensive residential level for safety.	**Intensity: 3** = Level III.1 clinically managed low-intensity residential services or Level III.3 or III.5. **LOC/Setting**: A temporary shelter, halfway house or "dual diagnosis" supportive living group home or residential services. For patients with a Dimension 3 Risk Rating of 2 to 3, psychiatric enhancement of addiction treatment services may be required. Such a patient also needs continuing mental health support in the living environment. Depending on the patient's Dimension 4 Risk Rating, the mental health supported living environment may be "wet" (continued active substance use is tolerated); "damp" (intoxication or recent use is tolerated); or "dry" (detoxification and abstinence are required). Appropriate case management and motivational enhancement therapies are provided.

Appendix B
Experimental Matrix for Matching Multidimensional Risk with Type and Intensity of Service Needs—Adolescent

The Work Group on Adolescent Criteria, in cooperation the Work Group on Co-Occurring Disorders, has developed an experimental approach to help the field move from a program-driven to an assessment-driven Matrix in the placement criteria for adolescents.

Before successfully moving through each developmental stage, the adolescent faces the complex nature of his/her involvement with family, school, work and friends and the need to meet certain social, educational and emotional requirements. Placing adolescents based on a diagnosis alone would not meet the more global biopsychosocial elements, which improve overall treatment outcomes for the adolescent patient.

The "future directions" Matrix seeks to reduce relapse and recidivism by basing placement on a thorough, consistent, biopsychosocial assessment that would provide clinicians a common language specific to adolescents. The severity of the risk ratings can be prioritized and ranked. The level of service is assigned to the highest ranked problem. Through continual monitoring on what is working or not, changes can be made to the treatment interventions to meet the needs of the patient more effectively. The Matrix format accompanies the criteria with "Risk Ratings" that can be matched with the types of services and modalities needed, as well as the intensity of services required and the treatment settings in which such services might appropriately be delivered.

The goal of the Matrix format is to promote improved assessment and treatment of adolescents, many of whom have co-occurring disorders. The Matrix adopts a more holistic, multidimensional approach that matches the adolescent's needs to specific treatment services, rather than to broader levels of care.

As with the Adult Matrix, the Adolescent Matrix is presented as a possible future direction for the field as a potential alternative or supplement to the traditional level of care criteria. As the field experiments with this format, the feedback received will assist in determining the usefulness of this approach in working with adolescents who may or may not have co-occurring mental and substance-related disorders. Because there have not been validity or reliability studies with this matrix, users should understand the piloting, field testing nature of this matrix and provide feedback and guidance accordingly.

For more information on the concepts underlying the Matrix, the rationale for the multidimensional risk profile, the characteristics of the Matrix, risk ratings, risk domains, and how to use the Matrix, see the introduction to the Adult Matrix.

Appendix B
Experimental Matrix for Matching Multidimensional Risk with Type and Intensity of Service Needs—Adolescent

Risk Rating and Description	Types of Services and Modalities Needed	Intensity of Service/ Level of Service/Setting
(Clinical descriptors of Risk Ratings 0 through 4)	*(Indicates which service(s) match the assessed risk rating)*	*(Indicates where the service can most safely and efficiently be delivered)*
Risk Rating: 0 = *Indicates full functioning; no severity; no risk in this dimension.*	*Indicates no need for specific services in this dimension.*	**Intensity: 0** = *Indicates no need for any intensity or level of service in this dimension.*
Risk Rating: 1-4 = *Indicates various levels of functioning and severity and the level of risk in this dimension.* (NOTE: *A higher number indicates a greater level of severity.*)	*Indicates the range of specific services needed in the treatment plan to match the patient's functioning and severity in this dimension.*	**Intensity: 1-4** = *Indicates the intensity or level of service that can deliver the service plan safely and efficiently in this dimension.* (NOTE: *A higher number indicates a greater level of intensity.*)

Dimension 1: Acute Intoxication/Withdrawal Potential
(DSM-IV Dependence Tolerance and Withdrawal Items; Abuse Items)

Risk Rating and Description (NOTE: A higher number indicates a greater level of severity or intensity.)	Types of Services and Modalities Needed	Intensity of Service/ Level of Service/Setting
Risk Rating: 0 = The patient is fully functioning and demonstrates good ability to tolerate and cope with withdrawal discomfort. No signs or symptoms of intoxication or withdrawal are present, or signs or symptoms are resolving.	No immediate intoxication monitoring or detoxification services are needed.	**Intensity: 0** = Does not affect the placement decision.
Risk Rating: 1 = The patient demonstrates adequate ability to tolerate and cope with withdrawal discomfort. Mild to moderate intoxication or signs and symptoms interfere with daily functioning, but do not pose an imminent danger to self or others. There is minimal risk of severe withdrawal (e.g., as a continuation of detoxification at other levels of service, or in the presence of heavy alcohol or sedative-hypnotic use with minimal seizure risk).	Low-intensity intoxication monitoring or detoxification services are needed.	**Intensity: 1** = Level I ambulatory detoxification without extended on-site monitoring. **Setting:** Outpatient primary care, addiction or mental health service.
Risk Rating: 2 = The patient has some difficulty tolerating and coping with withdrawal discomfort. Intoxication may be severe, but responds to support and treatment sufficiently that the patient does not pose an imminent danger to self or others. There are moderate signs and symptoms, with moderate risk of severe withdrawal (e.g., as a continuation of detoxification at other levels of service, or in the presence of heavy alcohol or sedative-hypnotic use with minimal seizure risk, or in the presence of many signs and symptoms of opiate or stimulant withdrawal, such as lethargy, agitation or depression).	Moderate-intensity intoxication monitoring or detoxification services are needed.	**Intensity: 2** = Level II.5 ambulatory detoxification with extended on-site monitoring. **Setting:** Outpatient primary care, addiction or mental health service.
Risk Rating: 3 = The patient demonstrates poor ability to tolerate and cope with withdrawal discomfort. Severe signs and symptoms of intoxication indicate that the patient may pose an imminent danger to self or others, and intoxication has not abated at less intensive levels of care. There are severe signs and symptoms or	Moderately high-intensity intoxication monitoring or detoxification services are needed. Nursing and medical monitoring may be needed for more severe withdrawal.	**Intensity: 3** = Level III.5 clinically managed residential detoxification or Level III.7 medically monitored inpatient detoxification.

Dimension 1: Acute Intoxication/Withdrawal Potential
(DSM-IV Dependence Tolerance and Withdrawal Items; Abuse Items)

Risk Rating and Description (NOTE: A higher number indicates a greater level of severity or intensity.)	Types of Services and Modalities Needed	Intensity of Service/ Level of Service/Setting
risk of severe but manageable withdrawal, or withdrawal is worsening despite detoxification at a less intensive level of care (e.g., as a continuation of detoxification at other levels of service, or in the presence of opiate withdrawal with cravings and impulsive behaviors). The patient may need opiate substitution therapy with titration.		**Setting:** General, addiction or mental health facility.
Risk Rating: 4 = The patient is incapacitated, with severe signs and symptoms. Severe withdrawal poses danger (e.g., seizures). Continued use poses an imminent threat to life (as through liver failure, a GI bleed, or fetal death). Drug overdose or intoxication has compromised the patient's mental status, cardiac function or other vital signs or functions.	High-intensity intoxication monitoring or detoxification services are needed, with monitoring and management more often than hourly.	**Intensity: 4** = Level IV medically managed intensive inpatient detoxification. **Setting:** General, addiction or mental health acute inpatient unit.

Dimension 2: Biomedical Conditions and Complications
(DSM-IV Axis III)

Risk Rating and Description (NOTE: A higher number indicates a greater level of severity or intensity.)	Types of Services and Modalities Needed	Intensity of Service/ Level of Service/Setting
Risk Rating: 0 = The patient is fully functioning and demonstrates good ability to cope with physical discomfort. No biomedical signs or symptoms are present, or biomedical problems are stable (e.g., stable asthma or stable juvenile arthritis).	No immediate biomedical services (except for long-term monitoring) are needed.	**Intensity: 0** = Does not affect the placement decision.
Risk Rating: 1 = The patient demonstrates adequate ability to tolerate and cope with physical discomfort. Mild to moderate signs or symptoms (such as mild to moderate pain) interfere with daily functioning.	Low-intensity biomedical services are needed, including case management to ensure further biomedical evaluation and treatment as part of a treatment plan.	**Intensity: 1** = Level I outpatient services. **Setting:** Outpatient primary care, addiction or mental health service
Risk Rating: 2 = The patient has some difficulty tolerating and coping with physical problems and/or has other biomedical problems that may interfere with recovery and mental health treatment. The patient neglects to care for serious biomedical problems. Moderately severe biomedical conditions and problems (which require non-urgent attention) are active, but manageable with easily accessible off-site care.	Moderate-intensity biomedical services are needed, including case management to ensure further biomedical evaluation and treatment as part of a treatment plan.	**Intensity: 2** = Level II.1 intensive outpatient or II.5 partial hospitalization services. **Setting:** Outpatient primary care, addiction or mental health service.
Risk Rating: 3 = The patient demonstrates poor ability to tolerate and cope with physical problems, or the patient's general health condition is poor. The patient has serious medical problems, which he or she neglects during outpatient or intensive outpatient treatment. Such problems are stable (e.g., asthma or diabetes is complicated or the patient is on a new treatment regimen).	Moderately high-intensity biomedical services are needed, including medical and nursing monitoring to ensure stabilization.	**Intensity: 3** = Level III.7 medically monitored inpatient services. **Setting:** General, addiction or mental health facility

Dimension 2: Biomedical Conditions and Complications
(DSM-IV Axis III)

Risk Rating and Description *(NOTE: A higher number indicates a greater level of severity or intensity.)*	Types of Services and Modalities Needed	Intensity of Service/ Level of Service/Setting
Risk Rating: 4 = The patient is incapacitated, with severe medical problems (e.g., extreme pain, uncontrolled diabetes, GI bleeding, or infection requiring IV antibiotics).	High-intensity biomedical services are needed for stabilization and medication management, including medical and nursing close observation and 24-hour management.	**Intensity: 4** = Level IV medically managed intensive inpatient services. **Setting:** General, addiction or mental health acute inpatient unit.

Dimension 3: Emotional/Behavioral/ Cognitive Conditions and Complications
(DSM-IV Dependence Impairment Items; Abuse Items; Axes IV and V)

Risk Rating and Description, by Risk Domains (a) (NOTE: A higher number indicates a greater level of severity or intensity and individuals need not match descriptions in all of the subdomains within any one risk category)	Types of Services and Modalities Needed (b)	Intensity of Service/ Level of Service/ Setting (c)
Risk Rating: 0 = *Dangerousness/Lethality:* The patient has good impulse control and coping skills. *Interference with Addiction Recovery Efforts:* The patient is able to focus on recovery, identify appropriate supports and reach out for help. *Social Functioning:* The patient is fully functioning in relationships with significant others, school, work, and friends. *Ability for Self-Care:* The patient is fully functioning, with good personal resources and skills to cope with emotional problems. *Course of Illness:* The patient has no emotional or behavioral problems, or any problems identified are stable (e.g., attention deficit hyperactivity disorder is stable and managed with medication). There is no recent serious or high-risk vulnerability.	No immediate mental health services are needed.	**Intensity: 0** = Does not affect the placement decision.
Risk Rating: 1 = *Dangerousness/Lethality:* The patient has adequate impulse control and coping skills to deal with any thoughts of harm to self or others. *Interference with Addiction Recovery Efforts:* The patient's emotional concerns relate to negative consequences and effects of addiction. He or she is able to view these as part of addiction and recovery. *Social Functioning:* The patient's relationships or spheres of social functioning (significant others, friends, school, work) are being impaired but not endangered by patient's substance use (for example, there is no imminent risk of expulsion from school or loss of job). The patient is able to meet personal responsibilities and maintain stable meaningful relationships despite the	Low-intensity mental health services are needed, including case management to coordinate addiction and mental health care, medication monitoring, psychoeducation about mental disorders and psychotropic medications, and self/mutual help support groups to deal with emotional aspects of recovery.	**Intensity: 1** = Level I outpatient services. **Setting:** Outpatient primary care, addiction or mental health service that incorporates specific services for "dual diagnosis" patients; addiction treatment services with psychiatric consultation/liaison; mental health care with addiction consultation/liaison.

Dimension 3: Emotional/Behavioral/ Cognitive Conditions and Complications
(DSM-IV Dependence Impairment Items; Abuse Items; Axes IV and V)

Risk Rating and Description, by Risk Domains (a)	Types of Services and Modalities Needed (b)	Intensity of Service/ Level of Service/ Setting (c)
(NOTE: A higher number indicates a greater level of severity or intensity and individuals need not match descriptions in all of the subdomains within any one risk category)		
mild symptoms experienced (e.g., mood or anxiety symptoms are subthreshold for *DSM-IV* diagnosis or, if they meet diagnostic criteria, the patient is able to continue in essential roles). *Ability for Self-Care:* The patient has adequate resources and skills to cope with emotional or behavioral problems. *Course of Illness:* The patient has mild to moderate signs and symptoms (e.g., dysphoria, relationship problems, work or school problems, or problems coping in the community), with good response to treatment in the past. Any past serious problems have a relatively long period of stability (e.g., serious depression and suicidal behavior four years ago) or past problems are chronic but not severe enough to pose any high-risk vulnerability (e.g., superficial wrist scratching, but no previous hospitalization or life-threatening behavior in a patient who has been able to contract for safety).		
Risk Rating: 2 = *Dangerousness/Lethality:* The patient has suicidal ideation or violent impulses (but without active behaviors or intent), which require more than routine outpatient monitoring. *Interference with Addiction Recovery Efforts:* The patient's emotional, behavioral or cognitive problems (e.g., memory problems associated with marijuana use) distract from recovery efforts. *Social Functioning:* The patient's relationships or spheres of social functioning (significant others, friends, school, work) are being impaired by substance use, and	Moderate-intensity mental health services are needed, including case management to ensure monitoring and evaluation of emotional, behavioral, and cognitive status as part of the treatment plan. Medication management and monitoring, and medical and nursing monitoring and management as needed.	**Intensity:** 2 = Level II.1 intensive outpatient or Level II.5 partial hospitalization services. **Setting:** Intensive mental health treatment with integrated addiction services, or "dual diagnosis" intensive outpatient services. Partial hospitalization mental health treatment with integrated

Dimension 3: Emotional/Behavioral/Cognitive Conditions and Complications
(DSM-IV Dependence Impairment Items; Abuse Items; Axes IV and V)

Risk Rating and Description, by Risk Domains (a) (NOTE: A higher number indicates a greater level of severity or intensity and individuals need not match descriptions in all of the subdomains within any one risk category)	Types of Services and Modalities Needed (b)	Intensity of Service/ Level of Service/ Setting (c)
may be linked to a psychiatric disorder (for example, a patient with depression or anxiety disorder is unable to sleep or socialize). Symptoms are causing moderate difficulty in managing relationships with significant others, social, work or school functioning, or coping in the community, but not to a degree that they pose a significant danger to self or others or cause the patient to be unable to manage activities of daily living or basic responsibilities in the home, work, school, or community. *Ability for Self-Care:* The patient has poor personal resources, with moderate or minimal skills to cope with emotional or behavioral problems. *Course of Illness:* The patient has frequent and/or intense symptoms (for example, frequent outbursts of disruptive behavior, suicidal or homicidal ideation with ability to contract for safety, vegetative signs, agitation or retardation, or inconsistent impulse control), with a history that indicates significant problems that are not well-stabilized (e.g., psychotic episodes with periods of decompensation). Acute problems pose some risk of harm to self or others, but the patient is not imminently dangerous (e.g., hallucinations and delusions invoke homicidal ideation, but the patient has no plan or means to harm others).	Parents or guardians must be willing and able to supervise the adolescent while at home during treatment	addiction services, or "dual diagnosis" partial hospitalization services. If problems in social functioning are causing severe impairment (e.g., inability to attend school due to depression, or trouble with the law for the first time, or school suspension or failure), the patient should be treated at a more intensive Level II.5. Occasional symptoms can be treated at Level II.1. Frequent and intensive symptoms should be treated at Level II.5
Risk Rating: 3 = *Dangerousness/Lethality:* The patient has frequent impulses to harm self or others, which are potentially destabilizing or chronic. However, the patient is not imminently dangerous in a 24-hour setting. For example, the patient has frequent suicidal ideation, but no plan and can contract for safety at Level III.5.	Moderately high-intensity mental health services are needed, including daily monitoring and ready access to medical management, and medication management if symptoms become acute but not dangerous.	**Intensity: 3** = Level III.5 clinically managed residential services or Level III.7 medically monitored inpatient services.

ASAM Patient Placement Criteria, Second Edition–Revised

Dimension 3: Emotional/Behavioral/ Cognitive Conditions and Complications
(DSM-IV Dependence Impairment Items; Abuse Items; Axes IV and V)

Risk Rating and Description, by Risk Domains (a) (NOTE: A higher number indicates a greater level of severity or intensity and individuals need not match descriptions in all of the subdomains within any one risk category)	Types of Services and Modalities Needed (b)	Intensity of Service/ Level of Service/ Setting (c)
The patient is no longer experiencing command hallucinations, is responding to medication but needs further stabilization at Level III.7. ***Interference with Addiction Recovery Efforts:*** Recovery efforts are negatively affected by the patient's emotional, behavioral or cognitive problems in significant and distracting ways, up to and including inability to focus on recovery. ***Social Functioning:*** The patient has significant functional impairment, with severe symptoms (e.g., disorganized thinking, depression with significant vegetative signs, agitation or retardation, and poor impulse control). Such symptoms seriously impair the patient's ability to function in family, social, work, or school settings, and cannot be managed at a less intensive level of service, or (in chronic populations) to function in shelters, homeless and other community situations (for example, an adolescent has had multiple attempts at property damage when unsupervised, has personality traits that are not severe but do require consistent boundary setting, or has a history of runaway behavior that requires 24-hour structured environment at Level III.5). ***Ability for Self-Care:*** The patient has insufficient or severe lack of capacity to cope with emotional or behavioral problems. His or her uncontrolled behavior, confusion or disorientation limit the patient's capacity for self-care, leading to inadequate ability to manage the activities of daily living. ***Course of Illness:*** Acute course of illness dominates the clinical presentation, with symptoms involving impaired reality testing, communication, thought processes, judgment, or attention to personal hygiene, which significantly compromise the patient's ability to adjust to life in the community. Alternatively,	Discharge planning for intensive case management and community outreach are needed for the severely and persistently mentally ill patient. Supportive living arrangements are needed, with 24-hour supervision.	**Setting:** Freestanding residential "dual diagnosis" service; subacute residential psychiatric unit with medical monitoring and integrated addiction services. If the adolescent is at risk for elopement, a locked unit may be necessary. If the adolescent has mild but stable emotional or behavioral problems but requires a less structured 24-hour environment, a Level III.1 setting may be used for placement (e.g., a homeless youth for whom monitoring of medications or assessment of psychiatric symptoms and behavior management can be provided through a concurrent Level I or II service).

Dimension 3: Emotional/Behavioral/Cognitive Conditions and Complications
(DSM-IV Dependence Impairment Items; Abuse Items; Axes IV and V)

Risk Rating and Description, by Risk Domains (a) *(NOTE: A higher number indicates a greater level of severity or intensity and individuals need not match descriptions in all of the subdomains within any one risk category)*	Types of Services and Modalities Needed (b)	Intensity of Service/ Level of Service/ Setting (c)
interventions at previous treatment levels have not achieved stabilization or complete remission of symptoms. Patient has limited ability to follow through with treatment recommendations, thus demonstrating risk of and vulnerability to dangerous consequences.		
Risk Rating: 4 = *Dangerousness/Lethality:* Severe psychotic, mood or personality disorders present acute risk to the patient, such as immediate risk of suicide, psychosis with unpredictable, disorganized or violent behavior, or gross neglect of self-care. *Interference with Addiction Recovery Efforts:* The patient is unable to focus on addiction recovery due to severe overwhelming mental health problems or regression and psychiatric symptoms due to continued alcohol or other drug use. *Social Functioning:* The patient is unable to cope with family, school, friends or work due to overwhelming mental health problems (such as a thought disorder of acute onset that places self and others at risk). Or the patient is manic and exchanges sex for drugs, or the patient engages in unsafe, sexually promiscuous behavior and is unable to stop the behavior. Symptoms indicate that the patient is at risk of harming self or others, or has a seriously impaired ability to function in family, school, social or work settings. *Ability for Self-Care:* The patient has developed a life-threatening condition that requires medical management (such as a severe eating disorder with significant malnutrition).	High-intensity mental health services are needed, including 24-hour medical and nursing monitoring and management, medication management, secure services, and close observation more often than hourly.	**Intensity:** 4 = Level IV medically managed intensive inpatient services. **Setting:** Psychiatric acute inpatient unit.

Dimension 3: Emotional/Behavioral/ Cognitive Conditions and Complications
(DSM-IV Dependence Impairment Items; Abuse Items; Axes IV and V)

Risk Rating and Description, by Risk Domains (a) (NOTE: A higher number indicates a greater level of severity or intensity and individuals need not match descriptions in all of the subdomains within any one risk category)	Types of Services and Modalities Needed (b)	Intensity of Service/ Level of Service/ Setting (c)
Course of Illness: The patient is at high risk, with significant vulnerability to dangerous consequences. He or she exhibits severe and acute life-threatening symptoms (for example, dangerous or impulsive behavior or cognitive functioning) that pose imminent danger to self or others. These might include symptoms of psychosis include command hallucinations or paranoid delusions. The patient's history of instability is such that high-intensity services are needed to prevent dangerous consequences (e.g., the patient is not responding to daily changes in medication at less intensive levels of service, with escalating psychosis).		

NOTES:

(a) Consider dangerousness/lethality, interference with addiction recovery efforts, social functioning, capacity for self-care, and course of illness (history of presenting illness—the pattern of symptoms and response to treatment up to, and including, the present illness—and the pattern of treatment response).

(b) Consider acute stabilization, medical management and monitoring, mental health consultation and integration of mental health and addiction services, skills training, multidimensional therapy (MDT), multisystemic therapy (MST), intensive in home outreach, assertive community outreach services; or other approaches to case management that highly coordinate intensive therapies across multiple systems; medication management and monitoring, and systems intervention and coordination.

(c) Consider traditional addiction and mental health services, as well as availability of addiction services coordinated with mental health services or mental health services coordinated with addiction treatment, integrated inpatient or outpatient "dual diagnosis" services.

Dimension 4: Readiness to Change

Risk Rating and Description (NOTE: A higher number indicates a greater level of severity or intensity.)	Types of Services and Modalities Needed	Intensity of Service/ Level of Care/Setting
Risk Rating: 0 = *Substance Use Disorders*: The patient is engaged in treatment as a proactive, responsible participant, and is committed to change his or her alcohol and/or other drug use. *Mental Disorders*: The patient is engaged in treatment as a proactive, responsible participant, and is committed to change his or her mental functioning and behavior.	No immediate engagement or motivational enhancement strategies or services are needed.	**Intensity: 0 =** Self/mutual help groups support referral into an appropriate addiction treatment service, depending on Risk Ratings in the other dimensions. For dual diagnosis patients with a Dimension 3 Risk Rating of 2 or higher at baseline, active addiction treatment may be integrated into a mental health setting, according to the intensity of service required by the patient's Risk Ratings in Dimensions 5 and 6.
Risk Rating: 1 = *Substance Use Disorders*: The patient is willing to enter treatment and to explore strategies for changing his or her substance use, but is ambivalent about the need for change. He or she is willing to explore the need for treatment and strategies to reduce or stop substance use (e.g., the patient views his or her substance use problem as caused by depression or another psychiatric diagnosis). Or the patient is willing to change his or her substance use, but believes it will not be difficult to do so, or will not accept full recovery treatment plans. *Mental Disorders*: The patient is willing to enter treatment and to explore strategies for changing his or her mental functioning, but is ambivalent about the need for change. He or she is willing to explore the need for treatment and strategies to deal with mental disorders. The patient's participation in mental health treatment is sufficient to avert mental decompensation (e.g., an adolescent who has attention deficit hyperactivity disorder is ambivalent about taking psychotropic medications, but generally follows through with treatment recommendations).	In any addiction or dual diagnosis setting, low-intensity engagement or motivational strategies are needed. These include education about the illness(es), education of family and significant others, and reinforcement of the need for treatment by the legal, work or school systems. For patients with impairment in Dimension 3, motivational enhancement is integrated into continuing care management at any degree of intensity, as well as into specific treatment episodes.	**Intensity: 1 =** Level I outpatient services for motivational enhancement strategies. **Setting:** An outpatient addiction or mental health service.

Dimension 4: Readiness to Change

Risk Rating and Description (NOTE: A higher number indicates a greater level of severity or intensity.)	Types of Services and Modalities Needed	Intensity of Service/ Level of Care/Setting
Risk Rating: 2 = *Substance Use Disorders*: The patient is reluctant to agree to treatment for substance use problems. He or she is able to articulate the negative consequences of substance use, but has a low level of commitment to change his or her use of alcohol or other drugs. The patient is assessed as having minimal readiness to change and is only passively involved in treatment, and is variably compliant with attendance at outpatient sessions or meetings of self/mutual help or other support groups. *Mental Disorders*: The patient is reluctant to agree to treatment for mental disorders. He or she is able to articulate the negative consequences of his or her mental health problems, but has low commitment to treatment. The patient is assessed as having minimal readiness to change and is only passively involved in treatment (e.g., the patient is variable in follow through with use of psychotropic medications or attendance at therapy sessions).	Moderate-intensity engagement or motivational strategies are needed, with active support from family, significant others, legal, work or school systems to set and follow through with clear, consistent limits and consequences. Multidimensional therapy (MDT), multisystemic therapy (MST), intensive in home outreach, assertive community outreach services; or other approaches to case management that highly coordinate intensive therapies across multiple systems may be needed. For patients who face legal consequences, court-mandated treatment (as through drug court) may be indicated. For patients with Dimension 3 baseline Risk Ratings of 2 or higher, intensive case management may be required to integrate motivational enhancement therapies and continuing mental health care.	**Intensity:** 1-2 = Level I outpatient services for motivational enhancement strategies, coupled with Level II services for assertive case management if the case management involves more than 6 hours per week. **Setting:** An outpatient addiction or mental health service. High-intensity residential addiction services are not recommended, unless appropriate legal consequences promote patient motivation. The patient may require outpatient motivational enhancement therapies in an addiction or mental health treatment setting, with coordinated mental health care (Dimension 3, Risk Rating 1), or outpatient motivational enhancement therapies and active treatment integrated into a mental health setting (Dimension 3, Risk Ratings 2 to 3).
Risk Rating: 3 = *Substance Use Disorders*: The patient exhibits inconsistent follow through and shows minimal awareness of his or her substance use disorder and need for treatment. He or she appears unaware of the need to change, and is unwilling or only partially able to follow through with treatment recommendations.	Moderately high-intensity engagement or motivational enhancement strategies are needed to engage the patient in treatment. Effort should be focused on any available systems leverage (family,	**Intensity:** 1-2 = Level I outpatient services for motivational strategies with families and significant others, and/or Level II services for education and engagement strategies and for

Dimension 4: Readiness to Change

Risk Rating and Description *(NOTE: A higher number indicates a greater level of severity or intensity.)*	Types of Services and Modalities Needed	Intensity of Service/ Level of Care/Setting
Mental Disorders: The patient exhibits inconsistent follow through and shows minimal awareness of his or her mental disorder and need for treatment. He or she appears unaware of the need to change, and thus is unwilling or only partially able to follow through with treatment recommendations.	If treatment reluctance is directly related to refractory ADHD or social anxiety disorder, multidimensional therapy (MDT), multisystemic therapy (MST), intensive in home outreach, assertive community outreach services; or other approaches to case management that highly coordinate intensive therapies across multiple systems may be needed. For patients with a Dimension 3 Risk Rating of 2 to 3, the following may be needed: increased medical management, multidimensional therapy (MDT), multisystemic therapy (MST), intensive in home outreach, assertive community outreach services; or other approaches to case management that highly coordinate intensive therapies across multiple systems	multidimensional therapy (MDT), multisystemic therapy (MST), intensive in home outreach, assertive community outreach services; or other approaches to case management that highly coordinate intensive therapies across multiple systems may be needed (if these services involve more than six hours per week). **Setting:** An outpatient addiction or mental health service, or an outpatient "dual diagnosis" service For the adolescent who is placed at a more intensive level of care based on Dimension 3 risk factors, the patient may require outpatient motivational enhancement therapies integrated into ongoing treatment.
4a (No immediate action required.) *Substance Use Disorders:* The patient is unable to follow through, has little or no awareness of substance use problems and any associated negative consequences, knows very little about addiction, and sees no connection between his/her suffering and	High-intensity of engagement or motivational strategies to try to engage the patient as a participant in treatment. Work with any systems leverage available (family, school, work, school, work, or legal system) to align incentives that promote treatment engagement and investment by the patient.	**Intensity:** 1-2 = Level I, Outpatient Services for motivational strategies with family and significant others; and/or Level II.1 services for education and engagement

Dimension 4: Readiness to Change

Risk Rating and Description (NOTE: A higher number indicates a greater level of severity or intensity.)	Types of Services and Modalities Needed	Intensity of Service/ Level of Care/Setting
substance use. He or she is not imminently dangerous or unable to care for self, is not willing to explore change, and is in denial regarding his or her illness and its implications (for example, he or she blames others for legal or family problems, and rejects treatment). *Mental Disorders:* The patient is unable to follow through, has little or no awareness of a mental disorder and any associated negative consequences, knows very little about mental illness, and sees no connection between his or her suffering and mental health problems. He or she is not imminently dangerous or unable to care for self, is not willing to explore change, and is in denial regarding his or her illness and its implications.	legal) to align incentives that promote treatment engagement and investment of patient. Any engagement and motivational strategies are practical multidimensional therapy or multisystemic interventions to develop leverage, rather than intensive therapy techniques aimed at breaking through denial.	strategies with the patient if necessary, and for multidimensional therapy (MDT), multisystemic therapy (MST), intensive in home outreach, assertive community outreach services; or other approaches to case management that highly coordinate intensive therapies across multiple systems may be needed (if these services involve more than six hours per week). **Setting:** Outpatient addiction or mental health service; outpatient dual diagnosis service
Risk Rating: 4b = (Immediate action required.) *Substance Use Disorders:* The patient is unable to follow through with treatment recommendations. As a result, his or her behavior represents an imminent danger of harm to self or others, or he or she is unable to function independently and to engage in self-care. For example, the patient repeatedly demonstrates inability to follow through with treatment and continues to use alcohol and/or other drugs and to become violent or suicidal or to act impulsively in runaway behavior. *Mental Disorders:* The patient is unable to follow through with treatment recommendations. As a result, his or her behavior poses an imminent danger of harm to self or others, or he or she is unable to function independently and to engage in self-care. For example, the patient refuses all medications and is overtly psychotic, so that his or her judgment and impulse control is severely impaired.	The patient needs containment for stabilization while imminently dangerous. If treatment resistance is caused by psychosis, involuntary commitment and placement in a secure unit may be necessary. If treatment resistance is caused by severe, acute intoxication, close observation may be needed until the patient is less toxic.	**Intensity:** 4 = Level IV medically managed intensive inpatient services, or Level III.5 clinically managed high-intensity residential services, or Level III.7 medically monitored intensive inpatient services may be required. **Setting:** A hospital-based acute care unit may be required if a secure unit is needed. The patient also may be placed in a freestanding residential dual diagnosis service or a subacute inpatient psychiatric unit with medical monitoring and integrated addiction services.

Adolescent Dimension 5: Relapse/Continued Use/Continued Problem Potential

Risk Rating and Description (NOTE: A higher number indicates a greater level of severity or intensity.)	Types of Services and Modalities Needed	Intensity of Service/Level of Care/Setting
Risk Rating: 0 = *Substance Use Disorders*: The patient has no potential for further substance use problems, or is at minimal risk of relapse and good coping skills. *Mental Disorders*: The patient is not at risk of further mental health problems, or has low risk and good coping skills.	No immediate relapse prevention services are needed. The patient may need self/mutual help or a non-professional support group.	**Intensity: 0** = Self/mutual help groups.
Risk Rating: 1 = *Substance Use Disorders*: The patient has minimal relapse potential, with some vulnerability, and has fair self-management and relapse prevention skills. *Mental Disorders*: The patient has minimal relapse potential, with some vulnerability, and has fair self-management and relapse prevention skills.	Low-intensity relapse prevention services are needed to reinforce coping skills until the patient is integrated into continuing care or a self/mutual help or non-professional group.	**Intensity: 1** = Level I outpatient services. **Setting:** An outpatient addiction or mental health service. For patients with a Dimension 3 Risk Rating of 2 to 4, these services may be provided in a mental health setting, or addiction treatment may be integrated into continuing care mental health services.
Risk Rating: 2 = *Substance Use Disorders*: The patient has impaired recognition and understanding of substance use relapse issues, but is able to self-manage with prompting. *Mental Disorders*: The patient has impaired recognition and understanding of mental illness relapse issues, but is able to self-manage with prompting.	Moderate-intensity relapse prevention services are needed to monitor and strengthen the patient's coping skills. The patient also needs relapse prevention education and help with integration into self/mutual help and community support groups, multidimensional therapy (MDT), multisystemic therapy (MST), intensive in home outreach, assertive community outreach services; or other approaches to case management	**Intensity: 2** = Level II.1 intensive outpatient services or Level II.5 partial hospitalization services for clinical care, coupled with multidimensional therapy (MDT), multisystemic therapy (MST), intensive in home outreach, assertive community outreach services; or other approaches to case management that highly coordinate intensive therapies across multiple systems

Adolescent Dimension 5: Relapse/Continued Use/ Continued Problem Potential

Risk Rating and Description *(NOTE: A higher number indicates a greater level of severity or intensity.)*	Types of Services and Modalities Needed	Intensity of Service/ Level of Care/Setting
	that highly coordinate intensive therapies across multiple systems Medication management may be needed (as with anti-craving, antidepressants, mood stabilizers or antipsychotic medications). The patient may need addiction treatment coupled with continuing outpatient mental health and/or addiction care (routine or intensive). For patients with a Dimension 3 Risk Rating of 1 to 2, continuing coordinated and integrated mental health care is required while intensive addiction treatment is provided. For patients with a Dimension 3 Risk Rating of 2 or (especially) 3, intensive case management services may be required to coordinate and integrate addiction treatment into continuing mental health care.	**Setting:** An outpatient addiction or mental health service or a partial hospital "dual diagnosis" service, coupled with multidimensional therapy (MDT), multisystemic therapy (MST), intensive in home outreach, assertive community outreach services; or other approaches to case management that highly coordinate intensive therapies across multiple systems. For patients with a Dimension 3 Risk Rating of 2 to 3, higher intensity addiction treatment services may be required (such as Level III residential services), or the patient may need psychiatrically enhanced services or to be integrated into a higher intensity mental health setting. Patients with a combination of addiction and mental impairments may require more intensive services than would either disorder alone.
Risk Rating: 3 = *Substance Use Disorders:* The patient has little recognition and understanding of substance use relapse issues, and has poor skills to cope with and interrupt addiction problems, or to avoid or limit relapse.	Moderately high-intensity relapse prevention services are needed, including structured coping skills training, motivational strategies, and	**Intensity: 2 or 3** = Level II.5 partial hospitalization services with Level III.1 clinically managed low-intensity residential services, combined

Adolescent Dimension 5: Relapse/Continued Use/ Continued Problem Potential

Risk Rating and Description (NOTE: A higher number indicates a greater level of severity or intensity.)	Types of Services and Modalities Needed	Intensity of Service/ Level of Care/Setting
Mental Disorders: The patient has little recognition and understanding of mental illness relapse issues, and has poor skills to cope with and interrupt mental health problems, or to avoid or limit relapse.	exploration of family and/or significant others' ability to align incentives to consolidate engagement in treatment and possible assistance in finding a supportive living environment. The patient also may need multidimensional therapy (MDT), multisystemic therapy (MST), intensive in home outreach, assertive community outreach services, or other approaches to case management that tightly coordinate intensive therapies across multiple systems. Medication management may be needed (as with anti-craving, antidepressants, mood stabilizer or antipsychotic medications). The patient may need addiction treatment coupled with continuing outpatient mental health and/or addiction care (routine or intensive). For patients with a Dimension 3 Risk Rating of 1 to 2, continuing coordinated and integrated addiction treatment and mental health care is required.	with coordinated outpatient mental health or addiction care. **Setting:** An outpatient addiction or mental health service or a partial hospital "dual diagnosis" service, coupled with a supportive living arrangement. For patients with a Dimension 3 Risk Rating of 2 to 3, these services need to be psychiatrically enhanced or integrated into an intensive mental health setting (such as Level II.5 or Level III.1 residential). Patients with a combination of addiction and mental impairments may require more intensive services than would either disorder alone.

Adolescent Dimension 5: Relapse/Continued Use/ Continued Problem Potential

Risk Rating and Description (NOTE: A higher number indicates a greater level of severity or intensity.)	Types of Services and Modalities Needed	Intensity of Service/ Level of Care/Setting
	For patients with a Dimension 3 Risk Rating of 2 to 3 at baseline multidimensional therapy (MDT), multisystemic therapy (MST), intensive in home outreach, assertive community outreach services; or other approaches to case management that highly coordinate intensive therapies across multiple systems may be required.	
Risk Rating: 4a = (No immediate action required.) *Substance Use Disorders*: Repeated treatment episodes have had little positive effect on the patient's functioning. He or she has no skills to cope with and interrupt addiction problems, or to prevent or limit relapse (for example, the patient has undergone repeated episodes of addiction treatment, but is unable to cope with continued cravings to use). However, the patient is not in imminent danger and is able to care for self. *Mental Disorders*: Repeated treatment episodes have had little positive effect on the patient's functioning. He or she has no skills to cope with and interrupt mental health problems, or to prevent or limit relapse (for example, the patient is severely and persistently mentally ill, with chronic dysfunction and inability to arrest psychotic episodes). However, the patient is not in imminent danger and is able to care for self.	Exploration of systems incentives to consolidate the patient's engagement in treatment is required. The patient needs motivational strategies, structured coping skills, assistance in finding supportive living arrangements, multidimensional therapy (MDT), multisystemic therapy (MST), intensive in home outreach, assertive community outreach services; or other approaches to case management that highly coordinate intensive therapies across multiple systems. Medication management may be needed (as with anti-craving, antidepressants, mood stabilizers or antipsychotic medications).	**Intensity: 1 to 3** = A range of levels, depending on the degree of danger the patient poses to self or others and his or her stage of readiness to change. These could involve Level I outpatient services for appropriate individual therapy, Level II services for clinical therapies and/or multidimensional therapy (MDT), multisystemic therapy (MST), intensive in home outreach, assertive community outreach services; or other approaches to case management that highly coordinate intensive therapies across multiple systems. Level III.1 clinically managed low-intensity residential services, or Level III.5.

Adolescent Dimension 5: Relapse/Continued Use/ Continued Problem Potential

Risk Rating and Description *(NOTE: A higher number indicates a greater level of severity or intensity.)*	Types of Services and Modalities Needed	Intensity of Service/ Level of Care/Setting
	The patient may need addiction treatment coupled with continuing outpatient mental health and/or addiction care (routine or intensive). For patients with a Dimension 3 Risk Rating of 2 or higher, coordinated and integrated addiction treatment and mental health case management and/or multidimensional therapy (MDT), multisystemic therapy (MST), intensive in home outreach, assertive community outreach services; or other approaches to case management that highly coordinate intensive therapies across multiple systems may be indicated.	**Setting:** An outpatient addiction or mental health service, or an outpatient dual diagnosis service, with multidimensional therapy (MDT), multisystemic therapy (MST), intensive in home outreach, assertive community outreach services; or other approaches to case management that highly coordinate intensive therapies across multiple systems, supportive living arrangements, and residential services. For patients who are ready to change, Level III.1, or III.5 services may be indicated, with a degree of mental health enhancement that reflects the patient's Dimension 3 Risk Rating. For patients who are at an early stage of readiness to change, continuing outpatient case management (at an intensity that reflects the patient's Dimension 3 Risk Rating) with motivational enhancement therapy is indicated, in a mental health/dual diagnosis outpatient setting or a more intensive mental health setting.

Adolescent Dimension 5: Relapse/Continued Use/ Continued Problem Potential

Risk Rating and Description *(NOTE: A higher number indicates a greater level of severity or intensity.)*	Types of Services and Modalities Needed	Intensity of Service/ Level of Care/Setting
Risk Rating: 4b = (Immediate action required.) ***Substance Use Disorders:*** The patient has no skills to arrest the addictive disorder, or to prevent relapse to substance use. His or her continued addictive behavior places the patient and/or others in imminent danger (e.g., the patient's continued drug use leads to impulsive, psychotic and aggressive behaviors). ***Mental Disorders:*** The patient has no skills to arrest the mental illness, or to prevent relapse to mental health problems. His or her continued psychiatric disorder places the patient and/or others in imminent danger (e.g., the patient's depression and feelings of hopelessness cause strong impulses to slash his or her wrists, or his paranoid delusions are accompanied by command hallucinations to harm others).	The patient needs containment for stabilization while imminently dangerous. If the relapse and/or dangerousness is due to psychosis, placement in a secure unit and/or involuntary commitment may be necessary. If continued use is due to severe, acute intoxication, close observation may be needed until the patient is less toxic. Medication management may be needed (as with anti-craving, antidepressants, mood stabilizers or antipsychotic medications). When the patient is stabilized, a supportive living arrangement will be needed. For patients with a Dimension 3 Risk Rating of 2 or higher at baseline, continuing mental health and addiction treatment with intensive case management also is required.	**Intensity: 4 =** Level IV medically managed intensive inpatient services (for the patient who needs psychiatric close observation because of dangerous, impulsive behavior), or III.5 clinically managed residential services (if the patient's degree of impulsivity requires 24-hour structure but not medical or psychiatric close observation). **Setting:** A hospital-based acute care unit if a secure setting is needed. If not, a free-standing residential "dual diagnosis" service for stabilization. Once the patient is stabilized, a supervised supportive living arrangement is appropriate.

Adolescent Dimension 6: Recovery Environment

Risk Rating and Description (NOTE: A higher number indicates a greater level of severity or intensity.)	Types of Services and Modalities Needed	Intensity of Service/ Level of Care/Setting
Risk Rating: 0 = *Substance Use Disorders*: The patient has a supportive environment or is able to cope with poor supports. *Mental Disorders*: The patient has a supportive environment or is able to cope with poor supports.	No immediate supportive living or skills training services are needed.	**Intensity: 0** = Self/mutual help groups allow the patient to access needed addiction or mental health treatment from his or her current living environment. For patients with severe mental impairment, Level III.1 residential support may assist with such access.
Risk Rating: 1 = *Substance Use Disorders*: The patient has passive support, or significant others are not interested in his or her addiction recovery, but he or she is not too distracted by this situation to be able to cope. *Mental Disorders*: The patient has passive support or significant others are not interested in an improved mental health environment, but he or she is not too distracted by this situation to be able to cope.	The patient needs assistance in finding a supportive living environment or skills training, support at school, vocational training, and transportation. For patients with a Dimension 3 Risk Rating of 1 or higher, coordination of mental health and addiction care may support functioning in the current recovery environment.	**Intensity: 1** = Level I outpatient services may allow the patient to live independently while obtaining needed treatment. **Setting:** An outpatient addiction or mental health service. For patients with severe mental impairment, mental health and case management support may be needed to structure access to and participation in treatment.
Risk Rating: 2 = *Substance Use Disorders*: The patient's environment is not supportive of addiction recovery but, with clinical structure, the patient is able to cope most of the time. *Mental Disorders*: The patient's environment is not supportive of good mental health but, with clinical structure, the patient is able to cope most of the time.	The patient needs assistance in finding a supportive living environment or skills training, support at school, vocational training, and transportation, multidimensional therapy (MDT), multisystemic therapy (MST), intensive in home outreach, assertive community outreach services; or other approaches to case	**Intensity: 1 to 3** = Level I outpatient services, Level II.1 intensive outpatient services, or Level II.5 partial hospitalization services, coupled with Level III.1 clinically managed low-intensity residential services.

Adolescent Dimension 6: Recovery Environment

Risk Rating and Description (NOTE: A higher number indicates a greater level of severity or intensity.)	Types of Services and Modalities Needed	Intensity of Service/Level of Care/Setting
	management that highly coordinate intensive therapies across multiple systems. The range of services needed depends on the interaction among Dimensions 3, 4 and 5. For example, an adolescent who has had one treatment episode for alcohol dependence is stable, back in school, and is ready for recovery and active in self/mutual help groups may need only individual or group counseling once a week. However, an adolescent who has had several treatment episodes; is involved with juvenile justice and also with gangs; is actively using Ecstasy and heroin; and who is not motivated for recovery and has few skills to cope with craving may need more intensive services.	**Setting:** An outpatient addiction or mental health service or a partial hospital "dual diagnosis" service, coupled with a supportive living environment, multidimensional therapy (MDT), multisystemic therapy (MST), intensive in home outreach, assertive community outreach services; or other approaches to case management that highly coordinate intensive therapies across multiple systems as needed. For patients with a Dimension 3 Risk Rating of 2 to 3, psychiatric enhancement of addiction treatment services may be required. Such a patient also needs continuing mental health support in the living environment. Appropriate case management and motivational enhancement therapies are provided.
Risk Rating: 3 = *Substance Use Disorders*: The patient's environment is not supportive of addiction recovery and he or she finds coping difficult, even with clinical structure. *Mental Disorders*: The patient's environment is not supportive of good mental health and he or she finds coping difficult, even with clinical structure.	The patient needs assertive assistance in finding a supportive living environment or skills training (depending on the patient's coping skills and impulse control), structured vocational rehabilitation, multidimensional therapy (MDT), multisystemic therapy (MST), intensive in home outreach, assertive community outreach services; or other	**Intensity:** 2 to 3 = Level II intensive outpatient services or Level II.5 partial hospitalization services, coupled with Level III.1 clinically managed low-intensity residential services, or equivalent support through case management and community outreach teams.

Adolescent Dimension 6: Recovery Environment

Risk Rating and Description (NOTE: A higher number indicates a greater level of severity or intensity.)	Types of Services and Modalities Needed	Intensity of Service/Level of Care/Setting
	approaches to case management that highly coordinate intensive therapies across multiple systems. The range of services needed depends on the interaction among Dimensions 3, 4 and 5, as described above.	**Setting:** A halfway house or "dual diagnosis" supportive living group home with multidimensional therapy (MDT), multisystemic therapy (MST), intensive in home outreach, assertive community outreach services; or other approaches to case management that highly coordinate intensive therapies across multiple systems as needed. For patients with a Dimension 3 Risk Rating of 2 to 3, psychiatric enhancement of addiction treatment services may be required. Such a patient also needs continuing mental health support in the living environment. Appropriate case management and motivational enhancement therapies are provided.
Risk Rating: 4a = (No immediate action required.) *Substance Use Disorders:* The patient's environment is not supportive and is chronically hostile and toxic to addiction recovery or treatment progress (for example, the patient has many drug-using friends, or drugs are readily available in the home environment, or there are chronic lifestyle problems but not acute conditions). The patient is unable to cope with the negative effects of such an environment on his or her recovery. *Mental Disorders:* The patient's environment is not supportive and is chronically hostile and toxic to good mental health (for example, there is persistent parental neglect and caretaking and adult supervision problems, but not acute conditions). The patient is unable to cope with the negative effects of this environment on his or her recovery.	The patient needs highly assertive assistance in finding a supportive living environment or skills training and impulse control services, or need for protection, multidimensional therapy (MDT), multisystemic therapy (MST), intensive in home outreach, assertive community outreach services; or other approaches to case management that highly coordinate intensive therapies across multiple systems.	**Intensity: 3** = Level III.1 clinically managed low-intensity residential services, or equivalent support through case management and community outreach teams. **Setting:** A halfway house or dual diagnosis supportive living group home with assertive case management, or multidimensional therapy (MDT), multisystemic therapy (MST), intensive in home outreach, assertive community outreach services; or other

Adolescent Dimension 6: Recovery Environment

Risk Rating and Description (NOTE: A higher number indicates a greater level of severity or intensity.)	Types of Services and Modalities Needed	Intensity of Service/ Level of Care/Setting
	The range of services needed depends on the interaction among Dimensions 3, 4 and 5, as described above. For example, an adolescent dependent on marijuana with persistent parental neglect who is motivated for recovery may need Level III.1 services, while a gang-involved, juvenile justice-involved, highly impulsive adolescent who drinks daily and lacks parental supervision and adult care taking may need multidimensional therapy (MDT), multisystemic therapy (MST), intensive in home outreach, assertive community outreach services; or other approaches to case management that highly coordinate intensive therapies across multiple systems than is available at Level III.1.	approaches to case management that highly coordinate intensive therapies across multiple systems. For patients with a Dimension 3 Risk Rating of 2 to 3, psychiatric enhancement of addiction treatment services may be required. Such a patient also needs continuing mental health support in the living environment. Appropriate case management and motivational enhancement therapies are provided.
Risk Rating: 4b = (Immediate action required.) *Substance Use Disorders*: The patient's environment is not supportive and is actively hostile to addiction recovery, posing an immediate threat to the patient's safety and wellbeing (for example, the patient lives with a parent who is a drug dealer and who offers drugs daily). *Mental Disorders*: The patient's environment is not supportive or is actively hostile to a safe mental health environment, posing an immediate threat to the patient's safety and wellbeing (for example, the patient lives with a physically abusive parent or adult caretaker).	The patient needs immediate separation from a toxic environment and placement in a temporary supportive living environment. The range of services needed depends on the interaction among Dimensions 3, 4 and 5, as described above.	**Intensity:** 3 = Level III.1 clinically managed low-intensity residential services or Level III.5. **Setting:** A temporary shelter, halfway house or "dual diagnosis" supportive living group home or residential services.

Adolescent Dimension 6: Recovery Environment

Risk Rating and Description (NOTE: A higher number indicates a greater level of severity or intensity.)	Types of Services and Modalities Needed	Intensity of Service/ Level of Care/Setting
	For example, a psychotic patient who is not motivated for recovery or an impulsive risk-taking adolescent with frequent cocaine use may need a more intensive residential level for safety.	For patients with a Dimension 3 Risk Rating of 2 to 3, psychiatric enhancement of addiction treatment services may be required. Such a patient also needs continuing mental health support in the living environment. Appropriate case management and motivational enhancement therapies are provided.

Appendix C
Dimension 5 Criteria:
Relapse, Continued Use or Continued Problem Potential

This section proposes a revised conceptual organization for Dimension 5 (Relapse, Continued Use or Continued Problem Potential), based on a review of the Dimension 5 constructs and criteria developed for earlier editions of the *ASAM Patient Placement Criteria*. The review included a decision analysis of the earlier Dimension 5 decision rules. Following that analysis, field data from the Massachusetts General Hospital (MGH)/Harvard ASAM Criteria Validity Study were analyzed for a large cohort of public and indigent patients in eastern Massachusetts.

After the validity and limitations of the earlier Dimension 5 decision rules were analyzed, the decision rules were rewritten to gain improved validity. This exercise revealed techniques that can and should be used to improve the discrimination of levels of care across all dimensions. Finally, the researchers expanded and refined the constructs that should compose a revised Dimension 5 to achieve a sequential and hierarchical list. The revised constructs offer face validity on several levels of basic and clinical research knowledge: behavioral pharmacology, behavioral psychology, learning theory and psychopathology.

While the present revision does not go so far as to propose final decision rules for Dimension 5, it does provide the framework for such a development in the next complete revision of the *ASAM Patient Placement Criteria*.

Previous Dimension 5 Constructs and Criteria

The first (1991) edition of the *ASAM Patient Placement Criteria* (*PPC-1*) described a Dimension 5 (then titled "Relapse Potential"). The dimension required assessment of several drinking-related factors, such as the risk of imminent danger, the risk of continued drinking or drug-taking behavior, the patient's understanding of the skills needed to prevent relapse, the severity of further distress if the patient failed to engage in treatment, the patient's awareness of relapse triggers, and the patient's skills for coping with cravings and controlling impulses.

In the second (1996) edition of the criteria (*ASAM PPC-2*), Dimension 5 was expanded to include assessment of continued use potential in patients who have not achieved any significant degree of abstinence beyond withdrawal and thus cannot meet the definition of "relapse." The *PPC-2* Dimension 5 required assessment across the continuum of service levels, as follows:

Level 0.5 (Early Intervention Services) was described as appropriate for the patient who needs an understanding of the risks of (or help in developing skills to change) current use patterns.

Level I (Outpatient Services) was described as appropriate for the patient who can control use or maintain abstinence with minimal support while pursuing recovery goals.

Level II (Intensive Outpatient Treatment) was deemed appropriate for the patient who is experiencing intensified addiction symptoms and functional deterioration despite participating in treatment at a less intensive level of care and despite efforts to revise the treatment plan. A distinction was made between Level II.1 (Intensive Outpatient Treatment) and Level II.5 (Partial Hospitalization). The latter was reserved for the patient who had failed to progress toward recovery at Level II.1 or for whom continued drinking or drug use or impending relapse is likely, and for whom less intensive treatment is judged be insufficient for stabilization.

Level III (Residential Services) was described as warranted, in general, when a patient's impending relapse or continued use is associated with *imminent danger* in the absence of 24-hour structured support. This circumstance might result from an inability to cope with environmental access to substances, difficulty in postponing immediate gratification or—in the event of Level III.3 (Clinically Managed Medium-Intensity Residential Treatment)—cognitive limitations, chronicity or intensity of substance use. In the less structured but still residential Level III.1 (Clinically Managed Low-Intensity Residential Treatment), the patient understands the nature of his or her problems, but is at risk because of an inability to apply recovery skills.

Opioid Maintenance Therapy (OMT) was defined as indicated on the basis of Dimension 5 for the opioid-dependent patient whose relapse is attributed to: (1) physiological craving, *or* (2) intensification of addiction symptoms, *or* (3) continued high-risk behaviors accompanied by deteriorating function, despite treatments other than opioid maintenance and efforts to adjust the treatment plan. Alternatively, OMT may be indicated for the patient who is at high risk of relapse because of lack of awareness of relapse triggers, difficulty in postponing immediate gratification or resistance to treatment.

Implementation of a Reliable Dimension 5 Assessment for Research

In the MGH/Harvard ASAM Criteria Validity Study, Dimension 5 was implemented for the *PPC-1* through use of selected items from the Recovery Attitude and Treatment Evaluator (RAATE) subscales A (Resistance to Treatment), B (Resistance to Continuing Care), and E (Environmental Factors Unsupportive of Recovery). These items provided a structured assessment of the patient's need for motivating strategies, relapse risk training and planning, recovery supports, high-risk social networks, impaired social skills, inadequate recreational activities and degree of unstructured daily routine. Additional questions to determine impulsivity were adopted from the Structured Clinical Interview for *DSM-IV* (SCID) Histrionic Personality Disorder Module. New items were developed to determine treatments within the preceding 90 days, to elicit information on any pattern of increasing addiction symptoms, and to obtain the interviewer's evaluation of whether the patient is in imminent danger of relapse.

Altogether, 18 question items were required to address the *PPC-1* decision rules for Dimension 5. *(The results presented below are drawn from an interim analysis and must be considered only preliminary until final sample size is accrued and data cleaning is completed; therefore, the empirical conclusions presented here should be considered illustrative and not final.)*

Decision Rule Problems

Of 586 subjects in the ASAM Criteria Validity Study, 107 subjects (18.3%) *did not qualify for any level of care* in Dimension 5. These patients were not necessarily at less risk of relapse than those who achieved a score, but they could not be scored into a level of care according to the existing decision rules.

Another problem was that nearly one-third of the subjects simultaneously *qualified for two or more levels of care*. Overall, 24.2% of subjects received simultaneous level of care scores for both Level II and Level III. Such overlap occurred when raters endorsed the Level II criterion "difficulty postponing immediate gratification" concurrently with the Level III criterion "unable to limit or control use if alcohol or drugs are present in the environment."

One solution to this apparent problem of overlap is to revise this dimension to achieve entirely discrete, non-overlapping criteria. While psychometrically preferable, this is not as easy as it sounds. Alternatively, a "highest intensity of service" default rule can be employed, so that patients who meet both the Level II and Level III criteria, for example, are automatically assigned to Level III. This is implied in the *PPC-1* and *PPC-2* and has been specifically confirmed as the intent of the criteria by an expert review group that included authors of the criteria.

Thus, some overlap may not represent a true shortcoming but rather a product of hierarchical clinical decision-making. Nevertheless, there is a challenge to write non-resolving and non-overlapping criteria. (To some degree, this is true of most dimensions of the ASAM criteria, not just Dimension 5.) Moreover, the issue occurs even more frequently in the *PPC-2* because of the subdivision of the levels of care.

Concurrent Validity of Dimension 5

Study subjects who required either partial hospitalization or residential treatment were recruited and assessed with the full Addiction Severity Index (ASI) as well as the ASAM *PPC-1* algorithm. (Subjects were men and women with various substance use disorders who presented in public sector settings in eastern Massachusetts.) Using a highest level of care default rule to resolve overlapping cases, 199 (34%) met the Dimension 5 criteria for Level II and 260 (44.4%) met the criteria for Level III.

Theoretically, patients rated on Dimension 5 as requiring Level III care should manifest higher ASI severity scores than patients who require Level II care. Of course, this is true only to the extent that Dimension 5 is consistent with the other dimensions with regard to severity. The nature of multi-dimensional assessment is that it is not linear. For example, an individual may not have a high ASI severity score, but may score well on readiness for change and engagement in recovery and may be well-suited to Level II. Another patient with a lower ASI severity score and good readiness to change on Dimension 4 may exhibit severe craving in Dimension 5 and thus need a Level III treatment program.

Study results indicate that patients who were rated on Dimension 5 as requiring Level III care did indeed have marginally greater composite severity scores on the ASI subscales for Alcohol, Employment, Family, and Legal problems. Only the ASI Drug and Psychiatric subscales failed to show this modest but consistent pattern. Baseline Global Assessment of Function (GAF) ratings also showed substantially worse functioning (average score of 55.1) for subjects rated on Dimension 5 as requiring Level III care, compared those rated as requiring Level II care (average score of 70.0). This is a clinically meaningful difference that supports concurrent validity.

Revising Dimension 5 for Discrete Thresholds

The MGH/Harvard group re-wrote the Dimension 5 decision rules to use the same items but combine them so as to avoid non-resolving or overlapping determinations. In some cases, this required setting discrete thresholds along a continuum. In others, it required use of a simplified hierarchy of combination rules. This eliminated the non-resolving determinations and resulted in a more balanced distribution of cases along Dimension 5: of the original 586 subjects, 27.5% were rated under the new rules as meeting the criteria for Level I care, 36.0% as Level II, and 36.5% as Level III.

Using the revised decision rules, preliminary results indicated that baseline Dimension 5 scores consistently grouped Level I, II, and III subjects in the expected staircase pattern of ascending ASI severity composite scores on the following subscales: Alcohol, Employment, Family, Legal and Psychiatric. (The Medical scores also were ascending but are not addressed in this analysis because medical exclusion criteria limited the range of the sample.)

The range of variance on each of the scales was somewhat greater with the revised rules. In baseline GAF scores, those who qualified for Level III were rated as least functional (56.2), followed by Level II (57.8), and Level I (rated the most functional at 68.0).

The revised method of scoring Dimension 5 also demonstrates some degree of near-term predictive validity. The interim sample for a baseline versus Month 1 comparison consisted of 271 subjects with complete data. Baseline categorization using revised Dimension 5 scoring was associated with a higher Month 1 ASI Alcohol composite score for Level III (.278 +/-.256 S.D.), compared to Level II (.187 +/-.212) and Level I (.180 +/-.231). This pattern was similar for the comparison of Month 1 ASI Drug composite severity for baseline Level III (.149 +/-.112) compared to both Level II (.121 +/-.109) and Level I (.126 +/-.111). These relationships were not consistently maintained, however, at Months 3 or 6 (for which there were smaller samples in the preliminary analysis). It may be too much to expect such extended predictive associations from a single criteria dimension, in any case.

Further Problems and Considerations

As noted above, scores on the ASI composite Medical Severity subscale were limited by the study's medical exclusion criteria. Naturalistic research is needed that will include patients who have severe medical problems. A theoretical problem here is the possibility that an acute medical crisis may temporarily decrease patients' subjective sense of relapse risk, but that once the medical problem subsides, the patient's relapse potential may increase dramatically. (This may be analogous to a depressed patient who poses minimal suicide risk during the most severe neurovegetative stage of depression but who, on initiation of effective pharmacotherapy, improves to the point of becoming capable of acting on suicidal urges.) A future revision thus will need to create decision rules to distinguish between an artificially low relapse risk due to short-term medical factors and a low intrinsic relapse risk.

Short-term confounds such as this may occur elsewhere and may include incarceration, coercion and family intervention—all acute circumstances (which should be assessed on Dimensions 4 and 6).that may change over time, releasing latent relapse risk.

Several variables are poorly assessed using current structured interview methods and, while considered important clinically, are difficult to measure reliably through conventional clinical interviewing. Two examples are the presence of acute coercive legal factors and approval-seeking response bias. Both may invalidate self-reports of a patient's intrinsic relapse potential. Also, temporal factors such as pregnancy may make relapse potential difficult to assess beyond the patient's delivery date.

Another concern is the mixing of constructs. A psychometrically coherent approach would initially isolate constructs for internal consistency, and subsequently combine them for a layer of cumulative decision rules. The following constructs are proposed to improve the psychometric coherence of Dimension 5:

Proposed Revised Constructs for Dimension 5:
Relapse, Continued Use or Continued Problem Potential

A. Historical Pattern of Use

   1. Chronicity of problem use

      How long and from what date has the individual had problem use or dependence and at what level of severity?

   2. Treatment or change response

      Has the individual managed brief or extended abstinence or reduction of use in the past?

B. Pharmacologic Responsivity

   1. Positive reinforcement (pleasure, euphoria)

   2. Negative reinforcement (withdrawal discomfort, fear)

C. External Stimuli Responsivity

   1. Reactivity to acute cues (trigger objects and situations)

   2. Reactivity to chronic stress (positive and negative stressors)

D. Cognitive and Behavioral Measures of Strengths and Weaknesses

   1. Locus of control and self-efficacy

      Is there an internal sense of self-determination and confidence that the individual can direct his or her own behavioral change?

   2. Coping skills (including stimulus control, other cognitive strategies)

   3. Impulsivity (risk-taking, thrill-seeking)

   4. Passive and passive/aggressive behavior

      Does the individual demonstrate active efforts to anticipate and cope with internal and external stressors, or is there a tendency to abdicate or assign responsibility to others?

These four domains are not inconsistent with the intent of the *PPC-2* version of Dimension 5, and offer a conceptually more clear *sequence of factors* that contribute to relapse potential. The sequence involves the historical phenomenon of relapse, the acute pharmacologic response to the substance(s), second-order behavioral responsivity that may mediate the preceding factors, and third-order personality or learned responses that may modify the preceding factors.

Constructs in Section A (historical pattern) may apply to use, abuse or dependence, depending on the patient's particular situation. A good number of studies show that demographic variables such as onset of alcohol or drug problems by age 25, never having been married, lacking a high school education, and being unemployed predict continued use or relapse. Clinical history variables, such as past treatment response, are good predictors of future relapse risk. Even if the patient has not previously experienced treatment, any past change efforts to reduce or cease substance use behavior are informative. This may apply to substances other than the one that is the current primary risk for the patient. For example, it may be helpful to know if the patient who must cease drinking has previously succeeded in quitting smoking.

In Section B, the term Pharmacologic Responsivity refers to internal stimuli at the neuronal level of the brain from reinforcing substances that produce either or both positive and negative reinforcement. The operative role here is the patient's expectation (that is, to what extent does the patient expect pleasure or euphoria [for positive reinforcement], or withdrawal discomfort and fear of withdrawal [for negative reinforcement]?) Negative reinforcement is not used here to represent the acute withdrawal symptoms themselves, as those are addressed in Dimension 1 (Intoxication/Withdrawal).

The constructs in section D differ from those in Dimension 3 (Emotional, Behavioral or Cognitive Conditions and Complications). Section D constructs are behavioral traits that are specific to relapse risk, although they may not be pathologic in other contexts. This distinguishes them from Dimension 3 constructs, which usually are psychiatric (*DSM-IV*) Axis I or II diagnoses that generalize to many behaviors and risk situations.

It is important to recognize that relapse risk is constantly changing. Therefore, the time frame for prediction is limited. In a given patient, each of the above constructs is highly variable; therefore, the patient requires frequent re-assessment as withdrawal subsides, a new treatment response is established, coping strengths are learned and tested, character traits grow and euphoric expectancies extinguish.

A Primary Versus Secondary Role for Relapse Potential in the Overall PPC Decision Tree

The importance of relapse potential is sufficient that the Committee seriously considered an alternate dimensional structure for the criteria: conceivably, all other dimensions could be assessed first, leaving relapse potential to be evaluated as a second-order, overarching, integrative dimension to solve the final level of care decision based on the pressure on relapse risk of all the other dimensions. Ultimately, this approach was discarded as reductionistic. After considering these options, the researchers resolved to maintain the six-dimensional model of assessment, with Relapse Potential separate from but equal to the other dimensions and considered concurrently with them. In keeping with this principle, the assessment of impulsivity and passivity was divided into two separate aspects: (1) general psychological pathology with potential for self-harm, as compared with (2) traits or coping characteristics that are more specific to substance use relapse and relapse prevention. The latter construct is retained in the proposed Dimension 5.

Prospects for Reliable Assessment

Structured assessments or subscales are available for most of the constructs. These are useful aids to implementation. Predictive relationships for individual constructs are relatively modest and the methodology is very much in need of further development (Finney et al., 1999). In the following list, selected measures are listed as examples after each construct heading. This list is incomplete and may omit valuable instruments, so clinicians and program administrators should investigate alternatives. The drafters invite submissions.

Criteria for assessment tools should include: good psychometric properties, shared face validity for the purpose for which the instrument was designed, brevity, and appropriateness for administration to a wide range of substance-abusing and substance-dependent populations. In the following list, citations are provided for both instruments and relevant descriptive papers. Some commercial or fee-based sources also are listed.

Suggested Instruments or Item Sources For Assessing Dimension 5

A. Historical Pattern of Use

   1. Chronicity of problem use

   How long and from what date has the individual had problem use or dependence and at what level of severity? (Finney & Moos, 1995)

   Measures:
   - Structured Clinical Interview for DSM-IV (SCID; First et al., 1997a, 1997b)
   - Substance Use Disorder Diagnostic Schedule (SUDDS; Davis et al., 1992; Buros Institute, 1999)

   2. Treatment or change response

   Has the individual managed brief or extended abstinence or reduction of use in the past?

   Measures that address both A.1 and A.2:
   - Addiction Severity Index Alcohol and Drug Severity Scales (ASI; McLellan et al., 1990, 1992)
   - Form 90 (U.S. Department of Health and Human Services, 1995)
   - Drinker Inventory of Consequences (DrInC; Miller et al., 1995)
   - Inventory of Drug Use Consequences (InDUC; Miller et al., 1995; based on the DrInC)
   - Alcohol Dependence Scale (ADS; Skinner & Horn, 1984)
   - Drug Use Questionnaire (DAST; Skinner, 1982)
   - Chemical Use, Abuse and Dependence Scale (CUAD frequency/amount/duration grid (McGovern & Morrison, 1992; modified for congruence with the *DSM-IV* by Rubin & Gastfriend, 1999).

B. Pharmacologic Responsivity

   1. Positive reinforcement (amount of pleasure or euphoria the individual obtains or expects from substance use). Expectancies, which may defined as the outcome(s) the individual anticipates from a particular behavior, have been shown to be related to substance use consumption and relapse.

   Measures:
   - Alcohol Effects Questionnaire (AEFQ) Global Positive subscale and Relaxation and Tension Reduction subscale (Rohsenow, 1983, 1995)
   - Alcohol Expectancies Questionnaire (AEQ; Brown et al., 1987; Brown, 1995)

   2. Negative reinforcement (amount of discomfort of negative effects the individual expects or fears from abstinence).

   Measures:
   - (Craving) Obsessive Compulsive Drinking Scale, item 11 (OCDS; Anton et al., 1996; Roberts et al., 1999)
   - Alcohol Dependence Scale, item 9 (ADS, aka Alcohol Use Questionnaire; Skinner & Horn, 1984)

C. External Stimuli Responsivity

Acute and chronic cues and stressors may include positive stressors, including vocational achievements, as well as negative stressors (such as social pressure situations or conflict situations, as well as ongoing environmental challenges such as homelessness, divorce and financial problems).

1. Reactivity to acute cues (reaction to trigger objects and situations, both in terms of strength of the reaction and the ubiquitous nature of the cues)

    Measures:
    - Inventory of Drinking Situations and Inventory of Drug Taking Situations (Annis et al., 1987, available from ARF; Turner et al., 1997)
    - Situational Confidence Questionnaire (SCQ; Annis & Graham, 1988)

2. Reactivity to chronic stress (positive and negative stressors; ability to manage ongoing environmental stressors that are not specific to substance use, such as homelessness, divorce or financial problems)

    Measures:
    Life Experiences Survey (Sarason, Johnson & Siegel, 1978)

D. Cognitive and behavioral measures of strengths and weaknesses

1. Locus of control and self-efficacy (is there an internal sense of self-determination and confidence that the individual can direct his or her own behavioral change?)

    Measures:
    - Recovery Attitude and Treatment Evaluator-Clinical Evaluation/Research Version, Scale B, Resistance to Continuing Care (RAATE-CE/R; Najavits et al., 1997; Mee-Lee et al., 1992; Gastfriend et al., 1995)
    - Drinking Related Locus of Control Scale (DRIE; Donovan & O'Leary, 1978, 1983; Lefcourt, 1991; Keyson & Janda, 1995). Also has been adapted for cigarette smokers (Bunch & Schneider, 1991) and cocaine abusers (Oswald et al., 1992).

2. Coping skills (including stimulus control and other cognitive strategies (Myers et al., 1993)

    Measures:
    - Recovery Attitude and Treatment Evaluator-Clinical Evaluation/Research Version, Scale B, Resistance to Continuing Care, and Scale E, Social/Family/Environmental Status (RAATE-CE/R; Najavits et al., 1997; Mee-Lee et al., 1992; Gastfriend et al., 1995)
    - URICA Action & Maintenance Scale Score (DiClemente & Hughes, 1990)
    - Coping Behaviors Inventory (CBI; Litman et al., 1983) and Effectiveness of Coping Behaviors Inventory (ECBI; Litman et al., 1984)
    - Ways of Coping (Lazarus & Folkman, 1984; Folkman, Lazarus et al., 1986)
    - Coping Resources Inventory (CRI; Moos et al., 1993, available from PAR)

3. Impulsivity (risk-taking, thrill-seeking or novelty-seeking states, rather than pathology, which is assessed in Dimension 3: Behavioral Conditions and Complications)

    Measures:
    - Personality Assessment Inventory: high scores on the Stimulus Seeking scale (PAI; Morey, 1992, available from PAR)
    - Temperament & Character Inventory (TCI; Cloninger et al., 1993)

4. Passive and passive/aggressive behavior

   Does the individual demonstrate active efforts to anticipate and cope with internal and external stressors, or is there a tendency to abdicate or assign responsibility to others? (These are traits rather than pathological conditions, which belong in Dimension 3.)

   Measures:
   - Personality Assessment Inventory: low scores in the Dominance scale indicate passivity (PAI; Morey, 1992, available from PAR)
   - See also Locus of Control (DRIE, above). External scores on any of the three subscales indicate that the individual assigns causality to events outside of his or her control and tends not to attempt to change the situation.
   - See also Coping Skills (CRI, above). High scores on Avoidant coping scales tend to suggest passive behavior.

References

American Psychiatric Association (1994). *Diagnostic and Statistical Manual of Mental Disorders, Fourth Edition (DSM-IV)*. Washington, DC: American Psychiatric Press.

Annis HM, Graham JM & Davis CS (1987). *Inventory of Drinking Situations*. Toronto, ON: Addiction Research Foundation.

Annis HM & Graham JM (1988). *Situational Confidence Questionnaire*. Toronto, ON: Addiction Research Foundation.

Anton RF, Moak DH & Latham PK (1996). The Obsessive Compulsive Drinking Scale: A new method of assessing outcome in alcoholism treatment studies. *Archives of General Psychiatry* 53:225-231.

Brown SA (1995). Alcohol Expectancy Questionnaire. In JP Allen & M Columbus (eds.) *Assessing Alcohol Problems: A Guide for Clinicians and Researchers* (Treatment Handbook Series, No. 4). Bethesda, MD: National Institute on Alcohol Abuse and Alcoholism, pp. 213-222.

Brown SA, Christiansen BA & Goldman MS (1987). The Alcohol Expectancy Questionnaire: An instrument for the assessment of adolescent and adult alcohol expectancies. *Journal of Studies on Alcohol* 48:483-491.

Bunch JM & Schneider HG (1991). Smoking-specific locus of control. *Psychological Reports* 69:1075-1081.

Buros Institute of Mental Measurements (1999). *Thirteenth Mental Measurements Yearbook*. Lincoln, NE: University of Nebraska.

Cloninger CR, Svrakic DM & Przybeck TR (1993). A psychobiological model of temperament and character. *Archives of General Psychiatry.* 50:975-990.

Davis LJ, Hoffmann NG, Morse RM & Luehr JG (1992). Substance use disorder diagnostic schedule (SUDDS): The equivalence and validity of a computer-administered and an interviewer-administered format. *Alcoholism: Clinical and Experimental Research* 16(2):250-254.

DiClemente CC & Hughes SO (1990). Stages of change profiles in outpatient alcoholism treatment. *Journal of Substance Abuse* 2:217-235.

DiClemente CC, Carbonari JP, Montgomery RPG & Hughes SO (1994). The Alcohol Abstinence Self-Efficacy Scale. *Journal of Studies on Alcohol* 55:141-148.

Donovan DM & O'Leary MR (1978). The drinking-related locus of control scale. *Journal of Studies on Alcohol* 39:759-784.

Donovan DM & O'Leary MR (1983). Control orientation, drinking behavior, and alcoholism. In HM Lefcourt (ed.) *Research with the Locus of Control Construct*. New York, NY: Academic Press, 2:107-154.

Finney JW & Moos RH (1995). Research report - Entering treatment for alcohol abuse: A stress and coping model. *Addiction* 90:1223-1240.

Finney JW, Moos RH & Humphreys K (1999). A comparative evaluation of substance abuse treatment: II. Linking proximal outcomes of 12-step and cognitive-behavioral treatment to substance use outcomes. *Alcoholism: Clinical and Experimental Research* 23:537-544.

First MB, Spitzer RL, Gibbon M & Williams JBW (1997a). *Structured Clinical Interview for DSM-IV Axis I Disorders, Clinician Version (SCID-CV)*. Washington, DC: American Psychiatric Press.

First MB, Spitzer RL, Gibbon M & Williams JBW (1997b). *Structured Clinical Interview for DSM-IV Axis I Disorders, Research Version, Patient Edition with Psychotic Screen (SCID-I/P W/ PSY SCREEN)*. New York, NY: Biometrics Research, New York State Psychiatric Institute.

Folkman S, Lazarus RS, Dunkel-Schetter C, DeLongis A & Gruen RJ (1986). Dynamics of a stressful encounter: Cognitive appraisal, coping, and encounter outcomes. *Journal of Personality and Social Psychology* 50:992-1003.

Gastfriend DR, Filstead WJ, Reif S, Najavits LM & Parella DP (1995). Validity of assessing treatment readiness in patients with substance use disorders. *American Journal on Addictions* 4:254-260.

Hsieh S, Hoffmann NG & Hollister CD (1998). The relationship between pre-, during-, and post-treatment factors and adolescent substance abuse behaviors. *The Journal of Addictive Behaviors* 23:1-12.

Hoffmann NG, DeHart SS & Gogineni A (1998). Alcohol dependence as a chronic health problem among older adults. *The Southwestern Journal on Aging* 14:57-64.

Hoffmann NG, Floyd AS, Zywiak WH & DeHart SS (1999). Strategies for Case-Mix Adjustments in Addictions Treatment Evaluations: Prognostic Indicators in Public Sector Populations. Report prepared for the State of Wisconsin under CSAT Contract 270-95-0023.

Hoffmann NG & Longabaugh R (1999). Final Report: Developing a Foundation for Outcomes Based Addictions Treatment. Submitted to the Robert Wood Johnson Foundation.

Keyson _ & Janda _ (1995). Drinking-Related Locus of Control Scale. In JP Allen & M Columbus (eds.) *Assessing Alcohol Problems: A Guide for Clinicians and Researchers* (Treatment Handbook Series, No. 4). Bethesda, MD: National Institute on Alcohol Abuse and Alcoholism.

Lazarus RS & Folkman S (1984). *Stress, Appraisal and Coping*. New York, NY: Springer Publishing.

Lefcourt HM (1991). Locus of control. In JP Robinson, PR Shaver, et al. (eds.) *Measures of Personality and Social Psychological Attitudes, Vol. 1: Measures of Social Psychological Attitudes.* San Diego, CA: Academic Press, pp. 413-489.

Litman GK, Stapleton J, Oppenheim AN & Peleg M (1983). An instrument for measuring coping behaviors in hospitalized alcoholics: Implications for relapse prevention and treatment. *British Journal of Addiction* 78:269-276.

Litman GK, Stapleton J, Oppenheim AN, Peleg M & Jackson P (1984). The relationship between coping behaviors, their effectiveness and alcoholism relapse and survival. *British Journal of Addiction* 79:283-291.

McGovern MP & Morrison DH (1992). The Chemical Use, Abuse and Dependence Scale (CUAD): Rationale, reliability and validity. *Journal of Substance Abuse Treatment* 9:27-38.

McLellan AT, Kushner H, Metzger D, Peters R, Smith I, Grissom G, Pettinati H & Argeriou M (1992). The fifth edition of the Addiction Severity Index. *Journal of Substance Abuse Treatment* 9:199-213.

McLellan AT, Parikh G, Bragg A, Cacciola J, Fureman B & Incmikoski R (1990). *Addiction Severity Index (5th ed.).* Philadelphia, PA: Penn-VA Center for Studies of Addiction.

Mee-Lee D, Hoffman NG & Smith MB (1992). *Recovery Attitude and Treatment Evaluator (RAATE) Manual (2nd ed.).* St. Paul, MN: CATOR/New Standards, Inc.

Miller WR (1996). Form 90: A structured assessment interview for drinking and related behaviors. In ME Mattson (ed.) *NIAAA Project MATCH Monograph Series* (Vol. 5). Bethesda, MD: National Institute on Alcohol Abuse and Alcoholism.

Miller WR, Tonigan JS & Longabaugh R (1995). *The Drinker Inventory Consequences: An Inventory for Assessing Adverse Consequences of Alcohol Abuse. Test Manual,* vol. 4 (Project MATCH Monograph Series). Bethesda, MD: National Institute on Alcohol Abuse and Alcoholism.

Moos RH, Brennan PL & Fondacaro MR (1990). Approach and avoidance coping responses among older problem and nonproblem drinkers. *Psychology of Aging* 5:31-40.

Morey L (1992). *PAI: An Overview of the Personality Assessment Inventory.* Odessa, FL: Psychological Assessment Resources.

Myers M, Brown S & Mott M (1993). Coping as a predictor of substance abuse treatment outcome. *Journal of Substance Abuse* 5:15-30.

Najavits LM, Gastfriend DR, Nakayama EY, et al. (1997). A measure of readiness for substance abuse treatment: Psychometric properties of the RAATE research interview. *American Journal of Addiction* 6:74-82.

Oswald LM, Walker GC, Reilly EL, Krajewski KJ, et al. (1992). Measurement of locus of control in cocaine abusers. *Issues in Mental Health Nursing* 13:81-94.

Roberts JS, Anton RF, Latham PK & Moak DH (1999). Factor structure and predictive validity of the Obsessive Compulsive Drinking Scale. *Alcoholism: Clinical and Experimental Research* 23:1484-1491.

Rohsenow DJ (1983). Drinking habits and expectancies about alcohol's effects for self versus others. *Journal of Consulting and Clinical Psychology* 51(5):752-756.

Rohsenow DJ (1995). Alcohol Effects Questionnaire. In JP Allen & M Columbus (eds.) *Assessing Alcohol Problems: A Guide for Clinicians and Researchers* (Treatment Handbook Series, No. 4). Bethesda, MD: National Institute on Alcohol Abuse and Alcoholism.

Sarason IG, Johnson JH & Siegel JM (1978). Assessing the impact of life changes: Development of the Life Experiences Survey. *Journal of Consulting and Clinical Psychology* 46:932-946.

Skinner HA (1982). *Drug Use Questionnaire*. Toronto, ON: Addiction Research Foundation.

Skinner HA & Horn HL (1984). *Alcohol Dependence Scale User's Guide*. Toronto, ON: Addiction Research Foundation.

Turner NE, Annis HM & Sklar SM (1997). Measurement of antecedents to drug and alcohol use: Psychometric properties of the Inventory of Drug-Taking Situations (IDTS). *Behaviour Research & Therapy* 35(5):465-483.

U.S. Department of Health and Human Services (1995). Form 90: A structured assessment interview for drinking and related behaviors. In WR Miller (ed.) Vol. 96-4004, Washington, DC: U.S. Government Printing Office.

Zywiak WH, Hoffmann NG & Floyd AS (1999). Enhancing alcohol treatment outcomes through aftercare and self-help groups. *Medicine & Health/Rhode Island* 82(3):87-90.

Sources

Measures listed as from the ARF (Addiction Research Foundation) may be obtained for a fee from:

Centre for Addiction and Mental Health
Addiction Research Foundation Division
Marketing and Sales Services
33 Russell Street
Toronto, Ontario
Canada M55 2S1
(1-800/661-1111)

Measures listed as available from PAR (Psychological Assessment Resources) may be obtained for a fee from:

Psychological Assessment Resources, Inc.
PO Box 998
Odessa, FL 33556
(1-800/331-TEST)

The ASI (Addiction Severity Index) may be obtained for a small copying fee from:

Treatment Research Institute
University of Pennsylvania
One Commerce Square
Suite 1120
2005 Market St.
Philadelphia, PA 19103
(215/665-2880)

The SCID-I/P Patient version and CV clinician version are obtained from:

SCID Central
Biometrics Research Department
New York State Psychiatric Institute
1051 Riverside Drive - Unit 60
New York, NY 10032
(212/543-5524)
http://cpmcnet.columbia.edu/dept/scid

The SUDDS and RAATE may be obtained for a fee from:

Evince Clinical Assessments
PO Box 17305
Smithfield, RI 02917
(1-800/755-6299)

Appendix D
Clinical Institute Withdrawal Assessment of Alcohol Scale, Revised (CIWA-Ar)

Many quantification instruments have been developed for monitoring alcohol withdrawal (Guthrie, 1989; Sullivan et al., 1989; Sellers & Naranjo, 1983). No single instrument is significantly superior to the others. What is clear is that there are significant clinical advantages to quantifying the alcohol withdrawal syndrome. Quantification is key to preventing excess morbidity and mortality in a group of patients who are at risk for alcohol withdrawal. Such instruments help clinical personnel recognize the process of withdrawal before it progresses to more advanced stages, such as *delirium tremens*. By intervening with appropriate pharmacotherapy in those patients who require it, while sparing the majority of patients whose syndromes do not progress to that point, the clinician can prevent over- and undertreatment of the alcohol withdrawal syndrome. Finally, by quantifying and monitoring the withdrawal process, the treatment regimen can be modified as needed.

The best known and most extensively studied scale is the Clinical Institute Withdrawal Assessment - Alcohol (CIWA-A) and a shortened version, the CIWA-A revised (CIWA-Ar). This scale has well-documented reliability, reproducibility and validity, based on comparison to ratings by expert clinicians (Knott, et al., 1981; Wiehl, et al., 1994; Sullivan, et al., 1989). From 30 signs and symptoms, the scale has been carefully refined to a list of 10 signs and symptoms in the CIWA-Ar (Wiehl, et al. 1994). It is thus easy to use and has been shown to be feasible to use in a variety of clinical settings, including detoxification units (Naranjo, et al., 1983; Hoey, et al., 1994), psychiatry units (Heinala, et al., 1990), and general medical/surgical wards (Young, et al., 1987; Katta, 1991). The CIWA-Ar has added usefulness because high scores, in addition to indicating severe withdrawal, are also predictive of the development of seizures and delirium (Naranjo, et al., 1983; Young, et al., 1987).

The CIWA-Ar scale can measure 10 symptoms. Scores of less than 8 to 10 indicate minimal to mild withdrawal. Scores of 8 to 15 indicate moderate withdrawal (marked autonomic arousal); and scores of 15 or more indicate severe withdrawal. The assessment requires 2 minutes to perform (Sullivan, et al, 1989).

CIWA-Ar categories, with the range of scores in each category, are as follows:

Agitation	(0-7)
Anxiety	(0-7)
Auditory Disturbances	(0-7)
Clouding of Sensorium	(0-4)
Headache	(0-7)
Nausea/Vomiting	(0-7)
Paroxysmal Sweats	(0-7)
Tactile Disturbances	(0-7)
Tremor	(0-7)
Visual Disturbances	(0-7)

The instrument also has been adapted for benzodiazepine withdrawal assessment (Clinical Institute Withdrawal Assessment-Benzodiazepine).

A study of the revised version of the CIWA predicted that those with a score of >15 were at increased risk for severe alcohol withdrawal (RR 3.72;95% confidence interval 2.85-4.85); the higher the score, the greater the risk. Some patients (6.4%) still suffered complications, despite low scores, if left untreated (Foy, et al., 1988).

References

Foy A, March S & Drinkwater V (1988). Use of an objective clinical scale in the assessment and management of alcohol withdrawal in a large general hospital. *Alcoholism: Clinical and Experimental Research* 12:360-364.

Guthrie SK (1989). The treatment of alcohol withdrawal. *Pharmacotherapy* 9(3):131-143.

Heinala P, Pieponen T & Heikkinen H (1990). Diazepam loading in alcohol withdrawal: Clinical pharmacokinetics. *International Journal of Clinical Pharmacology, Therapy and Toxicology* 28:211-217.

Hoey LL, Nahun A & Vance-Bryan K (1994). A retrospective review and assessment of benzodiazepines in the treatment of alcohol withdrawal in hospitalized patients. *Pharmacotherapy* 14:572-578.

Katta BB (1991). Nifedapine for protracted withdrawal syndrome. *Canadian Journal of Psychiatry* 36:155.

Knott DH, Lerner D, Davis-Knott T & Fink RD (1981). Decision for alcohol detoxification: A method to standardize patient evaluation. *Postgraduate Medicine* 69:65-76.

Naranjo CA, Sellers EM, Chater K, Iversen P, Roach C & Sykora K (1983). Nonpharmacologic intervention with acute alcohol withdrawal. *Clinical Pharmacology and Therapeutics* 34:214-219.

Sellers EM & Naranjo CA (1983). New strategies for the treatment of alcohol withdrawal. *Psychopharmacology Bulletin* 22:88-91.

Sullivan JT, Sykora K, Schneiderman J, Naranjo CA & Sellers EM (1989). Assessment of alcohol withdrawal: The revised Clinical Institute Withdrawal Instrument for Alcohol Scale (CIWA-Ar). *British Journal of Addiction* 84:1353-1357.

Young GP, Rores C, Murphy C & Dailey RH (1987). Intravenous phenobarbital for alcohol withdrawal and convulsions. *Annals of Emergency Medicine* 16:847-850.

Wiehl WO, Hayner G & Galloway G (1994). Haight Ashbury Free Clinics drug detoxification protocols, Part 4: Alcohol. *Journal of Psychoactive Drugs* 26:57-59.

Addiction Research Foundation
Clinical Institute Withdrawal Assessment for Alcohol, Revised (CIWA-Ar)

Patient: _____ Pulse or heart rate, taken for 1 minute: _____

Date: _____ Time: _____ Blood pressure: _____

Nausea and Vomiting: Ask, "Do you feel sick to your stomach? Have you vomited?" Observation:

0 No nausea and no vomiting
1 Mild nausea with no vomiting
2
3
4 Intermittent nausea with dry heaves
5
6
7 Constant nausea, frequent dry heaves and vomiting

Tremor: Arms extended and fingers spread apart. Observation:

0 No tremor
1 Not visible but can be felt fingertip to fingertip
2
3
4 Moderate, with patient's arm extended
5
6
7 Severe, even with arms not extended

Paroxysmal Sweats: Observation:

0 No sweat visible
1
2
3
4 Beads of sweat obvious on forehead
5
6
7 Drenching sweats

Tactile Disturbances: Ask, "Have you any itching, pins and needles sensations, any burning, any numbness, or do you feel bugs crawling under your skin?" Observation:

0 None
1 Very mild itching, pins and needles, burning or numbness
2 Mild itching, pins and needles, burning or numbness
3 Moderate itching, pins and needles, burning or numbness
4 Moderately severe hallucinations
5 Severe hallucinations
6 Extremely severe hallucinations
7 Continuous hallucinations

Auditory Disturbances: Ask, "Are you more aware of sounds around you? Are they harsh? Do they frighten you? Are you hearing anything that is disturbing to you? Are you hearing things you know are not there?" Observation:

0 Not present
1 Very mild harshness or ability to frighten
2 Mild harshness or ability to frighten
3 Moderate harshness or ability to frighten
4 Moderately severe hallucinations
5 Severe hallucinations
6 Extremely severe hallucinations
7 Continuous hallucinations

Visual Disturbances: Ask, "Does the light appear to be too bright? Is the color different? Does it hurt your eyes? Are you seeing anything that is disturbing to you? Are you seeing things you know are not there?" Observation:

0 Not present
1 Very mild sensitivity
2 Mild sensitivity
3 Moderate sensitivity
4 Moderately severe hallucinations
5 Severe hallucinations
6 Extremely severe hallucinations
7 Continuous hallucinations

ASAM Patient Placement Criteria, Second Edition–Revised

Addiction Research Foundation
Clinical Institute Withdrawal Assessment for Alcohol, Revised (CIWA-Ar)

Patient: _____ **Pulse or heart rate, taken for 1 minute:** _____

Date: _____ **Time:** _____ **Blood pressure:** _____

Anxiety: Ask, "Do you feel nervous?" Observation:

0 No anxiety, at ease
1 Mildly anxious
2
3
4 Moderately anxious, or guarded, so anxiety is inferred
5
6
7 Equivalent to acute panic states, as seen in severe delirium or acute schizophrenic reactions

Agitation: Observation:

0 Normal activity
1 Somewhat more than normal activity
2
3
4 Moderately fidgety and restless
5
6
7 Paces back and forth during most of the interview, or constantly thrashes about

Headache, Fullness in Head: Ask, "Does your head feel different? Does it feel like there is a band around your head?" Do not rate dizziness or lightheadedness. Otherwise, rate severity.

0 Not present
1 Very mild
2 Mild
3 Moderate
4 Moderately severe
5 Severe
6 Very severe
7 Extremely severe

Orientation and Clouding of Sensorium: Ask, "What day is this? Where are you? Who am I?" Observation:

0 Oriented and can do serial additions
1 Cannot do serial additions or is uncertain about date
2 Disoriented for date by no more than 2 calendar days
3 Disoriented for date by more than 2 calendar days
4 Disoriented for place and/or person

Total CIWA-Ar Score _____
(maximum possible score = 67)

Rater's Initials _____

Patients scoring less than 10 do not usually need additional medication for withdrawal.

Note: The CIWA-Ar is not copyrighted and may be used freely. Source: Sullivan JT, Sykora K, Schneiderman J, Naranjo CA & Sellers EM (1989). Assessment of alcohol withdrawal: The revised Clinical Institute Withdrawal Assessment for Alcohol scale (CIWA-Ar). *British Journal of Addiction* 84:1353-1357.

Appendix E
Glossary of Terms Used in the Second Edition-Revised

A glossary of terms used in the *ASAM PPC-2R* is given here to help the reader interpret the criteria. Terms are defined as follows:

[Note: an asterisk denotes a definition that has been formally adopted by ASAM's Board of Directors.]

*Abstinence
Non-use of a specific substance. In recovery, non-use of any addictive psychoactive substance. May also denote cessation of an addictive behavior, such as gambling, over-eating, etc.

*Abuse
Harmful use of a specific psychoactive substance. The term also applies to one category of psychoactive substance-related disorders. While recognizing that "abuse" is part of present diagnostic terminology, ASAM recommends that an alternative term be found for this purpose because of the pejorative connotations of the word "abuse."

Acceptance/Resistance
See Readiness to Change.

*Addiction
A primary, chronic, neurobiologic disease, with genetic, psychosocial and environmental factors influencing its development and manifestations. It is characterized by behaviors that include one or more of the following: impaired control over drug use, compulsive use, continued use despite harm, and craving.

*Addictionist
Also, "addictionologist." A physician who specializes in addiction medicine.

Addiction-Only Services (AOS)
Services directly solely at the treatment of addictive disorders. Such services are not directed at co-occurring mental disorders: for example, an AOS program typically would not accept an individual who needs psychotropic medications, and mental health issues generally would not be addressed in treatment planning or content.

Admission
That point in an individual's relationship with an organized treatment service when the intake process has been completed and the individual is entitled to receive the services of the treatment program.

Adolescent
As used in the *ASAM PPC-2R*, an individual aged 13 through 18. The term also frequently applies to young adults aged 18 to 21, who may be in need of adolescent-type services rather than adult-type services. (Many states classify individuals up to age 21 as adolescents.)

*Alcoholics Anonymous
"A fellowship of men and women who share their experience, strength and hope with each other that they may solve their common problem and help others recover from alcoholism. The only requirement for membership is a desire to stop drinking" (from the *Alcoholics Anonymous Preamble*).

Alcoholism
A general but not diagnostic term, usually used to describe alcohol dependence, but sometimes used more broadly to describe a variety of problems related to the use of beverage alcohol.

Ambulatory Detoxification
Detoxification that is medically monitored but that does not require admission to an inpatient, medically or clinically monitored or managed setting.

Assessment
Those procedures by which a program evaluates an individual's strengths, weaknesses, problems and needs, and determines priorities so that a treatment plan can be developed.

Assertive Community Treatment (ACT)
Active outreach to persons, usually with serious and persistent mental illness, who need a support system that facilitates living and functioning adequately in the community. ACT involves comprehensive services designed to engage and retain patients in treatment and assist them in managing daily living, obtaining work, building and strengthening family and friendship networks, managing symptoms and crises and preventing relapse.

Biomedical
Biological and physiological aspects of a patient's condition and thus of the assessment and treatment of the patient. In addiction treatment, biomedical problems may be the direct result of a substance use disorder or be independent of and interactive with them, thus affecting the total treatment plan and prognosis.

*Blackout
Acute anterograde amnesia with no formation of long-term memory, resulting from the ingestion of alcohol or other drugs; i.e., a period of memory loss for which there is no recall of activities.

Bundling
An approach to treatment that ties or "bundles" several treatment services together, often delivering them in a specific treatment setting. Because this approach often overlooks a patient's individual needs and can lead to inappropriate and unnecessary services, the current trend is toward "unbundled" services.

Case Management
Case management is a collaborative process which assesses, plans, implements, coordinates, monitors and evaluates the options and services to meet an individual's health needs, using communication and available resources to promote quality, cost-effective outcomes. (Definition of the National Case Management Task Force; reprinted from the *CCM Certification Guide*, CIRSC/Certified Case Manager, Rolling Meadows, IL, 1993.)

*Chemical Dependency
A generic term relating to psychological or physical dependency, or both, on one or more psychoactive substances.

Client
An individual who receives treatment for alcohol or other drug problems. The terms "client" and "patient" sometimes are used interchangeably, although staff in medical settings more commonly use "patient," while staff of non-medical residential or outpatient settings refer to "clients."

Clinically Managed Services
Clinically managed services are directed by non-physician addiction specialists rather than medical personnel. They are appropriate for individuals whose primary problems involve emotional, behavioral or cognitive concerns, readiness to change, relapse, or recovery environment, and whose problems in Dimension 1 (intoxication/withdrawal) and Dimension 2 (biomedical concerns), if any, are minimal or can be managed through separate arrangements for medical services.

Clinical Necessity
Synonymous with "medical necessity" (see below). Sometimes used to broaden inappropriately narrow definitions of medical necessity.

Coalition for National Clinical Criteria
A multidisciplinary group of individuals involved in alcohol and other drug treatment, research, reimbursement, professional associations, and state and federal government. The Coalition formed in November 1992 to assess support for the adoption of national patient placement criteria and to determine methods of garnering the support of the treatment field for such criteria.

Co-Occurring Disorders
Concurrent substance-related and mental disorders. Other terms used to describe co-occurring disorders include "dual diagnosis," "dual disorders," "mentally ill chemically addicted" (MICA), "chemically addicted mentally ill" (CAMI), "mentally ill substance abusers" (MISA), "mentally ill chemically dependent" (MICD), "coexisting disorders,"

"comorbid disorders," and "individuals with co-occurring psychiatric and substance symptomatology" (ICOPSS). Use of the term carries no implication as to which disorder is primary and which secondary, which disorder occurred first, or whether one disorder caused the other.

Continued Service Criteria
In the process of patient assessment, certain problems and priorities are identified as justifying admission to a particular level of care. Continued Service Criteria describe the degree of resolution of those problems and priorities and indicate the intensity of services needed. The level of function and clinical severity of a patient's status in each of the six assessment dimensions is considered in determining the need for continued service.

Continuing Care
The provision of a treatment plan and organizational structure that will ensure that a patient receives whatever kind of care he or she needs at the time. The treatment program thus is flexible and tailored to the shifting needs of the patient and his or her level of readiness to change. [This term is preferred to "aftercare."]

Continuum of Care
An integrated network of treatment services and modalities, designed so that an individual's changing needs will be met as that individual moves through the treatment and recovery process.

*Cross-tolerance
Tolerance, induced by repeated administration of one psychoactive substance, that is manifested toward another substance to which the individual has not been recently exposed.

*Decriminalization
Removal of criminal penalties for the possession and use of illicit psychoactive substances.

*Dependence
Used in three different ways: (1) physical dependence is a state of adaptation that is manifested by a drug class specific withdrawal syndrome that can be produced by abrupt cessation, rapid dose reduction, decreasing blood level of the drug, and/or administration of an antagonist; (2) psychological dependence is a subjective sense of need for a specific psychoactive substance, either for its positive effects or to avoid negative effects associated with its abstinence; and (3) one category of psychoactive substance use disorder.

*Detoxification
A process of withdrawing a person from a specific psychoactive substance in a safe and effective manner.

Dimension
A term used in the *ASAM Patient Placement Criteria* to refer to one of six patient problem areas that must be assessed in making a placement decision.

Discharge/Transfer Criteria
In the process of patient assessment, certain problems and priorities are identified as justifying treatment in a particular level of care. Discharge/Transfer Criteria describe the degree of resolution of those problems and priorities and thus are used to determine when a patient can be treated at a different level of care or discharged from treatment. Also, the appearance of new problems may require services that can be provided effectively only at a more or less intensive level of care. The level of function and clinical severity of a patient's status in each of the six assessment dimensions is considered in determining the need for discharge or transfer.

*Drug Intoxication
Dysfunctional changes in physiological functioning, psychological functioning, mood state, cognitive process, or all of these, as a consequence of consumption of a psychoactive substance; usually disruptive, and often stemming from central nervous system impairment.

Dual Diagnosis
Refers to the patient who has signs and symptoms of concurrent substance-related and mental disorders. Other terms used to describe such co-occurring disorders include "co-occurring disorders," "dual disorders," "mentally ill chemically addicted" (MICA), "chemically addicted mentally ill" (CAMI), "mentally ill substance abusers" (MISA), "mentally ill chemically dependent" (MICD), "coexisting

disorders," "comorbid disorders," and "individuals with co-occurring psychiatric and substance symptomatology" (ICOPSS).

Dual Diagnosis Capable (DDC)
Treatment programs that address co-occurring mental and substance-related disorders in their policies and procedures, assessment, treatment planning, program content and discharge planning are described as "Dual Diagnosis Capable" (DDC). Such programs have arrangements in place for coordination and collaboration with mental health services. They also can provide psychopharmacologic monitoring and psychological assessment and consultation, either on site or through coordinated consultation with off site providers. Program staff are able to address the interaction between mental and substance-related disorders and their effect on the patient's readiness to change—as well as relapse and recovery environment issues—through individual and group program content. Nevertheless, the primary focus of DDC programs is the treatment of substance-related disorders.

Dual Diagnosis Enhanced (DDE)
Describes treatment programs that incorporate policies, procedures, assessments, treatment and discharge planning processes that accommodate patients who have co-occurring mental and substance-related disorders. Mental health symptom management groups are incorporated into addiction treatment. Motivational enhancement therapies specifically designed for those with co-occurring mental and substance-related disorders are more likely to be available (particularly in outpatient settings) and, ideally, there is close collaboration or integration with a mental health program that provides crisis back-up services and access to mental health case management and continuing care. In contrast to Dual Diagnosis Capable services, Dual Diagnosis Enhanced services place their primary focus on the integration of services for mental and substance-related disorders in their staffing, services and program content.

Early Intervention
Services that explore and address any problems or risk factors that appear to be related to use of alcohol and other drugs and that help the individual to recognize the harmful consequences of inappropriate use. Such individuals may not appear to meet the diagnostic criteria for a substance use disorder, but require early intervention for education and further assessment.

*Enabling
Any action by another person or an institution that intentionally or unintentionally has the effect of facilitating the continuation of an individual's addictive process.

Facility
The physical structure (building or portions thereof) in which treatment services are delivered.

Failure (as in treatment failure)
Lack of progress and/or regression at any given level of care. Such a situation warrants a reassessment of the treatment plan, with modification of the treatment approach. Such situations may require changes in the treatment plan at the same level of care or transfer to a different (more or less intensive) level of care to achieve a better therapeutic response. Sometimes used to describe relapse after a single treatment episode—an inappropriate construct in describing a chronic disease or disorder.

*Familial Alcoholism
A pattern of alcoholism occurring in more than one generation within a family, due to either genetic or environmental factors, or both.

*Family Intervention
A specific form of intervention, involving family members of an alcoholic/addict, designed to benefit the patient as well as the family constellation.

Habilitation
The development, for the first time in an individual's life, of an optimum state of health through medical, psychological and social interventions (also see "Rehabilitation").

Harm Reduction
Policies and programs whose primary goal is to reduce the adverse health, social, legal and economic consequences of drug use, without necessarily reducing or eliminating such use.

Imminent Danger
Three components constitute imminent danger: (a) a high probability that certain behaviors (such as continued alcohol or drug use or relapse) will occur; (b) the likelihood that such behaviors will present a significant risk of serious adverse consequences to the individual and/or others (as in a consistent pattern of driving while intoxicated); and (c) the likelihood that such adverse events will occur in the very near future. The concept of imminent danger *does not* encompass all the possible things that may happen, but is restricted to the combination of the three factors listed above. On the other hand, the interpretation of imminent danger should not be restricted to acute suicidality, homicidality, or medical or psychiatric problems that create an immediate, catastrophic risk.

*Impairment
A dysfunctional state resulting from use of psychoactive substances, or mental, emotional or cognitive problems.

Individualized Treatment
Treatment designed to meet a particular patient's needs, guided by a treatment plan that is directly related to a specific, unique patient assessment.

Intensity of Service
The number, type and frequency of staff interventions and other services (such as consultation, referral or support services) provided during treatment at a particular level of care.

Intensive Case Management
Intensive case management is a comprehensive community service that includes evaluation, outreach and support services, usually provided on an outpatient basis. The case manager (or management team) advocates for the patient with community agencies and arranges services and supports. He or she also may teach community living and problem-solving skills, model productive behaviors and the patient become self-sufficient. (Adapted from Moss S (1998). *Contracting for Managed Substance Abuse and Mental Health services: A Guide for Public Purchasers* (Technical Assistance Publication Series No. 22). Rockville, MD: Center for Substance Abuse Treatment, pp. 217-237).

Intensive Outpatient Treatment
An organized service delivered by addiction professionals or addiction-credentialed clinicians, which provides a planned regimen of treatment, consisting of regularly scheduled sessions within a structured program, for a minimum of 9 hours of treatment per week for adults and 6 hours of treatment per week for adolescents.

Interdisciplinary Team
A group of clinicians trained in different professions, disciplines or service areas (such as physicians, counselors, psychologists, social workers, nurses, and certified substance abuse counselors), who function interactively and interdependently in conducting a patient's biopsychosocial assessment, treatment plan and treatment services.

*Intervention
A planned interaction with an individual who may be dependent on one or more psychoactive substances, with the aim of making a full assessment, overcoming denial, interrupting drug-taking behavior, or inducing the individual to initiate treatment. The preferred technique is to present facts regarding psychoactive substance use in a caring, believable and understandable manner.

*Legalization
Removal of legal restrictions on the cultivation, manufacture, distribution, possession and/or use of a psychoactive substance.

Length of Service
The number of days (for inpatient care) or units/visits (for outpatient care) of service provided to a patient, from admission to discharge, at a particular level of care.

Level of Care
As used in the *ASAM Patient Placement Criteria*, this term refers to a discrete intensity of clinical and environmental support services bundled or linked together and available in a variety of settings.

Level of Function
An individual's relative degree of health and freedom from specific signs and symptoms of a mental or substance-related disorder, which determine whether the individual requires treatment.

Level of Service
As used in the *ASAM Patient Placement Criteria*, this term refers to broad categories of patient placement, which encompass a range of clinical services such as early intervention, detoxification, or opioid maintenance therapy
services and levels of care such as intensive outpatient treatment or clinically managed medium-intensity residential treatment.

*Loss of Control
The inability to consistently limit the self-administration of psychoactive substance.

Matching
A process of selecting treatment resources to conform to an individual patient's needs and preferences, based on careful assessment. Matching has been shown to increase treatment retention and thus to improve treatment outcome. It also improves resource allocation by directing patients to the most appropriate level of care and intensity of services.

Medically Managed Treatment
Services that involve daily medical care, where diagnostic and treatment services are directly provided and/or managed by an appropriately trained and licensed physician.

Medically Monitored Treatment
Services that are provided by an interdisciplinary staff of nurses, counselors, social workers, addiction specialists and other health care professionals and technical personnel, under the direction of a licensed physician. Medical monitoring is provided through an appropriate mix of direct patient contact, review of records, team meetings, 24-hour coverage by a physician, and quality assurance programs.

Medical Necessity
Pertains to essential care for biopsychosocial severity; defined by the extent and severity of problems identified in a multidimensional assessment of the individual.

*Misuse
Any use of a prescription drug that varies from accepted medical practice.

Modality
A specific type of treatment (technique, method or procedure) that is used to relieve symptoms or induce behavior change. Modalities of addiction treatment include, for example, detoxification or antagonist medication, motivational interviewing, cognitive behavioral therapy, group therapy, social skills training, vocational counseling, and self/mutual help groups.

Motivational Enhancement Therapy
A patient-centered counseling approach for initiating behavior change by helping patients to resolve ambivalence about engaging in treatment and stopping substance use. This approach employs strategies to evoke rapid and internally motivated change in the patient, rather than guiding the patient stepwise through the recovery process. (Adapted from *Principles of Drug Addiction Treatment—A Research Based Guide*, National Institute on Drug Abuse, 1999).

Multidimensional Family Therapy
Outpatient family-based substance abuse treatment for adolescents. Multidimensional Family Therapy views adolescent drug use in terms of a network of influences (individual, family, peer, community) and suggests that reducing unwanted behavior and increasing desirable behavior occur in multiple ways in different settings. Treatment includes individual and family sessions held in the clinic, in the home, or with family members at the family court, school, or other community locations. (Adapted from *Principles of Drug Addiction Treatment—A Research Based Guide*, National Institute on Drug Abuse, 1999).

Multisystemic Therapy
Addresses factors associated with serious antisocial behavior in children and adolescents who have substance-related disorders. Such factors include characteristics of the adolescent (such as favorable attitudes toward drug use), the family (involving poor discipline, family conflict or parental drug abuse, for example), the school (such as early school-leaving or poor academic performance) and the neighborhood (a criminal subculture, for example). Multisystemic therapy

emphasizes intensive treatment in natural environments (such as home, school and neighborhood settings). (Adapted from *Principles of Drug Addiction Treatment—A Research Based Guide*, National Institute on Drug Abuse, 1999).

Outpatient Detoxification
See "ambulatory detoxification."

Outpatient Service
An organized non-residential service, delivered in a variety of settings, in which addiction treatment personnel provide professionally directed evaluation and treatment for substance-related disorders.

Outpatient Treatment
An organized service, delivered in a variety of settings, in which treatment staff provide professionally directed evaluation and treatment of substance-related disorders.

*Overdose
The inadvertent or deliberate consumption of a dose much larger than that either habitually used by the individual or ordinarily used for treatment of an illness, and likely to result in a serious toxic reaction or death.

Patient
As used in the *ASAM Patient Placement Criteria*, an individual receiving alcohol/other drug treatment. The terms "client" and "patient" sometimes are used interchangeably, although staff in non-medical settings more commonly refer to "clients."

Partial Hospitalization
A generic term encompassing day, night, evening and weekend treatment programs that employ an integrated, comprehensive and complementary schedule of recognized treatments. Commonly referred to as "day treatment." A partial hospitalization program does not need to be attached to a licensed hospital.

Placement
Selection of an appropriate level of service, based on assessment of a patient's individual needs and preferences.

*Polydrug Dependence
Concomitant use of two or more psychoactive substances in quantities and with frequencies that cause the individual significant physiological, psychological and/or sociological distress or impairment.

Polysubstance Dependence
A *DSM-IV* diagnosis (304.80) reserved for behavior during the same 12-month period in which the individual was repeatedly abusing at least three groups of substances (excluding caffeine and nicotine), but no single substance predominated. Such use met the dependence criteria for substances as a group, but not for any specific substance. (Adapted from the *Diagnostic and Statistical Manual of Mental Disorders, Fourth Edition*, American Psychiatric Association, 1994.)

*Prevention
Social, economic, legal, medical and/or psychological measures aimed at minimizing the use of potentially addicting substances, lowering the dependence risk in susceptible individuals, or minimizing other adverse consequences of psychoactive substance use. Primary prevention consists of attempts to reduce the incidence of addictive diseases and related problems in a general population. Secondary prevention aims to achieve early detection, diagnosis and treatment of affected individuals. Tertiary prevention seeks to diminish the incidence of complications of addictive diseases.

*Problem Drinking
An informal term describing a pattern of drinking associated with life problems prior to establishing a definitive diagnosis of alcoholism. Also, an umbrella term for any harmful use of alcohol, including alcoholism. ASAM recommends that the term not be used in the latter sense.

Program
A generalized term for an organized system of services designed to address the treatment needs of patients.

Readiness to Change
An individual's emotional and cognitive awareness of the need to change, coupled with a commitment to change. When applied to addiction treatment and particularly assessment

Dimension 4, "Readiness to Change" describes the patient's degree of awareness of the relationship between his or her alcohol or other drug use or mental health problems, and the adverse consequences of such use, as well as the presence of specific readiness to change personal patterns of alcohol and other drug use.

Recognize, Understand and Apply
The distinction in the criteria is made between an individual's ability to *recognize* an addiction problem, *understand* the implications of alcohol and other drug use on the individual's life, and *apply* coping and other recovery skills in his/her life to limit or prevent further alcohol or other drug use. The distinction is in the difference between an intellectual awareness and more superficial acknowledgment of a problem (recognition) and a more productive awareness of the ramifications of the problem for one's life (understanding); and the ability to achieve behavior change through the integration of coping and other relapse prevention skills (application).

Recovery
A process of overcoming both physical and psychological dependence on a psychoactive substance, with a commitment to sobriety. As used in the *ASAM Patient Placement Criteria*, "recovery" refers to the overall goal of helping a patient to achieve overall health and well-being.

Recovery Environment
As used in Dimension 6 of the *ASAM Patient Placement Criteria*, encompasses the external supports for recovery. The quality and extent of services (such as child care, transportation, crisis and transitional housing, and other "wrap around" services), all of which influence treatment outcome.

*Rehabilitation
The restoration of an optimum state of health by medical, psychological and social means, including peer group support, for an alcoholic or addict, a family member or a significant other.

*Relapse
Recurrence of psychoactive substance-dependent behavior in an individual who has previously achieved and maintained abstinence for a significant period of time beyond withdrawal.

Relapse, Continued Use or Continued Problem Potential
As used in Dimension 5 of the ASAM *Patient Placement Criteria*, the patient's attitudes, knowledge and coping skills, as well as the likelihood that the patient will relapse from a previously achieved and maintained abstinence and/or stable and healthy mental health function. If an individual has not yet achieved abstinence and/or stable and healthy mental health function, this dimension assesses the likelihood that the individual will continue to use alcohol or other drugs and/or continue to have mental health problems.

Resident
A patient in one of the clinically managed, residential levels of care.

Setting
A specific place in which treatment is delivered. Settings for alcohol/other drug treatment include hospitals, methadone clinics, community mental health centers, and prisons or jails.

Severity of Illness
Specific signs and symptoms for which a patient requires treatment, including the degree of impairment and the extent of a patient's support networks.

*Sobriety
A state of complete abstinence from psychoactive substances by an addicted individual, in conjunction with a satisfactory quality of life.

Social Support System
The network of relationships that surround an individual. A health social support system—involving family members, friends, employers, members of mutual support groups and others—tends to support an individual's recovery efforts and goals. What these individuals have in common is that their relationship with the individual is current and that the individual is comfortable contacting them in times of distress.

Stages of Change
This refers principally to the work of Prochaska and DiClemente, who described how individuals progress and regress through various levels of

awareness of a problem, as well as the degree of activity involved in a change in behavior. While their original work studied individuals who changed from smokers to non-smokers, the concept of stages of change subsequently has been applied to a variety of behaviors.

Subdomain

A subdomain is an assessment subcategory within Dimension 3 (Emotional, Behavioral or Cognitive Problems), as described below:

- *Dangerousness/Lethality*. This subdomain describes how impulsive an individual may be with regard to homicide, suicide or other behaviors that pose a risk of harm to self or others and/or to property. The seriousness and immediacy of the individual's ideation, plans and behavior—as well as his or her ability to act on such impulses—determine the patient's severity and the type and intensity of services needed.

- *Interference with Addiction Recovery Efforts*. This subdomain describes the degree to which a patient is distracted from addiction recovery efforts by emotional, behavioral and/or cognitive problems and, conversely, the degree to which a patient is able to focus on addiction recovery.

- *Social Functioning*. This subdomain describes the degree to which an individual's relationships (that is, ability to cope with friends, significant others or family, or vocational or educational demands, or ability to meet personal responsibilities) are affected by his or her substance use and/or other emotional, behavioral and cognitive problems.

- *Ability for Self-Care*. This subdomain describes the degree to which an individual's ability to perform activities of daily living (such as personal grooming and obtaining food and shelter) is affected by his or her substance use and/or other emotional, behavioral or cognitive problems.

- *Course of Illness*. This subdomain employs the history of the patient's illness and response to past treatment to help interpret the patient's current signs, symptoms and presentation and predict the patient's likely response to future treatment. Thus, the domain assesses the interaction between the chronicity and severity of the patient's current difficulties. A determination of high severity is warranted when the individual is assessed as at significant risk for dangerous consequences, either because of severe or acute symptoms and/or because a history of instability suggests that high-intensity services are needed to prevent dangerous consequences.

For example, a patient who recently discontinued antipsychotic medications may present with medication compliance problems. If such a patient has a history of rapidly decompensating into acute psychosis when medication is stopped, he or she is assessed as at high severity. However, if in the past he or she slowly became isolated, without any rapid deterioration, when medication was stopped, the severity is assessed as lower.

The key lies in using the patient's past course of illness to predict his or her future course of illness. For example, a patient with medication compliance problems may present after having recently discontinued antidepressant medication. If the patient has a history of rapid decompensation with suicidal depression when medication is stopped, then his or her severity is high in the "course of illness" subdomain. However, if the patient has a history of gradual recurrence of mood disorder and social isolation when medication is stopped, then the "course of illness" severity is lower. Another example is a patient who presents with a recent lapse/relapse and who has a history of cycles of remission and relapse. If the patient has had grave difficulties in the past with a rapidly deteriorating pattern of substance dependence, his or her severity would be much higher than if he or she has a history of a slower pattern of relapse.

Substance Dependence

Substance dependence is marked by a cluster of cognitive, behavioral and physiological symptoms indicating that the individual continues to use alcohol or other drugs despite significant related problems. The cluster of symptoms can include tolerance, withdrawal or use of a substance in larger amounts or over a longer period of time than intended; persistent desire or unsuccessful efforts to cut down or control substance use; a great deal of time spent in activities related to obtaining or using substances or to recover from their effects; relinquishing important social, occupational or recreational activities because of substance use; and continuing alcohol or drug use despite knowledge of having a persistent or recurrent physical or psychological problem that is likely to have been caused or exacerbated by such use. Specific diagnostic criteria are given in the *Diagnostic and Statistical Manual of Mental Disorders, Fourth Edition (DSM-IV)* of the American Psychiatric Association.

Substance-Induced Disorders
Substance-Induced Disorders include Substance Intoxication, Substance Withdrawal and other disorders that cause symptoms characteristic of other mental disorders. These include delirium, persisting dementia, persisting amnestic disorder, psychotic disorder, mood disorder, anxiety disorder, sexual dysfunction and sleep disorder. Specific diagnostic criteria are given in the *Diagnostic and Statistical Manual of Mental Disorders, Fourth Edition (DSM-IV)* of the American Psychiatric Association. In the *ASAM PPC-2R*, Substance-Induced Disorder is part of the diagnostic criteria for admission for several of the levels of service.

Substance-Related Disorders
Substance-Related Disorders include disorders related to the taking of alcohol or another drug of abuse, to the side effects of a medication and to toxin exposures. They are divided into two groups: the Substance Use Disorders and the Substance-Induced Disorders, as defined in the *Diagnostic and Statistical Manual of Mental Disorders, Fourth Edition (DSM-IV)* of the American Psychiatric Association. In the *ASAM PPC-2R*, the broader diagnostic category of Substance-Related Disorders is used when the criteria involve both diagnostic subgroups. When the criteria relate only to one of the diagnostic subgroups or disorders within that subgroup, that specific diagnostic group or disorder is used in the diagnostic admission criteria.

Substance Use Disorders
Substance Use Disorders include Substance Dependence and Substance Abuse, according to the specific diagnostic criteria given in the *Diagnostic and Statistical Manual of Mental Disorders, Fourth Edition (DSM-IV)* of the American Psychiatric Association. Substance Use Disorders are one of two subgroups of the broader diagnostic category of Substance-Related Disorders. In the *ASAM PPC-2R*, the specific subgroup or disorder is used in the diagnostic criteria for admission to certain levels of care.

Support Services
Support services are those readily available to the program through affiliation, contract or because of their availability to the community at large (for example, 911 emergency response services). They are used to provide services beyond the capacity of the staff of the program and which will not be needed by patients on a routine basis or to augment the services provided by staff.

*Tolerance
A state of adaptation in which exposure to a drug induces changes that result in diminution of one or more of the drug's effects over time.

Transfer
Movement of the patient from one level of service to another, within the continuum of care.

*Treatment
Application of planned procedures to identify and change patterns of behavior that are maladaptive, destructive and/or injurious to health; or to restore appropriate levels of physical, psychological and/or social functioning.

Triage
As used in the *ASAM Patient Placement Criteria*, decisionmaking at the conclusion of an initial assessment process to determine the specific assignment of the patient to a level of care or service.

Twenty-Three Hour Observation Bed
Admission for no more than 23 hours for assessment and stabilization to determine the need for inpatient versus outpatient care. Such a "bed" may be located in an inpatient or an outpatient setting (such as a hospital emergency department).

Unbundling
An approach to treatment that seeks to provide the appropriate combination of specific services to match a patient's needs. The goal of unbundling is to provide an array of options for flexible individualized treatment, which can be delivered in a variety of settings. The intensity of clinical services are determined independently of the individual's need for supportive living arrangements and other environmental supports.

*Withdrawal Syndrome
The onset of a predictable constellation of signs and symptoms following the abrupt discontinuation of, or rapid decrease in, dosage of a psychoactive substance.

Appendix F
Contributors to the Development of the ASAM PPC-2R

Key stages in the development of the ASAM *PPC-2R* included the following:

- Responses to questionnaires, roundtable discussions, meetings of the Coalition for National Clinical Criteria and general feedback from the field since 1991 led to the identification of a variety of gaps and areas of potential improvement in the *ASAM Patient Placement Criteria.*

- Work Groups of the Coalition for National Clinical Criteria developed first drafts of revised and new sections for the *ASAM PPC-2R.*

- The draft material was subjected to an exhaustive field review.

- Comments and suggestions from the field reviewers were incorporated in the draft by a small Steering Committee on the *ASAM PPC-2R.*

- The final draft of the *ASAM PPC-2R* was submitted to review by a group of experts from the field and the leadership of the American Society of Addiction Medicine.

Steering Committee

David Mee-Lee, M.D. (Chair)
Chair, Coalition on National Clinical Criteria
Davis, CA

Candace Baker, M.S.W.
Clinical Affairs Manager
National Association of Alcoholism and
Drug Abuse Counselors (NAADAC)
Arlington, VA

James F. Callahan, D.P.A.
Executive Vice President/CEO
American Society of Addiction Medicine (ASAM)
Chevy Chase, MD

Marc Fishman, M.D.
Department of Psychiatry and Behavioral Sciences
The Johns Hopkins University School of Medicine
Baltimore, MD

David R. Gastfriend, M.D.
Associate Professor of Psychiatry,
Harvard Medical School
Director, Addiction Research Program
Massachusetts General Hospital
Boston, MA

Julia Harris Griffith, M.A., CPHQ
Managed Care Quality Assessment
and Improvement Division
Michigan Department of Community Health
Lansing, MI

Roger W. Hartman
Office of the Assistant Secretary of Defense
(Health Affairs)
TRICARE Management Activity
Falls Church, VA

Ronald J. Hunsicker, D.Min., FACATA
President/CEO
National Association of Addiction Treatment Providers
Lititz, PA

Ric Ohrstrom
National Council on Alcoholism and
Other Drug Dependence
Greenwich, CT

Lawrence W. Osborn, M.D.
Aetna-U.S. Healthcare
Blue Bell, PA

Sam R. Segal, LPC, LADC, CBHE
Senior Clinical Officer and
Director, Addiction Services Policy Connecticut
Department of Mental Health and Addiction Services
Hartford, CT

Gerald D. Shulman, M.A., FACATA
Training & Consulting in Behavioral Health
Jacksonville, FL

Bonnie B. Wilford, M.S.
Editor, ASAM Publications
Arlington, VA

Work Group on Adolescents

Marc Fishman, M.D. (Chair)
Department of Behavioral Sciences
The Johns Hopkins University
School of Medicine
Baltimore, MD

Hoover Adger, M.D.
Department of Pediatrics
The Johns Hopkins Hospital
Baltimore, MD

Marie Armentano, M.D. (Associate Chair)
(ASAM Committee on Adolescents)
Chelsea Memorial Health Center
Chelsea, MA

Lori A. Berkes-Nelson
Administrator
Rosecrance on Alpine
Rockford, IL

Sandra A. Brown, Ph.D.
Professor of Psychology and Psychiatry
University of California at San Diego
San Diego, CA

George Comerci, M.D. (Associate Chair)
(American Academy of Pediatrics)
Tucson, AZ

John Courshon
Gateway Foundation, Inc.
Lake Villa, IL

Anthony Dekker, D.O.
Phoenix Indian Medical Center
Phoenix, AZ

Michael L. Dennis, Ph.D.
Senior Research Psychologist
Chestnut Health Systems
Bloomington, IL

Bernie Glos, Ph.D.
Gateway Foundation, Inc.
Chicago, IL

Bobbe J. Kelley, D.O.
Maple Grove Center
Henry Ford Hospital
West Bloomfield, MI

L. Darnell Lee-Redish
Alcohol/Drug Abuse
Services Administration
Washington, DC

John G. Looney, M.D.
Durham, NC

Robert P. Milin, M.D. (Associate Chair)
(American Academy of Addiction Psychiatry)
Clinical Director, Child Psychiatry
Royal Ottowa Hospital
Ottawa, Ontario

Allison Minugh
Abt Associates Inc.
Cambridge, MA

Carol Regier, R.N., CCDC III
Executive Director
Keystone Treatment Center
Canton, SD

D. Paul Robinson, M.D. (Associate Chair)
(Society for Adolescent Medicine)
Director, Division of Adolescent Medicine
Children's Hospital of Missouri
Columbia, MO

Deborah Simkin, M.D. (Associate Chair)
(Chair, Committee on Adolescent
Substance Abuse
American Academy of Child
and Adolescent Psychiatry)
Emerald Coast Psychiatric Care
Fort Walton Beach, FL

Ramon Solhkah, M.D.
(ASAM Committee on Adolescents)
Massachusetts General Hospital
Boston, MA

Julian M. Somers, Ph.D.
Clinic Director
Department of Psychology
University of British Columbia
Vancouver, BC

Sharon S. Sweede, M.D. (Associate Chair)
(American Academy of Family Physicians)
JFK Alcohol and Drug Treatment Center
Black Mountain, NC

Ken Winters, Ph.D.
General Pediatrics and Adolescent Health
University of Minnesota
Minneapolis, MN

Work Group on Co-Occurring Disorders

David Mee-Lee, M.D. (Chair)
Davis, CA

Hugh Biggar, M.A., C.A.P., ICADC
Regional Addictions Services Manager
MCC Behavioral Care
Grand Island, FL

Dennis Bouffard, Ph.D. (Subgroup Consultant)
Program Manager
Addiction Services Division
Connecticut Valley Hospital
Middletown, CT

Dennis Carroll
Director, Addiction Services Division
Connecticut Valley Hospital
Middletown, CT

Dorynne Czechowicz, M.D.
Treatment Research Branch
National Institute on Drug Abuse
Rockville, MD

Stephen L. Dilts, M.D., Ph.D.
(President, American Academy
of Addiction Psychiatry)
Morrison, CO

Lisa Dixon, M.D.
Columbia, MD

Karen Downey, Ph.D.
Associate Professor
Department of Psychiatry
Wayne State University
Detroit, MI

R. Jeffrey Goldsmith, M.D.
Department of Veterans Affairs
Veterans Healthcare System of Ohio
Cincinnati, OH

Brian Heatherton, M.S., LCPC
Doctoral Resident
BroMenn Healthcare
Normal, IL

Ronald M. Kadden, Ph.D. (Subgroup Chair)
Professor of Psychiatry
University of Connecticut Health Center
Farmington, CT

Edward J. Khantzian, M.D.
Associate Chief of Psychiatry
Tewksbury Hospital
Tewksbury, MA

Bobbe J. Kelley, D.O.
Maple Grove Center
Henry Ford Hospital
West Bloomfield, MI

John Lord, Ph.D., Director
Behavioral Health
Baton Rouge, LA

Barbara Marin, Ph.D.
Walter Reed Army Medical Center
Bethesda, MD

Norman S. Miller, M.D., FASAM
Department of Psychiatry
Michigan State University
East Lansing, MI

Ken Minkoff, M.D. (Subgroup Consultant)
Medical Director
Choate Health Management
Woburn, MA

Joe Morrison, M.A., LPC, LPCDS
Laramie, WY

Patrice Muchowski, Ed.D. (Subgroup Chair)
Clinical Director
AdCare Hospital of Worcester
Worcester, MA

Edgar P. Nace, M.D.
(Past President, American Academy
of Addiction Psychiatry)
Dallas, TX

Lisa Najavits, Ph.D.
Associate Psychologist
McLean Hospital
Belmont, MA

C.C. Nuckols, Ph.D.
Apopka, FL

Edward V. Nunes, M.D. (Subgroup Chair)
NYS Psychiatric Institute
New York, NY

Patricia Penn, Ph.D.
La Frontera Center
Tucson, AZ

Richard K. Ries, M.D. (Subgroup Consultant)
Harborview Medical Center
Outpatient Programs
Seattle, WA

Richard N. Rosenthal, M.D. (Associate Chair)
(American Academy of Addiction Psychiatry)
Beth Israel Medical Center
New York, NY 10003

Bruce Rounsaville, M.D.
Connecticut Mental Health Center
New Haven, CT

Stanley Sacks, Ph.D.
National Development and Research Institute
New York, NY

Terry K. Schultz, M.D., FASAM
Arlington, VA

Richard T. Suchinsky, M.D.
Department of Veterans Affairs
Washington, DC

Roger Weiss, M.D.
McLean Hospital
Alcohol and Drug Program
Belmont, MA

Douglas Ziedonis, M.D.
Robert Wood Johnson School of Medicine
Princeton, NJ

Jo Ann Ziegler, M.A.
Director of Dual Diagnosis Services
Southeast Wyoming Mental Health Center
Laramie, WY

Joan Zweben, Ph.D. (Subgroup Chair)
Clinical Professor of Psychiatry
University of California at San Francisco
Berkeley, CA

Work Group on Level 0.5/Level I

Julia Harris Griffith, M.A., CPHQ (Chair)
Managed Care Quality Assessment
and Improvement Division
Michigan Department of Community Health
Lansing, MI

Carolyn Barrett-Ballinger
Bureau of Medicine and Surgery
Washington, DC

Dorynne Czechowicz, M.D.
Treatment Research Branch
National Institute on Drug Abuse
Rockville, MD

Diane DePietro
Wheeler Clinic, Inc.
Plainville, CT

Michael L. Fox, D.O.
Farmington Hills, MI

Frank Fleming, Ed.D.
Vice President of Clinical Services
Merit Behavioral Care Corporation
Maryland Heights, MO

Sandor Genser, M.D.
Clinical Medicine Branch
National Institute on Drug Abuse
Rockville, MD

Roger W. Hartman
Office of the Assistant Secretary of Defense
(Health Affairs)
TRICARE Management Activity
Falls Church, VA

Gina Hayden, M.D.
Westport, CT

William Miller, Ph.D.
Department of Psychology
University of New Mexico
Albuquerque, NM

Howard B. Moss, M.D.
CEDAR-University of Pittsburgh
School of Medicine
Pittsburgh, PA

David R. Selden, President
Enterprise Health Solutions
Salem, MA

Steven Thayer, Clinical Director
Insight, Inc.
Detroit, MI

Janet Zwick, Director
Iowa Division of Substance Abuse
and Health Promotion
Des Moines, IA

Work Group on Level III

Gerald D. Shulman, M.A., FACATA (Chair)
Training & Consulting Services
in Behavioral Health
Jacksonville, FL

Dennis Bouffard, Ph.D. (Associate Chair)
Program Manager
Addiction Services Division
Connecticut Valley Hospital
Middletown, CT

Michael F. Boyle III, D.O., FASAM
Maple Grove Center
Henry Ford Hospital
West Bloomfield, MI

John Hamilton
Vice President for Clinical Services
Liberation Programs, Inc.
Stamford, CT

Ronald J. Hunsicker, D.Min., FACATA
(Associate Chair)
President/CEO
National Association of Addiction
Treatment Providers
Lititz, PA

Pat Riehl, President
Association of Halfway House PNA
Lake Hopatcong, NJ

Bruce Roberts, M.D.
Highland Park, IL

Frank Sadlack, Ph.D.
La Hacienda Treatment Center
Hunt, TX

Mona L. Sumner, M.H.A., ACATA
Chief Operations Officer
Rimrock Foundation
Billings, MT

Linda R. Wolf-Jones, D.S.W. (Associate Chair)
Executive Director
Therapeutic Communities of America
Washington, DC

Steve Zellmer, M.S., LPC (Associate Chair)
Director of Behavioral Healthcare Management
APS Healthcare
Missoula, MT

Work Group on Dimension 5

David R. Gastfriend, M.D. (Chair)
Associate Professor of Psychiatry,
Harvard Medical School
Director, Addiction Research Program
Massachusetts General Hospital
Boston, MA

Raymond F. Anton, M.D.
Medical University of South Carolina
Charleston, SC

Dennis M. Donovan, Ph.D.

Richard Fuller, M.D.
Deputy Director
National Institute on Alcohol Abuse
and Alcoholism
Bethesda, MD

Terence Gorski, Ph.D.
CENAPS
Homewood, IL

Norman Hoffman, Ph.D.
President, Evince Clinical Assessments
Clinical Associate Professor of Community Health
Brown University
Providence, RI

Alan Marlatt, Ph.D.
University of Washington
Seattle, WA

Steven Maisto, Ph.D.
Syracuse University
Syracuse, NY

Amy Rubin, Ph.D.
Massachusetts General Hospital
Boston, MA

Terry K. Schultz, M.D., FASAM
Arlington, VA

Estee Sharon, Psy.D.
Massachusetts General Hospital
Boston, MA

Gerald D. Shulman, M.A., FACATA
Training & Consulting in Behavioral Health
Jacksonville, FL

Kingsley H. Turner, B.S.
Massachusetts General Hospital
Boston, MA

Winston M. Turner, Ph.D.
University of Maine
Orono, ME

Field Reviewers

Gregg Benson, M.A., CADC
Program Administrator
St. Clare's Hospital
Adult/Adolescent Chemical Dependency Services
Boonton Township, NJ

Audrey Blankfeld, M.S., CCS, MAC
Treatment Program Advisor
Maryland Alcohol and Drug Abuse
Administration
Baltimore, MD

Sheila B. Blume, M.D., CAC, FASAM
Sayville, NY

Sandra A. Brown, Ph.D.
Professor of Psychology & Psychiatry
University of California at San Diego
La Jolla, CA

Joseph Buttacci, M.A., CAC
Manager
Blue Cross of Northeastern PA
Wilkes-Barre, PA

Barbara Cimaglio, Director
Oregon Office of Alcohol & Drug Abuse
Programs
Salem, OR

Carol Coley, M.S.
Senior Public Health Advisor
Center for Substance Abuse Treatment
Rockville, MD

Stephanie W. Colston
Vice President
Johnson, Bassin & Shaw, Inc.
Silver Spring, MD

Mark Disselkoen
Program Specialist
Nevada Bureau of Alcohol and Drug Abuse
Las Vegas, NV

Paul Earley, M.D., FASAM
Program Director
Adult Addiction Medicine
Smyrna, GA

Janice Embree-Bever
Alcohol & Drug Abuse Division
Colorado Department of Human Services
Denver, CO

Jennifer Fiedelholtz
Public Health Analyst
Substance Abuse and Mental Health
Services Administration
Rockville, MD

Timothy L. Fischer, D.O.
Medical Director
TCCADA
Orangeburg, SC

Luceille Fleming, Director
Ohio Department of Alcohol
and Drug Addiction Services
Columbus, OH

Michael L. Fox, D.O.
Farmington Hills, MI

Mark G. Fuller, M.D.
Vice President
Highmark Blue Cross-Blue Shield
Pittsburgh, PA

Robert J. Gallati
Chief of Service Research
New York State Office of
Alcohol and Substance Abuse Services
Albany, NY

Sue A. Garfinckel, M.S., CADC
Director, Addiction Services
Bayonne Hospital
Bayonne, NJ

Lee Gartner, Planner
Minnesota Department of Human Services
St. Paul, MN

Stuart Gitlow, M.D., M.P.H.
Addiction Psychiatry Consultant
CORE, Inc.
Providence, RI

Sue Green
Washington Division of Alcohol
and Substance Abuse
Olympia, WA

James M. Heckler
Coordinator of Managed Care/Treatment
New York State Office of
Alcohol and Substance Abuse Services
Albany, NY

Richard B. Heyman, M.D.
Suburban Pediatric Associates
Cincinnati, OH

Arnold J. Hill, M.D., FASAM
Marlboro Medical Center
Marlborough, MA

Elizabeth F. Howell, M.D.
Atlanta, GA

M. Kay Keller, M.P.A., SSW
Senior Human Services Program Specialist
Florida Department of Children & Families
Tallahassee, FL

Thomas A. Kirk, Jr., Ph.D.
Deputy Commissioner
Connecticut Department of Mental Health
and Addiction Services
Hartford, CT

Jonathan Krejci, Ph.D.
Department of Psychiatry
University of Medicine and Dentistry
of New Jersey
Robert Wood Johnson Medical School
New Brunswick, NJ

Barry W. Lovgren
Program Specialist
Nevada Bureau of Alcohol and Drug Abuse
Carson City, NV

Robert I. Lynn, Ed.D.
NCADD-NJ
Hamilton, NJ

Dennis W. Malmer
Certification Specialist
Washington Division of Alcohol
and Substance Abuse
Olympia, WA

Ruby J. Martinez, R.N., Ph.D., CS
Assistant Professor
University of Colorado
School of Nursing
Denver, CO

Michael M. Miller, M.D., FASAM
Director, Meriter Behavioral Services
Meriter Hospital
Madison, WI

Raymond Miller, M.A., CCDC, CCS
Treatment Program Advisor
Maryland Alcohol and Drug Abuse
Administration
Baltimore, MD

Robert B. Millman, M.D.
Professor of Public Health & Psychiatry
Cornell University Medical College
New York, NY

Bobbi Nelson, M.A., CSAC
Clinical Coordinator
Casa De Vida
Tucson, AZ

Lt. Col. Dick Newsome
Medical Inspector
Air Force Inspection Agency

Mary K. O'Sullivan
Director, The Center
ETP, Inc.
East Hartford, CT

Alan Petroski, Ph.D.
Director, Behavioral Healthcare
Blue Cross of Northeastern PA
Wilkes-Barre, PA

David J. Powell, Ph.D.
Chairman, ETP
East Hartford, CT

Larry D. Raper
Director, Office of Program Compliance
Arkansas Bureau of Alcohol & Drug Abuse Prevention
Little Rock, AR

Peter D. Rogers, M.D., M.P.H., FASAM
Children's Hospital
Cincinnati, OH

Bonnie Saltzman, M.S.W., J.D.
Signal Behavioral Health Network
Denver, CO

Robin Schor, M.D.
Associate Medical Director
United Behavioral Health
Philadelphia, PA

Karen Schrock
Executive Director
Adult Well-Being Services
Detroit, MI

Tracie Scott
Michigan Bureau of Substance Abuse Services
Lansing, MI

David R. Selden
President
Enterprise Health Solutions
Salem, MA

Dan Shaffer, M.D.
ValueHealth, Inc.

Steven J. Sheldon
Behavioral Health Administrator
Ann Arbor, MI

David E. Smith, M.D., FASAM
Founder & Medical Director
Haight Ashbury Free Clinics
San Francisco, CA

James W. Smith, M.D., FASAM
Medical Director
Shick-Shadel Hospital
Seattle, WA

John G. Soffe, M.A., M.Div., CPC
Chief, Treatment Services
Maryland Alcohol and Drug Abuse Administration
Baltimore, MD

Wesley E. Sowers, M.D.
Chief Clinical Officer
Center for Addiction Services
St. Francis Medical Center
Pittsburgh, PA

Shelley Steenrod, Ph.D.
Reading, MA

CDR Richard Stoltz, Ph.D., ABPP
Department of the Navy
Bureau of Medicine & Surgery
Health Care Operations
Washington, DC

Erik Stone
Clinical Director
Signal Behavioral Health Network
Denver, CO

David Timken, Ph.D.
Senior Research Scientist
Timken and Associates
Boulder, CO

Rochelle Turner
Missouri Division of Alcohol
and Drug Abuse
Jefferson City, MO

Stephanie White-Perry, M.D.
Assistant Commissioner
Tennessee Department of Health
Bureau of Alcohol & Drug Abuse Services
Nashville, TN

Ken Willinger, Ph.D.
Hawaii Alcohol & Drug Abuse Division
Kapolai, HI

Janet Wood
Director
Colorado Alcohol and Drug Abuse Division
Denver, CO

Steven P. Zellmer, M.S., LPC
Director
Behavioral Health Care Management
APS Healthcare
Missoula, MT

Douglas Ziedonis, M.D., M.P.H.
Director, Division of Addiction Psychiatry
Robert Wood Johnson Medical School
University of Medicine & Dentistry
of New Jersey
Piscataway, NJ

Marc Zimmerman, Ph.D.
Baton Rouge, LA

Janet Zwick, Director
Iowa Division of Substance Abuse
and Health Promotion
Des Moines, IA